"Social justice has been a primary concern i
This book presents a collection of essays that opens new avenues for the
contemporary bioethical debate. It goes beyond the usual fixation on
individual autonomy and addresses vulnerability, social responsibility, and
solidarity. The authors also take the implications of globalization seriously
while at the same time focusing on specific issues such as gun violence,
human trafficking, racial disparities, just workplaces, outsourcing, and the
environment. The book demonstrates how an 'old' tradition of ethical concern
can be revitalized in a new context."

> —Henk ten Have
> Professor of Healthcare Ethics
> Center for Healthcare Ethics
> Duquesne University, Pittsburgh

"A welcome addition to the growing call for a Catholic bioethics that is richly
informed by Catholic social thought. Theoretically sophisticated yet grounded
in the daily practice of Catholic health care, this collection breaks out of the
traditional locus for bioethics in the clinic and at the bedside to give voice to
marginalized communities and invisible populations. Here justice is not an
afterthought or a fourth principle but the lens through which we question
everything from how we weigh social investments in health care to what counts
as a moral issue. Required reading for anyone concerned with the social
construction of health, health care, and health policy and anyone who has ever
wondered what bioethics from an option for the poor would look like."

> —Maura A. Ryan
> John Cardinal O'Hara, CSC, Associate Professor of Christian Ethics
> University of Notre Dame

"In one adroit volume, M. Therese Lysaught and Michael McCarthy bring
together the rich tradition of Catholic social thought, a fresh reading of the
Ethical and Religious Directives for Catholic Health Care Services, and key
interdisciplinary thought leaders in service of the most pressing ethical issues
health care faces today.

"*Catholic Bioethics and Social Justice* is a gift not only for ethicists,
theologians, and mission leaders, but for anyone interested in the integrity of
Catholic health care."

> —Michael Miller, Jr.
> System Vice President, Mission & Ethics
> SSM Health

"The twenty-four essays in this book, along with the helpful introduction to Catholic social thought, spark the reader's imagination to reconstruct and reconsider the nature of Catholic bioethics. The 'traditional' questions will never leave us, but considered by themselves, they simply do not do justice to the range of moral issues facing Catholic health care providers and institutions. This book pushes us. It is a creative project that is bound to shape what we do in Catholic bioethics."

—Bernard Brady
University of Saint Thomas

"We talk about micro- and macroethics, clinical and social dimensions of health care ethics, but the specific clinical aspects—especially those around sex and reproduction—continue to absorb a disproportionate amount of ethicists' attention. This volume shows both the social context of health care ethics and the influence that social factors have on clinical issues we face. Reading this volume is almost like zooming out on a GPS so that you see not just the street corner, but the surrounding terrain and how we got to the street corner in the first place.

"This book is an important advance in our efforts to understand how social factors—violence, racism, mental illness, ecology, gender, and business practices—affect health status and outcomes. It is a contribution to our ongoing efforts to make the person, 'fully and adequately considered' the heart of our ethical undertaking."

—Charles E. Bouchard, OP, STD
Senior Director, Theology and Ethics
The Catholic Health Association of the United States

"In an eloquent methodological shift, *Catholic Bioethics and Social Justice* offers a renewed vision of Christian bioethics rooted in Catholic social teaching, praxis, and the key of liberation. Bridging theological bioethics with interdisciplinary and clinical expertise, this volume provides a fresh ethical perspective from within marginalized communities and real-life complexities that daily challenge health care delivery in a US context. A must-read for undergraduate and graduate students interested in theological bioethics, as well as religious leaders and clinicians engaging the general underrepresentation within Christian health care debates concerning justice, the preferential option, and diverse participation across a range of emerging issues."

—Autumn Alcott Ridenour, PhD
Assistant Professor
Religious and Theological Studies
Merrimack College

Catholic Bioethics and Social Justice

The Praxis of US Health Care in a Globalized World

Edited by
M. Therese Lysaught
and
Michael McCarthy

Foreword by
Lisa Sowle Cahill

LITURGICAL PRESS
ACADEMIC

Collegeville, Minnesota
www.litpress.org

Cover design by Monica Bokinskie. The cover photos are courtesy of Loyola University Chicago and Dr. Judith Jennrich. The top photo was taken in a health clinic in Corozal, Belize, through a partnership between Dr. Jennrich (not pictured) and the clinic in Corozal. The bottom photo captures a "White Coats for Black Lives" protest, demonstrating the medical community's recognition of the importance of advocacy efforts on behalf of their patients and bringing awareness to the effects of marginalization on the health of individuals and communities.

Scripture quotations are from New Revised Standard Version Bible © 1989 National Council of the Churches of Christ in the United States of America. Used by permission. All rights reserved worldwide.

Excerpts from documents of the Second Vatican Council are from *Vatican Council II: Constitutions, Decrees, Declarations; The Basic Sixteen Documents*, edited by Austin Flannery, OP, © 1996. Used with permission of Liturgical Press, Collegeville, Minnesota.

1   2   3   4   5   6   7   8   9

Library of Congress Cataloging-in-Publication Data

Library of Congress Control Number: 2018951941

ISBN 978-0-8146-8455-9   ISBN 978-0-8146-8479-5 (e-book)

To

Kevin D. O'Rourke, OP, and
Dean Brackley, SJ,

*who taught us Catholic bioethics and the
Catholic social tradition at their best*

Contents

PART FIVE

PART SIX

Foreword

Catholic Bioethics and Social Justice captures the vision of two accomplished Catholic theological ethicists, Therese Lysaught and Michael McCarthy, who have broad and deep experience in the practical side of bioethics through their teaching and research roles at Loyola University Chicago Stritch School of Medicine. Their vision is a bioethics that puts the common good in global perspective, is committed to a gospel option for the poor, integrates faith and action, and provides practical wisdom and concrete strategies to make change happen for the underserved and overlooked.

With this book, Catholic bioethics moves decisively out of the confines of traditional act-oriented "moral theology," and into a challenging new world of domestic and global health disparities; health care economics; and the "intersectionality"[1] of factors such as race, class, and gender in creating the moral realities and dilemmas of mission-driven health care today. Among the many strengths of this collection are its attention to emerging priorities such as the environmental repercussions of medical care, the responsibilities of Catholic health care institutions and leaders trying to achieve sustainability in a market environment, and the relation of US care providers, recipients, and researchers to populations in the Global South for whom basic conditions of good health are a very scarce resource.

---

[1] The term intersectionality was coined three decades ago to capture the way multiple variables of race, class, sex, gender, and economics interact to create the realities of disadvantaged persons or groups, especially African-American women. See Kimberlé Crenshaw, "Demarginalizing the Intersection of Race and Sex: A Black Feminist Critique of Antidiscrimination Doctrine, Feminist Theory and Antiracist Politics," *University of Chicago Legal Forum*, vol. 1989, issue 1, 139–67. As the editors of *Catholic Bioethics and Social Justice* remark in introducing part II, "marginalization in health care can take place in a number of ways—race, education level, economics, gender."

The introduction of a Catholic social teaching lens will be welcomed by any reader familiar with more standard approaches that focus primarily on physician-patient decisions, on patient autonomy and consent, or on the standing Catholic preoccupation with avoiding personal or institutional entanglement in "intrinsically immoral acts" (associated primarily with sterilization, abortion, the use of reproductive technologies, and euthanasia). (See Jorge José Ferrer's analysis of the models and methodologies this volume aims to replace.) A particular asset of *Catholic Bioethics and Social Justice* is that its twenty-first-century justice optic illumines bioethics' connection to social challenges that were, until recently, regarded as occupying distinct spheres, such as environmental degradation, immigration, human trafficking, and gun violence. Another is that it takes the "business ethics" side of Catholic health care past the still-important questions of internal labor practices, and into mission-destabilizing phenomena such as jobs outsourcing and the pressure to get immediate return on investment from community outreach and partnerships. A striking innovation of this volume is the dedication of several chapters to ecology as a bioethical concern (in chapters by Cristina Richie, Ron Hamel, and Andrea Vicini and Tobias Winright; with Cory D. Mitchell, Armand Andreoni, and Lena Hatchett applying Pope Francis's concept of "integral ecology" to the integration of health care with community health and well-being more broadly understood).

The strengths of this volume can be displayed just as well by the attention it gives to justice concerns that are hardly new but, at least until now, rarely well served by Catholic health care ethics: gender and race. The 2018 sixth edition of the *Ethical and Religious Directives for Catholic Health Care Services* (like its 2009 predecessor) does highlight that surrogate motherhood "denigrates the dignity of women, especially the poor" (no. 42); that pastoral and physical care should be given to those who have suffered "the trauma of abortion" (no. 46); and that rape victims deserve "compassion and understanding" (no. 36). Nevertheless, as Hille Haker shows in her chapter on the social repercussions of genetics, the salient concern of most Catholic teaching documents on bioethics is to protect the procreative purpose of the so-called marital act, and "centers around the Vatican's teaching on sexual ethics, leaving little room to engage in social ethics questions," including the ways infertility, pregnancy, and birth impinge particularly on women, and draw into the moral picture bigger questions of gender inequality in resources, social opportunities, agency, and respect. The 2018 edition of the *Ethical and Religious Directives* also gives brief recognition to "racial minorities" (no. 3). But although it calls for special attention to "the health care needs of the poor, the uninsured, and the underinsured" (part 1, introduction), it gives no intersectional analysis of the ways a variety of social conditions conspire to uphold what multiple authors in this volume refer to as "structures of sin" that keep entire communities at the margins of what Charles M. A. Clark calls the "social good" of health care.

Jana Bennett offers a discouraging "roadmap" to the disadvantages women in particular face in trying to access compassionate and successful health care, and many other chapters confirm her assessment, whether or not gender is their main concern. The chapter on human trafficking stresses that the majority of trafficked persons are forced laborers, including domestic workers, but also reveals how women, girls, and disadvantaged racial-ethnic groups can be especially vulnerable (Alan Sanders, Kelly R. Herron, and Carly Mesnick). Aana Marie Vigen directly addresses the intersection of gender with race in her analysis of how pregnant women can be disempowered by an impersonal and paternalistic medical system that plies its skills and technologies on them rather than with them. Michael McCarthy stresses similar virtues of presence, empathy, attention, flexibility, and respect on the part of medical professionals serving gender nonconforming young people—rather than being fixated on how identities, lifestyles, and potential treatments do or do not comply with Catholic tradition's normative sexual ethics. These same virtues of compassion, respect, and attention come into play in offering appropriate end-of-life options to African Americans, so often excluded by and thus mistrustful of the "White spaces" of medical care (Sheri Bartlett Browne and Christian Cintron).

Unsurprisingly, gender and racial-ethnic differences coalesce in disadvantageous ways when global health concerns are on the table too. With consequences for maternal-child health, among other needs, Brian Medernach and Antoinette Lullo, Bruce Compton, and Dónal O'Mathúna take distinct approaches that together mount a powerful case that "global health systems" and humanitarian interventions can only function well if they function as partnerships among international providers and local communities.

Gender and racial disparities challenge the ethics of heath care from the provider side as well, a fact already marked on Jana Bennett's roadmap. As Bennett points out, only 34 percent of physicians are women, while women pack the ranks of nurses, nurses' aides, speech therapists, occupational therapists, audiologists, and midwives. Unionization (Daniel P. Dwyer) and the outsourcing of jobs and services (M. Therese Lysaught and Robert DeVita) are of special significance for workers on the lower end of the status, job security, and pay structure (disproportionately women and "minorities"). Readers will be edified and inspired by a safety-net community hospital in Chicago, serving a 97 percent Black patient population, that has made a conscious and conscientious effort to diversify its workforce to better correspond to the racial identities of those it serves (Robert Gordon). This hospital, St. Bernard's, was founded by a religious congregation of women, the Religious Hospitallers of St. Joseph, who pledged Christian service to and solidarity with the poor and vulnerable.

A very important dimension of *Catholic Bioethics and Social Justice* is that virtually every chapter goes beyond outlining ideals, norms, and desiderata. With the editors, the other individual authors share a firm footing in health care education or practice. They realize what normative claims and critiques signify at the practical level, and they know the strategies required to reduce inequities and bring real-life health access closer to Catholic social tradition's ideals of common good, personal dignity, affirmative inclusion of "the poor," and global health justice. The bioethics they offer is not only grounded and practical, it is hopeful and transformative.

Lisa Sowle Cahill, PhD
J. Donald Monan Professor
Theology Department
Boston College

Acknowledgments

Books like this usually require equal doses of serendipity, collaboration, hard work, patience, and forbearance on the part of many. It began with serendipity when Mark Kuczewski, director of the Neiswanger Institute for Bioethics & Healthcare Leadership at Loyola University Chicago Stritch School of Medicine, suggested that we team-teach a course entitled "Catholic Bioethics and Social Justice" for our graduate programs in Bioethics and Health Care Mission Leadership. We went looking for a text for the class and could not find one, so we decided to write one. Thank you, Mark!

We are equally grateful to the students in Loyola Chicago's graduate programs in Bioethics and Health Care Mission Leadership who braved the course, especially the first time we taught it in Fall 2016 and were (almost) building the plane in the air, as they say. They, along with the students who took the course in Spring 2018, helped us to pilot, develop, field test, and refine this material. Our thanks go to Skya Abbate, Lezley Anderson, Larry Beaumont, Jill Boerstler, Linda Bollenbach, Alexis Chamtcheu, John Charnock, Marc Guillemette, Bill Hennessey, Travis Kahle, Leslie Kuhnel, Alex Lescher, Francine Lynch, David Mann, Megan McGuire, Cory Mitchell, Isioma Odum, Mark Polak, Grace Stark, Scott Stiegemeyer, Miriam Arizpe Paredes, Karla Ashenhurst, Sheri Browne, Cecilia Bustamante Pixa, Julie Carter, Daniel Casey, Mary Cohen, Mary Donnelly, Donna Ewy, Valerie Garrick, Mary Kelly, Sr. Hosea Lee, Tim Morgan, Teresa Morris, Patrice Nerone, Holli Oliver, Jennifer Ramseyer, Gina Santori, Esme Strydom, Greg Webster, John Halstead, Jennifer Kuchemba-Hunter, Jeannette Martin, and Ann McDonald.

We are also grateful for the collaborators who provided podcasts for the class or journeyed with us on the project, including John Hardt, Philip Boyle, Fr. Jack MacCarthy, Shawnee Daniels-Sykes, Dr. Marsha Griffin, John Swinton, Richard Payne, and Michael Seifert.

We owe a debt of gratitude to Hans Christoffersen at Liturgical Press who not only patiently waited for the manuscript, but who also had the vision to see that this was an innovative and important project. We applaud Liturgical Press for being one of the few theological presses that seeks to cross over from the academy to Catholic health care, recognizing the need and desire for quality theological publications in this important ministry of the church. Perhaps it was, again, serendipity—or grace—that located the Liturgical Press booth just down from ours at the 2017 Catholic Health Association Assembly, leading to this fruitful collaboration. We are also grateful to our production editor at Liturgical Press, Stephanie Lancour, for her hard work on this manuscript.

And, of course, we are endlessly grateful for the patience, forbearance, and support of our colleagues and friends as we lassoed this book into being. We particularly thank our colleagues Dan Rhodes, timone davis, Jean-Pierre Fortin, Marian Diaz, Gina Lopez, Mark Bersano, Mirta Garcia, Kelly Johnson, Clara Villatoro, Laura Brock, Emily Anderson, Katie Wasson, David Cook, Kayhan Parsi, and Lena Hatchett and, most especially, our families—Bill, Meg, and Sam Riker, and Ginny, Cate, Libby, and Jack—who—at different times and in different ways—graciously asked, "Are you still working on that book?!"

Introduction

Catholic Bioethics Meets Catholic Social Thought: The Problematic, a Primer, and a Plan

The Problematic

An eight-year-old girl is rushed through the door of the emergency department (ED), collateral damage in the ongoing gang violence that plagues her neighborhood. An elderly African-American man with end stage renal disease lies unconscious in the ICU, tethered to an array of machines. His family is refusing to sign a DNR order, calling it a "death warrant" and saying the health care team has given up on him. A volcanic eruption in Guatemala has the cafeteria abuzz with passionate associates making plans to aid in disaster relief. A dedicated yet disillusioned physician is looking to leave your hospital in light of a board decision to discontinue a comprehensive care management program for low-income patients with complex medical and social needs.

Such challenges are nothing new for health care delivery. Mission leaders, ethicists, physicians, and others who work in Catholic health care face scenarios like these and more. Again and again, they are presented with complex situations that reverberate with ethical resonances. These situations call not just for a medical decision, not just procedural clarification—they press for a moral response. However, the bioethics texts that line our bookshelves are largely not helpful. The principle of double effect does not apply to the ED patient who presents after being the latest victim of gun violence. Little progress can be made in the meeting with the African-American family when

1

you try to explain the distinction between ordinary and extraordinary treatment, because underneath their grief is an inherent mistrust of the medical system. The phrase "global health" does not appear in the *Ethical and Religious Directives* (ERDs).[1] While there is great vigilance in Catholic health systems and academic writing around moral concerns related to women's health, tubal ligations, contraceptive practices, and abortion, little ethical reflection exists around discernments for closing the free clinic, responding to the community crises that perpetuate gun violence, disparate infant mortality rates, and food insecurity, or the reality of structural racism that plagues health care in the United States. Yet each of these scenarios falls squarely within the purview of Catholic bioethics.

Injustices taking place within the communities in which Catholic health care institutions operate affect the health of individuals who become patients. These patients are then transferred back into the environments that have had adverse effects on their health, raising further bioethical questions. Catholic bioethics remains a critical discipline for assisting mission leaders, health care practitioners, institutions, and patients in navigating the knotty and dynamic realities of contemporary health care delivery. Yet in the face of these aforementioned issues, Catholic bioethics has very little to say.

Historically, Catholic bioethics has been limited in a number of ways. First, it is constrained by a particular philosophical methodology that is largely inadequate in the face of the complex realities of twenty-first-century health care. Catholic bioethics continues primarily to use categories and concepts drawn from pre-Vatican II moral theology. This tradition was developed for a very specific purpose: to help priests hear confessions. Thus, it has always focused on specific acts undertaken by individuals.[2] Secondly, Catholic bioethics weds

---

[1] United States Conference of Catholic Bishops, *Ethical and Religious Directives for Health Care Services*, 6th ed. (Washington DC: USCCB, 2018).

[2] For histories of the development of Catholic moral theology and bioethics, see James F. Keenan, *A History of Catholic Moral Theology in the Twentieth Century: From Confessing Sins to Liberating Consciences* (New York: Continuum, 2010); Benedict M. Ashley, Jean DeBlois, and Kevin D. O'Rourke, *Health Care Ethics: A Catholic Theological Analysis*, 5th ed. (Washington, DC: Georgetown University Press, 2006); and John Mahoney, *The Making of Moral Theology: A Study of the Roman Catholic Tradition* (New York: Oxford University Press, 1987).

this pre-Vatican II method with the principlist approach of secular bioethics, which likewise relies on an individual act-based approach to decision-making, focusing primarily on clinical issues related to the beginning and end of life.[3] Finally, Catholic bioethics also remains captured by the institution of medicine, focusing primarily on issues encountered and addressed within the clinical setting. Thus, anything that happens before or after a clinical encounter falls outside the established framework.

Pull any Catholic bioethics book off your shelf. You will find that it likely engages a finite set of clinically-oriented issues. These issues center on questions at the beginning of life (procreation/contraception, reproductive technologies, marriage, abortion). Other books focus on the end of life (withholding and withdrawing treatment, medically assisted nutrition and hydration, persistent vegetative state, euthanasia, physician-assisted suicide, futility, pain management). Others take-up more specific issues: organ donation, research with human subjects, stem cells, culture wars, conscience, and genetics.[4] However, the bioethical scope is confined to questions that are asked and answered within the domain of health care, or health research, itself. Due to their histories and methods, both traditional Catholic moral theology and secular bioethics share a significant blind spot: neither has developed the conceptual tools necessary for engaging the social dynamics, largely fraught with injustices, that shape almost every aspect of health care delivery in the US.

---

[3] Tom L. Beauchamp and James F. Childress, *Principles of Biomedical Ethics*, 7th ed. (New York: Oxford University Press, 2013).

[4] See, for example, Jason T Eberl, *Contemporary Controversies in Catholic Bioethics* (Cham, Switzerland: Springer, 2017); Willem Jacobus Cardinal Eijk, Lambert Hendriks, J.A. Raymakers, and John Fleming, eds., *Manual of Catholic Medical Ethics: Responsible Healthcare from a Catholic Perspective* (Australia: Connor Court Publishing, 2014); William E. May, *Catholic Bioethics and the Gift of Human Life* (Huntington, IN: Our Sunday Visitor, 2000/2013); Nicanor P.G. Austriaco, *Biomedicine and Beatitude: An Introduction to Catholic Bioethics* (Washington, D.C: Catholic University of America, 2011); Anthony Fisher, *Catholic Bioethics for a New Millennium* (New York: Cambridge University Press, 2011); D. Brian Scarnecchia, *Bioethics, Law, and Human Life Issues* (Lanham, Maryland: Scarecrow Press, 2010); David F. Kelly, Gerard Magill, and Henk ten Have, *Contemporary Catholic Health Care Ethics* (Washington, DC: Georgetown University Press, 2004); and Peter J. Cataldo and Albert S. Moraczewski, eds., *Catholic Health Care Ethics: A Manual for Ethics Committees* (Boston: The National Catholic Bioethics Center, 2001).

Yet a rich resource exists for doing so, namely, the tradition of Catholic social thought (CST). Troublingly, fifty years after the close of Vatican II, there is still little rapprochement between Catholic bioethics and CST. Although formally part of the Catholic tradition for over 125 years, these two resources for ethical analysis and formation in the Catholic tradition have remained largely siloed. Catholic bioethics has remained virtually silent—with a few notable exceptions around inequalities in accessing health care services and HIV/AIDS— with respect to social determinants of health, environmental effects on health, and broader questions in global health.[5] It rarely incorporates resources, categories, or concepts of the Catholic social tradition, beyond an occasional reference to the common good or a focus on human dignity. At the same time, while many theologians have engaged social inequalities by drawing on CST, those who work in this area have rarely taken up questions at the intersection of social realities and health care.[6]

---

[5] See, for example, Jacquineau Azetsop, ed., *HIV and AIDS In Africa: Christian Reflection, Public Health, Social Transformation* (Maryknoll, NY: Orbis Press, 2016); Agbonkhianmeghe Orobator, ed., *AIDS, 30 Years Down the Line: Faith-Based Reflections About the Epidemic in Africa* (Nairobi, Kenya: Pauline Publications Africa, 2012); Mary Jo Iozzio, Elsie M. Miranda, and Mary M. Doyle Roche, eds., *Calling for Justice Throughout the World: Catholic Women Theologians on the HIV/AIDS Pandemic* (New York: Continuum Books, 2009); Agbonkhianmeghe Orobator, *From Crisis to Kairos: The Mission of the Church in the Time of HIV/AIDS, Refugees and Poverty* (Nairobi, Kenya: Pauline Publications Africa, 2005); Agbonkhianmeghe Orobator, "Ethics of HIV/AIDS Prevention: Paradigms of a New Discourse from an African Perspective," in *Applied Ethics in a World Church: The Padua Conference*, ed. Linda Hogan (Maryknoll, NY: Orbis, 2008), 147–54; and James F. Keenan, Jon Fuller, Lisa Sowle Cahill, and Kevin T. Kelly, *Catholic Ethicists on HIV/AIDS Prevention* (New York: Continuum, 2000).

[6] For a few emerging voices who do explore the interface between health care and CST, see John A. Gallagher, "Pope Francis' Potential Impact on American Bioethics," *Christian Bioethics* 21, no. 1 (2015): 11–34; Brenda Margaret Appleby and Nuala P. Kenny, "Relational Personhood, Social Justice and the Common Good: Catholic Contributions Toward a Public Health Ethics," *Christian Bioethics* 16, no. 3 (2010): 296–313; Daniel J. Daly, "Unreasonable Means: Proposing a New Category for Catholic End-of-Life Ethics," *Christian Bioethics* 19, no. 1 (2013): 40–59; Christian Spiess, "Recognition and Social Justice: A Roman Catholic View of Christian Bioethics of Long-term Care and Community Service," *Christian Bioethics* 1, no. 3 (2007): 287–301; and Michael Jaycox, "Coercion, Autonomy, and the Preferential Option for the Poor in the Ethics of Organ Transplantation," *Developing World Bioethics* 12, no. 3 (2012): 135–47.

This book seeks to take a step forward in breaking down these siloes. It argues that CST can and should serve as a primary resource for Catholic bioethics. It considers the ways in which Catholic social thought illuminates new issues within the concrete practice of health care and provides new tools of analysis for bioethics. This move is timely for a number of reasons. First, given its constant engagement with social realities, Catholic health care remains one of the key places where the church embodies its social teaching. In many ways, the praxis of Catholic health care—from the early church through monastic medicine to the Sisters who founded Catholic health care in the US—preceded the official beginning of the Catholic social tradition, which is often marked in the late 1800s with the promulgation of Leo XIII's, *Rerum Novarum*. Thus, Catholic health care has, from its inception, been committed to the promotion of human dignity, the common good, the preferential option for the poor, subsidiarity, and more.

Furthermore, since the Second Vatican Council, the Catholic social tradition has experienced exponential growth both within the academy and magisterial writings. From Paul VI to Pope Francis, with bishops' conferences and curial offices, the magisterium has advanced, deepened, championed, and witnessed to the centrality of this integral component of Catholic theology. The doctrinal status of Catholic social thought was solidified by the Pontifical Council for Justice and Peace in 2004, when they entitled their integrated summation of the tradition, the *Compendium of the Social Doctrine of the Catholic Church*. Although Catholic moral theology and Catholic social teaching developed on what might be called parallel tracks throughout the first half of the twentieth century, Catholic social teaching can no longer be considered optional for the work of moral theology or its subdiscipline, Catholic bioethics.

Third, the scope of Catholic health care positions a Catholic social perspective for bioethics as a model for bioethics more broadly. Catholic health care is a robust player in the health care infrastructure of the United States, comprising roughly 15 percent of inpatient care per year (via a variety of measures) and providing an outsize proportion of ancillary care delivery, particularly in long-term care and behavioral health. Globally, the Roman Catholic church operates as the largest nongovernmental provider of health care services, managing an estimated 26 percent of the world's health care facilities, including 5,500 hospitals, 65 percent of which are outside the usual geography of bioethics, namely, the US and Europe.[7] Catholic health care fulfills its mission in an environment that regularly encounters questions of injustice. Such questions arise from both the infrastructure for health care delivery and finance in the US and from the ways that many patients bear the effects of social injustices.

Fourth, the social embeddedness of Catholic bioethics is discussed in an oft-overlooked place: the *Ethical and Religious Directives for Catholic Health Care Services* (ERDs). Each iteration of the ERDs, published by the United States Conference of Catholic Bishops, develops from collaborative efforts between theologians, bishops, health care leaders, and practitioners.[8] Front and center and framing the entire document stands part I, "The Social Responsibility of Catholic Health Care Services." Here, the document specifically names the key principles of the Catholic social tradition—human dignity, preferential option for the poor, common good, and subsidiarity. It foregrounds fundamental issues, such as promoting the health of *communities* via dialogue and participation; a just and participative working environment for associates (employees); and more. In so doing, the ERDs privilege social issues as integral to Catholic bioethics, while likewise suggesting that the social tradition can and should serve as a lens through which the issues in subsequent sections (patient-provider relationships, beginning of life, end of life, and partnerships) should be interpreted.

In this book, we seek to take this guidance seriously in order to broaden the scope of what constitutes Catholic bioethics. In so doing, we turn to the practice of US-based Catholic health care examined through a lens informed by the Catholic social tradition broadly construed. The Catholic social tradition draws on social analyses, personalist philosophical traditions, social encyclicals, liberation theology, liturgy, science, social science, and the work of disciples and activists who accompany the poor in solidarity. How might these

---

[7] See Robert Calderisi, *Earthly Mission: The Catholic Church and World Development* (New Haven, CT: Yale University Press, 2013), 40.

[8] Kevin O'Rourke, Thomas Kopfensteiner, and Ron Hamel, "A Brief History: A Summary of the Development of the Ethical and Religious Directives for Catholic Health Care Services," *Health Progress* 82, no. 6 (2001): 18–21.

methodological resources transform how we *see* and *understand* the practice of health care? How might they *illuminate* issues that were previously invisible? What practical options for *action* might they open up?

Envisaging Catholic bioethics in light of Catholic social thought requires a shift in epistemological locus. It will not necessarily begin in the clinical setting with a problem defined by the parameters and power structures of medicine. Rather, grounded in the preferential option for the poor, who in bioethical parlance are referred to as vulnerable populations, it takes as its starting point the realities and concerns of those who have been marginalized within the US context, analyzing the places where these persons encounter Catholic health care and the ethical issues these encounters present. These persons in these places provide Catholic bioethics with knowledge essential to its work that can only be gained by listening carefully to them. Here, issues of race, health care disparities, immigration status, social determinants of health, and gender inequality emerge as deeply intertwined with traditional issues of patient care and health care systems. Such issues simultaneously point to social challenges that undermine the common good, expanding the array of issues encompassed within Catholic bioethics to include environmental degradation, unions, health care financing, and so forth. By engaging the Catholic social tradition, a more complete approach to bioethics emerges that enables those who work in Catholic health care to attend to the complexities of basic issues while expanding our ability to recognize and engage the full range of moral and ethical dimensions of the Catholic health care ministry.

We are not the first to sense a need to integrate Catholic social thought into Catholic bioethics. A small but growing cadre of theologians and ethicists has been working at the interface of Catholic bioethics and social justice since the 1970s.[9] Yet to date, this work

---

[9] See M. Therese Lysaught and Michael McCarthy, "A Social Praxis for US Health Care: Revisioning Catholic Bioethics via Catholic Social Thought," *Journal for the Society of Christian Ethics* 38, no. 2 (Fall/Winter 2018). This article reports the results of a literature review on the interface of Catholic bioethics and social justice. This review unearthed approximately seventy-five publications from 1980 to 2017, most of which focused on a single social concern. The topics most frequently addressed pertain to access to health care and HIV/AIDS with occasional attention to end-of-life issues, reproductive issues, genetics, global poverty, and recently *Laudato Si'*.

remains sparsely scattered throughout the literature in obscure places, infrequently finding its way to the bookshelves of Catholic health care mission leaders and ethicists.

The one exception is Lisa Sowle Cahill's book, *Theological Bioethics*.[10] Cahill moves the conversation forward in important ways. She demonstrates the role that theological voices have played in shaping the issues addressed in both secular and Catholic bioethics. Moreover, she pushes the tradition further by pointing to the sociopolitical contexts in which many bioethical debates are played out. Thus, her argument both draws attention to the Catholic roots of the discipline of bioethics and raises key issues in which theology needs to further participate in shaping the discourses in bioethics that have shifted to a primarily secular perspective.

While her contributions are significant and lay the groundwork for this book, her approach is distinctly different from the one taken here. The main lens of *Theological Bioethics* is not the *integration* of Catholic health care ethics and Catholic social thought *per se*. Rather, Cahill seeks to augment the framework of secular bioethics using insights from the Catholic social tradition, developing a notion of "participatory bioethics." Thus, her main interlocutor is academic, secular, and theological bioethicists rather than those involved in the day-to-day realities of Catholic health care ethics although they, too, may benefit. What is more, Cahill continues to focus on traditional issues in bioethics: end of life, reproduction, access to health care, and genetics. While she demonstrates the explicit ways in which social ethics and CST bear upon each of these particular topics, her analysis does not shed light on new bioethical issues that can be illuminated by exploring the social inequalities that manifest themselves in a variety of health care settings.

Thus, in a certain sense, the logic of this volume operates in reverse of Cahill's *Theological Bioethics*. Cahill takes up issues that have already been analyzed within the tradition and are readily apparent in the clinical setting, reflecting on them in light of CST and social ethics. In other words, her social analysis sheds new light on old questions. Our approach, however, uses CST as a lens to illuminate

---

[10] Lisa Sowle Cahill, *Theological Bioethics: Participation, Justice, and Change* (Washington, DC: Georgetown University Press, 2005).

new issues for bioethics. It asks what bioethical issues result from social inequalities and injustices, that is, what questions pertain directly to the health and well-being of individuals and communities but have been rarely considered by Catholic bioethics. *Catholic Bioethics and Social Justice* brings these analyses together in order to attend systematically to the clinical, organizational, and policy implications of Catholic social thought in health care.

Catholic Social Thought and Liberation Theology: A Brief Primer

The Catholic social tradition is often referred to as the church's "best kept secret." Thus, to understand what this lens entails, we offer here a general overview of CST.[11] Many Catholics as well as those from other denominations may have only glancing familiarity with the Catholic social tradition, if at all. Papal encyclicals provide a normative source for CST, and from those, a number of principles of CST have been distilled that can be explored and drawn upon in a variety of contexts. Liberation theology provides the most vibrant articulation of the tradition in response to global realities. We will comment briefly on each of these. While encyclicals are foundational to the tradition, it is important to note that CST is a living tradition

---

[11] Our intention here is not to provide a comprehensive overview of CST. Rather, we offer a general overview and direct the reader to additional sources that provide a more detailed focus on CST. For those who wish to know more, a rich array of accessible sources are available. One of the best introductions to the Catholic social tradition is Bernard V. Brady's *Essential Catholic Social Thought,* 2nd ed. (Mahwah, NJ: Orbis Books, 2017). Other useful primers include Kenneth R. Himes and Lisa Sowle Cahill eds., *Modern Catholic Social Teaching: Commentaries and Interpretations* (Washington, DC: Georgetown University Press, 2018); Thomas Massaro, *Living Justice: Catholic Social Teaching in Action,* 3rd ed. (Rowman and Littlefield, 2015); Kenneth Himes, *Responses to 101 Questions on Catholic Social Teaching,* 2nd ed. (New York: Paulist Press, 2013); David Matzko McCarthy, *The Heart of Catholic Social Teaching: Its Origin and Contemporary Significance* (Brazos, 2009); and Charles Curran, *Catholic Social Teaching, 1891-Present: A Historical, Theological, and Ethical Analysis,* Moral Traditions Series (Washington, DC: Georgetown University Press, 2002).

Useful websites include Education for Justice, https://educationforjustice.org /resources; Catholic Charities of St. Paul/Minneapolis, https://www.cctwincities .org/education-advocacy/catholic-social-teaching/; and the USSCB, http://www .usccb.org/beliefs-and-teachings/what-we-believe/catholic-social-teaching/.

that informs and is informed by the changing landscape of the reality in which we live.

The roots of CST are found in Scripture, tradition, and urgent threats to the well-being of persons and the common good. While Scripture's constant attention to the poor and marginalized and ceaseless call for justice may be easy to understand, the role of tradition and experience bears further explanation. Tradition and experience mutually inform each other: the tradition develops from the historical response to needs presented within and outside the church. As Meghan J. Clark notes, CST developed "through direct and systematic engagement with new social problems through a series of papal encyclicals, conciliar and synodical documents, and episcopal statements."[12] From the oppressive working conditions of early capitalism, atomic threats to peace, the increasing economic inequities between the global north and south, continued threats to labor in the 1980s, the global economic crash of the early twenty-first century, and the current ecological crisis, the urgent realities of human oppression have provided opportunities for the church to hone, expand, and bear witness to its social doctrine.

Encyclicals

The official start of CST begins in 1891 with the promulgation of Pope Leo XIII's encyclical *Rerum Novarum* (On the Condition of Labor), which took on the egregious conditions experienced by workers in the Industrial Revolution of the late 1800s.[13] This document is considered foundational for Catholic social teaching and is referred to frequently both within the tradition and by many of the authors in this book. As Thomas Shannon notes, *Rerum Novarum* sets up many of the foundational questions addressed in the whole of CST, including "the relation between capital and labor, employee and employer,

---

[12] Meghan J. Clark, *The Vision of Catholic Social Thought: The Virtue of Solidarity and the Praxis of Human Rights* (Minneapolis, MN: Fortress Press, 2014), 4.

[13] For a list of documents that comprise Catholic social teaching, see http://www.usccb.org/beliefs-and-teachings/what-we-believe/catholic-social-teaching/foundational-documents.cfm. One shortcoming of many sites on Catholic social teaching is that they list only documents written by Vatican officials and US bishops, omitting key documents authored by the Latin American bishops' conferences, particularly the documents known as *Medellin* and *Puebla*.

the wealthy and the poor."[14] This encyclical, then, launched and informed much of the rest of the tradition. There are few documents in the tradition of Catholic social thought that do not reference it. It catalyzed decades of Catholic activism to work for social change while living Christian charity in solidarity with the poor, and it continues to speak to questions of social inequality today.

Over the next seventy years or so, only two major encyclicals emerge. The second major encyclical of the Catholic social tradition is *Quadragesimo Anno* by Pius XI (1931) and was issued to mark the fortieth anniversary of *Rerum Novarum*. It moves the tradition along by introducing the principle of subsidiarity. This principle, promulgated in the midst of a global economic depression and the rise of totalitarian regimes, encourages actions and solutions to be developed and enacted by the people most closely affected by the issue when possible.[15] It was another thirty years before the next encyclical, *Mater et Magistra,* was issued in 1961, followed two years later by *Pacem in Terris,* a document focused on peace, the nuclear arms race, and human rights. Both documents were written by Pope John XXIII and emerged prior to the Second Vatican Council (1963–67).

The church, prior to Vatican II, had been primarily concerned with internal reform and the social encyclicals reflect this. Up until the Second Vatican Council, the encyclicals, first and foremost, were addressed to the Catholic hierarchy and only spoke to so-called faithful Catholics in their concluding sections. With the Second Vatican Council, we see a marked shift in language of magisterial documents. Most notably, as John O'Malley, SJ, notes, the documents of Vatican II represent a shift in style: "The Text explicitly addresses, 'not only the sons and daughters of the church and all who call upon the name of Christ but the whole of humanity as well.' *Gaudium et Spes* [GS] is an instruction but also an invitation writ large."[16] The invitation of GS, the final document of the council, to "read the signs of the times" and to respond to them in light of the Gospel is issued to all of humankind. Thus, GS places the church squarely in the public sphere and

---

[14] Thomas A. Shannon, "Commentary on *Rerum Novarum* (The Condition of Labor)," in *Modern Catholic Social Teaching*, 2nd ed. (Washington, DC: Georgetown University Press, 2018), 133.

[15] Massaro, *Living Justice*, 93.

[16] John W. O'Malley, *What Happened at Vatican II?* (Cambridge, MA: Harvard University Press, 2008), 267.

calls it to move beyond magisterial teaching and engage in social analysis. This opening of the church to the modern world, as David Hollenbach notes, is done through a "dialogic universalism . . . acknowledge[ing] that reason is embedded in history."[17] Thus, the reading of the signs of the times turns not only to the wisdom of the church but toward history, science, economics, politics, and social theory.

Liberation Theology

It is with this turn to history and socio-economic theory that local bishops' conferences, particularly those in Latin America, began to shape CST's commitment to poor and marginalized communities. That it was the Latin American bishops who took the lead here is not accidental. Liberation theology grew, in part, out of the egregious violence, oppression, and persecution suffered by the Latin American poor—particularly people of indigenous descent—especially through the twentieth century, though certainly stretching back to the beginning of colonization.[18] Two landmark events that gave ecclesial life to liberation theology in response to GS's call to read the signs of the times are the Medellin Conference in 1968 and the Puebla conference in 1979—both sponsored by the Latin American bishops. Medellin marked the significance and the challenge of taking up GS's call to read the sign of the times. Medellin distinguishes between types of poverty and claims that "all members of the church are called to live in evangelical poverty, but not all in the same way."[19] Dom Helder Camara, another seminal figure in the development of liberation theology, makes clear the connection between poverty and violence—not the usual claim that those who are poor are more violent, but rather the claim that poverty itself is a form of violence against the poor.[20]

---

[17] David Hollenbach, "*Gaudium et Spes* (Pastoral Constitution on the Church in the Modern World)," in *Modern Catholic Social Teaching*, 2nd ed. (Washington, DC: Georgetown University Press, 2018), 287.

[18] For a sobering history of these centuries of oppression, see Eduardo Galeano, *Open Veins of Latin America: Five Centuries of Pillage of a Continent* (Monthly Review Press, 1997).

[19] Brady, *Essential Catholic Social Thought*, 158.

[20] Ibid., 162.

Thus, in addressing this challenge, the 1979 Latin American Bishops' conference in Puebla, Mexico, coins the phrase "preferential option for the poor."[21] The preferential option for the poor describes a theological locus, a place from which one begins analyzing the reality of the world from the perspective of those "marked by God's love and predilection for the weak and abused of human history."[22] Thus, the poor ought to be sought out and listened to first, as a starting place for addressing any theological or ethical question. They give us privileged insight into what it means to be a person and how the world works. The perspective of the poor also should be reflected in the conclusion of any social analysis: How does the solution impact those who are poor? Are there people who remain disadvantaged, marginalized, or unable to participate fully? Therefore, the option for the poor and the signs of the times point us not solely to a theoretical starting point for doing Catholic bioethics but to a praxis-based method that reflects critically on social realities in light of the reign of God.

While liberation theology has had its critics—including, initially, John Paul II who ultimately incorporated the option for the poor in his writings—the preferential option for the poor has become a dominant theme throughout papal encyclicals in the remainder of the twentieth- and start of the twenty-first century.[23] Subsequent to the work of the Latin American bishops and the development of liberation theology,

---

[21] Conference of Latin American Bishops, *Evangelization in Latin America's Present and Future*, 1979, sec. 733.

[22] Gustavo Gutiérrez, "Option for the Poor," in *Mysterium Liberationis: Fundamental Concepts of Liberation Theology*, ed. Ignacio Ellacuria and Jon Sobrino (Maryknoll, NY: Orbis Books, 1993), 240.

[23] Due to associations made between liberation theology and Marxism—some legitimate, some not—there were tensions between the Vatican and liberation theologians in the early 1980s. A 1984 document issued by the Congregation for the Doctrine of the Faith under Cardinal Ratzinger was entitled "Instruction on *Certain* Aspects of the Theology of Liberation," http://www.vatican.va/roman_curia/congregations/cfaith/documents/rc_con_cfaith_doc_19840806_theology-liberation_en.html. These tensions have largely receded over time, so much so that in 2012, Cardinal Gerhard Mueller—the then-head of the Congregation for the Doctrine of the Faith—co-authored a book with Gustavo Gutiérrez; see Gustavo Gutiérrez and Cardinal Gerhard Ludwig Müller, trans. Robert Anthony Krieg and James B. Nickoloff, *On the Side of the Poor: The Theology of Liberation* (Maryknoll, NY: Orbis Books, 2015). Thus, the Vatican has definitively refuted those who wish to refer to liberation theology as a heresy.

the CST has continued to grow exponentially in the writings of the papacy.

Throughout his enormous corpus of writing and encyclicals, John Paul II never failed to give labor priority over capital, to give persons priority over money. This priority of labor and the value of work for the dignity of the human person is a key theme throughout the Catholic social tradition since *Rerum Novarum*. Perhaps John Paul II's most important encyclical is *Sollicitudo Rei Socialis* (On Social Concern) promulgated in 1987. *Sollicitudo* is a reflection, thirty years later, on the work of Paul VI's *Populorum Progressio* (On the Development of Peoples) and builds on some of the themes included in John Paul II's first encyclical *Laborem Exercens* (1981). He continues Paul VI's concern about international economic development and the "development of peoples" rooted in solidarity. He also here explores for the first time in a papal document the notion of "structural sin."

Themes of economics, interdependence, and solidarity—all of which build off of a preferential option for the poor—are echoed in the social encyclicals authored by the latest two popes: Benedict XVI and Francis. Benedict XVI's *Caritas in Veritate* and Pope Francis's *Laudato Si'* both draw on a broad array of sources—economic, social scientific, scientific, philosophical, and the experiences of the poor—to describe the social challenges facing the church in the midst of the twenty-first century. Benedict's *Caritas in Veritate* finds itself addressing yet another global economic crisis, much like the crisis faced by Leo XIII. Benedict reiterates the importance of justice and encourages a reform of international economic systems rooted in ethics, charity, and truth. In highlighting the inequality in economic structures, he points to the violation of solidarity and friendship that results in environmental degradation and a disordering of relationships within society and the world.[24] Benedict's essay foreshadows themes presented in Pope Francis's *Laudato Si'*, which calls for an integral ecology acknowledging that "everything is connected" and draws on foundational principles of CST.[25]

---

[24] Meghan J. Clark, "*Caritas in Veritate* (On Integral Human Development in Charity and Truth)," in *Modern Catholic Social Teaching*, 2nd ed. (Washington, DC: Georgetown University Press, 2018), 496.

[25] Thomas Massaro, *Mercy in Action: The Social Teachings of Pope Francis* (Lanham, MD: Rowman and Littlefield, 2018), 69–95.

The Principles of Catholic Social Teaching

Francis's integral ecology fits well with the established principles of CST. These principles distill the tradition into a manageable list of themes interwoven and developed throughout these documents. Currently, there is no one definitive list of principles. As one visits various sites or reads different authors, one will find overlapping and still-developing sets of principles. They draw deeply, but differently, on various documents, Scripture, and the tradition, serving as guidelines for responding to the variety of human experiences in a global context. The principles include:

Human Dignity

Common Good

Preferential Option for the Poor

Rights and Responsibilities

Subsidiarity

Solidarity

Participation and Association

Rights of Labor and Dignity of Work

Care for Creation

Peacemaking and Nonviolence

Gratuitousness

Human dignity and common good jostle for priority in the tradition. One could argue that in *Rerum Novarum* and throughout much of the twentieth century, the principle of the common good was the primary principle of the CST; but with the Second Vatican Council, and particularly the encyclicals of John Paul II, the principle of human dignity has moved to the fore. Either way, both are still the primary foundational principles for every component of the Catholic social tradition. Summaries of the above principles can be found on various websites.[26] Throughout the chapters in this volume, the authors will reference encyclicals, principles, and social challenges raised with CST and their implications for Catholic bioethics.

---

[26] See, for example, https://www.cctwincities.org/wp-content/uploads/2017/05 /Key-10-Principles-of-CST-1-pager-2017.pdf.

The Plan of the Book

While human dignity is foundational to the socio-ethical analysis in almost every chapter of this book, our starting point is grounded in the insights of liberation theology, the preferential option for the poor, and a praxis-based approach. Informed by those who seek to do "bioethics in a liberationist key," the contributions to this book shift the *locus* or starting point for Catholic bioethics to the impoverished, marginalized, and those at risk of disadvantage.[27] Doing so fundamentally reshapes the scope of issues that fall within the purview of Catholic bioethics. While not eliminating any of the issues that have occupied Catholic bioethics to date, starting from the place of those pushed to the margins incorporates a wider spectrum of voices into deliberation about questions in bioethics. It creates a dialogical process that empowers the excluded to participate in the social and political arena. What is more, it not only invites the poor to the table of bioethics, a table that remains within the walls of the hospital; the insight of liberationist bioethics is that the table itself must be moved. A Catholic social perspective requires bioethicists to leave the hospital and "to join with the poor and marginalized to share their lives and see reality from their perspective."[28] Such a move establishes a different set of priorities for bioethics and requires a physical shift in "our network of social relationships, the people to whom we attribute importance, the necessities or problems to which we give priority."[29] Thus, a Catholic social bioethics is not only cognizant of social relationships, but it privileges relationships with individuals and communities overlooked in the provision and organization of Catholic health care.

---

[27] Marcio Fabri dos Anjos, "Bioethics in a Liberationist Key," in *Matter of Principles? Ferment in Bioethics*, ed. Edwin R. DuBose, Ronald P. Hamel, and Laurence J. O'Connell (Valley Forge, PA: Trinity Press International, 1994), 130–47; Marie J. Giblin, "The Prophetic Role of Feminist Bioethics," *Horizons* 24, no. 1 (1997): 37–39; Shawnee Daniels-Sykes, "Code Black: A Black Catholic Liberation Bioethics," *The Journal of the Black Catholic Theological Symposium* 3 (2009): 29–61; and Alexandre A. Martins, "Healthy Justice: A Liberation Approach to Justice in Health Care," *Health Care Ethics USA* (Summer 2014).

[28] Martins, "Healthy Justice," 1.

[29] Ibid.

This framework shapes the twenty-four chapters that follow. The book starts from this place of vulnerability, integrates Catholic social thought into bioethics, and via this lens brings new issues to the forefront, making visible the myriad ways that injustice intersects with Catholic health care. It seeks consistently to view each issue from both the perspective of health care associates as well as the perspective of marginalized persons and communities, recursively moving back and forth between them. Integrating Catholic social thought into bioethical method also challenges the current boundaries between clinical ethics, organizational ethics, and political advocacy, making clear that every issue encompasses all three. For example, what might seem on its face to be a clinical issue—racial disparities in end of life—is equally an issue of diversity in staffing of our organizations and an issue which calls for advocacy with regard to lack of access to health care for underserved African-American citizens.

The chapters have been divided into six sections that address an array of social challenges facing those engaged in frontlines of Catholic health care. The six sections have been ordered so as to follow issues as they emerge in a health care setting, moving from the community through the door of the emergency room, into physicians' offices, to the staff room, the board room, and then to places where hospital associates cross international borders, and future concerns. At these various interfaces, Catholic health care encounters the needs and realities of local communities and vulnerable persons, and powerful—yet often invisible or unspoken—ethical issues emerge. We close this introduction by sketching the overarching structure of the volume; a more detailed précis of each chapter and the logic underlying the chapter groupings may be found in the short introductions to each section of the book.

Part I, "Accompanying Vulnerable Communities," opens in the emergency room, where Catholic health care institutions come face-to-face with the injustices embedded in the communities that immediately surround many of our facilities. In chapter 1, "Health Care Providers on the Frontline: Responding to the Gun Violence Epidemic," Michelle Byrne, Virginia McCarthy, Abigail Silva, and Sharon Homan explore the reality of gun violence in the US, which continues to produce too many victims. When these victims can be saved, however, they are immediately placed back in the community where the violence persists, their lives compounded by other vulnerabilities. Chapter 2, "Catholic Bioethics and Invisible Problems: Human Trafficking, Clinical Care, and Social Strategy," explores another set of patients who may appear in the ED, victims of human trafficking. From sex trafficking to labor trafficking, Alan Sanders, Kelly R. Herron, and Carly Mesnick address ethical conundrums in caring for victims, outline how to support them, and marshal key partners in collaborating to address this global challenge on a local level. Chapter 3, "Far from Disadvantaged: Encountering Persons with Mental Illness," draws out a population that has been historically neglected and maligned yet is increasing exponentially in the twenty-first century, namely, persons with mental health issues. Abraham Nussbaum, a psychiatrist, explores the dearth of options for mental health patients in many Catholic health care institutions beyond treating an emergent medical need, a new reality that contradicts a key historical feature of the Catholic health care tradition. The final contribution to part I, chapter 4, "Integral Ecology in Catholic Health Care: A Case Study for Health Care and Community to Accelerate Equity," reverses the flow through the hospital entrance and asks how a Catholic health care institution might work in partnership with local communities to stem the impacts of structural violence. Detailing the health burdens imposed by lack of food, education, and meaningful work, Cory Mitchell, Armand Andreoni, and Lena Hatchett detail a form of community-building designed to address structural injustice at its roots, thereby mitigating negative health outcomes.

Part II, "Countering Injustice in the Patient-Physician Encounter," explores the concerns of patients whose social marginalization is compounded when they engage with health care professionals. In chapter 5, "Neglected Voices at the Beginning of Life: Prenatal Genetics and Reproductive Justice," Aana Marie Vigen begins by recounting the disparities in infant and maternal mortality rates between Black women and children, when compared to their white peers. She argues for an understanding of reproductive justice that includes the prenatal challenges that many Black women face at the beginning of life. Once life begins, the complex challenges do not stop. Michael McCarthy, in chapter 6, "Bewildering Accompaniment: The Ethics of Caring for Gender Non-Conforming Children and Adolescents," explores the myriad of challenges faced by pediatric gender-questioning patients and the deadly effects of being rejected in a health care setting. He argues that greater attention needs to be paid to caring for this expanding and vulnerable patient population. Chapters 7 and 8 take two different approaches to questions at the end of life. Cristina Richie, in chapter 7, "Greening the End of Life: Refracting Clinical Ethics through an Ecological Prism," looks at the increasing awareness of patients about the environmental impact of treatments at the end of life. She offers a proposal for patients and families who might be interested in incorporating attention to ecological questions when developing advanced care plans. Chapter 8, "Racial Disparities at the End of Life and the Catholic Social Tradition," explores disparities at the end of life, highlighting ongoing tensions that often exist between Black patients and (usually) White caregivers. Sheri Bartlett Browne and Christian Cintron argue for the need to develop greater relationships of trust between Catholic health care institutions and Black communities that have had historically negative interactions within the "White space" of health care.

While parts I and II focus on patients' engagement with health care, part III, "Incarnating a Just Work Place," explores the organizational decisions that shape the ways both patients and professionals experience Catholic health care. Each chapter in this section brings CST's constant focus on questions of labor and meaningful work for integral human development to bear on how Catholic health care organizations structure the work-life of their associates. In chapter 9, "Unions in Catholic Health Care: A Paradox," Daniel P. Dwyer describes the process of unionization in Catholic health care and the ironic resistance to this process from most Catholic health care leadership. Chapter 10, "Inviting the Neighborhood into the Hospital: Diversifying Our Health Care Organizations," examines the importance of staffing an organization by looking at a model hospital on the Southside of Chicago, a story told by Robert Gordon. This hospital, St. Bernard Hospital and Health Center, has prioritized hiring practices that reflect the racial diversity of the surrounding community and the important role Catholic health care plays in shaping local economies. For Catholic health care, whose physician and executive leadership trends heavily White, this is an important chapter for demonstrating that achieving such diversity and community-engaged outcomes are possible. Jana Marguerite Bennett, in chapter 11, "The

Rocky Road of Women and Health Care: A Gender Roadmap," examines the equally difficult road faced by women in navigating the landscape of health care. She sketches a "gender roadmap" in the hope of providing equity in how women are cared for and employed within Catholic health care. The final chapter of the section, chapter 12, "Continuing the Ministry of Mission Doctors," reflects on the critical role played by women and men religious in providing health care via Catholic missions throughout the world. With a decline in the number of vowed religious and the surge in global health interest among medical students and residents, physicians Brian Medernach and Antoinette Lullo ask if now is the time for Catholic health care to organize their institutions to facilitate the next generation of mission doctors.

Where part III examined the interface between social realities and the staff room, part IV, "Leading for Social Responsibility," explores issues where social realities interface with the board room. Health care leadership is critical in establishing an organizational agenda that grounds the mission of Catholic health care in justice. Ron Hamel, in chapter 13, "A Call to Conversion: Toward a Catholic Environmental Bioethics and Environmentally Responsible Health Care," asks whether health care leadership understands the environmental impact of health care and what responsibility it has in promoting environmentally responsible health care. While Hamel asks about our responsibility to the environment, Mark Kuczewski, in chapter 14, "DACA and Institutional Solidarity," asks about our responsibility to immigrants. Globally, immigrants have more recently been maligned, marginalized, and isolated through nationalistic rhetoric that deprives them of access to communities, resources, and security. Many immigrants, such as recipients of the Deferred Action for Childhood Arrivals (DACA) program, have recently been offered a path forward, only now to have it threatened. For a church that has consistently stood on the side of vulnerable migrants, Catholic health care has a responsibility to likewise organize on behalf of these vulnerable immigrants who are their patients and associates. Chapter 15, "Reframing Outsourcing," asks a different kind of justice question with respect to mission and the outsourcing of service lines—aka, jobs. M. Therese Lysaught and Robert DeVita wrestle with how an accepted business practice might align with or undermine the mission and identity of a Catholic health care institution. The final chapter in this section, chapter 16, "Population Health: Insights from Catholic Social Thought," describes the need for health care organizations to shift their practices from a fee-for-service model to one that focuses on the health of communities and populations. Michael Panicola and Rachelle Barina draw on the principles of human flourishing, justice, and the common good to describe why efforts directed toward population health align better with CST.

The penultimate section of the book, part V, "Embodying Global Solidarity," recognizes the growing interest in global health emerging within Catholic health systems and examines the places where this interest leads our institutions to interface with global realities of oppression and injustice. The first two chapters in this section emphasize the importance of developing authentic partnerships when working outside of a US context. Brian Volck's "Body Politics: Medicine, the Church, and the Scandal of Borders" (chapter 17) narrates his experiences as a pediatrician working in Honduras. Recognizing the global context in which health care is practiced, he reframes one's sense of social responsibility that reveals, what he calls, a scandal of artificial borders particularly for those who understand themselves to be members of the Body of Christ. Bruce Compton's subsequent chapter, "Creating Partnerships to Strengthen Global Health Systems" (chapter 18), builds on Volck's argument, drawing on the resources of the Catholic Health Association to establish a framework for creating partnerships that prioritizes the health needs of local communities in the Global South. The final two chapters address health issues that call for further response through collaborative efforts between the Global North and the Global South. Alexandre Martin, in chapter 19, "Non-Communicable and Chronic Diseases: Putting Palliative Care on the Global Health Agenda," describes the rise in noncommunicable and chronic diseases throughout the Global South. Due to lack of resources or access to treatment, greater efforts at expanding palliative care resources to the Global South are needed to better attend to the health needs of those in pain or dying. The final chapter addresses a different type of crisis. Dónal O'Mathúna, in chapter 20, "Humanitarian Ethics: From Dignity and Solidarity to Response and Research," tackles the thorny issue of humanitarian crises that elicit responses from health care and the global community. However, these responses tend not to yield long-term or desired effects because of the underlying structural inequalities that accompany natural and human-made disasters. O'Mathúna turns to the work of Jon Sobrino to reflect on how a framework for justice and solidarity can better establish evidence-based responses in the midst of humanitarian crises.

The final section, part VI, "Re-Imagining the Frontiers of Catholic Bioethics," raises questions that lie at the boundaries of a variety of disciplines—research, reproductive genetic technology, the environment, and the economics of health care—all of which have significant consequences for health and health outcomes. However, there has been little sustained reflection on the social dimensions of each of these topics, particularly within Catholic bioethics. Jorge José Ferrer, in chapter 21, "Research as a Restorative Practice: Catholic Social Teaching and the Ethics of Biomedical Research," examines how CST has had very little impact on establishing justice in research priorities. He considers how research can function as a restorative practice and what role it should have in shaping that practice. Pope Francis's ethical imagination lies at the heart of chapter 22, "Environmental Ethics as Bioethics," by Andrea Vicini and Tobias Winright. Their chapter draws on the practice of contemplation, inviting readers to imagine the environmental degradation that exists globally and how CST offers resources to reimagine the important intersection between environmental ethics and bioethics that has been too long neglected. Hille Haker's chapter, "A Social Bioethics of Genetics" (chapter 23), is likewise interested in how to shape practices around the development and use of new genetics technology, in particular CRISPR technology. While CRISPR technology may hold much medical promise, she is cautious about its implementation and turns to an interdisciplinary model of social bioethics put forward by Alfons Auer after the Second Vatican Council that she sees being utilized, again, in the teaching of Pope Francis. The final chapter also explores an area that receives too little attention in Catholic bioethics yet underlies almost every issue in this book, namely, the economics of health care. While economics arises frequently with questions of access to health care, Charles M. A. Clark's chapter, "For-Profit Health Care: An Economic Perspective," analyzes the difference between a profit and nonprofit model of health care, the dominant model in Catholic health care.

His economic analysis asks an important question: What, financially, is asked of Catholic health care in taking responsibility for social injustices facing health care institutions?

❖ ❖ ❖ ❖ ❖

In conclusion, this book seeks to break down the siloes that too often constrain our field. We tackle here not only the siloes between Catholic bioethics and CST, but the artificial siloes between clinical ethics, organizational ethics, and policy advocacy. Moreover, the interdisciplinary nature of the authorships strives to identify points of dialogue between the theological academy and those engaged in the daily challenges of Catholic health care. In that vein, twenty-five of the thirty-five contributors to the volume hail from Catholic health care or Catholic academic medical centers.

While the range of issues covered in this volume is significant, we realize that these twenty-four topics do not begin to exhaust the issues the lie at the intersection of Catholic bioethics and social justice. By engaging with these authors, however, we hope to spur dialogue within Catholic health care about the social responsibilities entailed in living out the mission of this ministry and to catalyze future work in this area. Certainly, we hope that others will expand this work by identifying an array of new issues in need of analysis and discussion. We want this book to serve as an invitation to scholars to continue to explore the methodological issues entailed in integrating CST into the traditional methodology of bioethics and to engage in further analysis of justice questions that rest at the heart of bioethics.

PART ONE

Accompanying Vulnerable Communities

The Catholic social tradition challenges Catholic bioethics to "move the table," changing the place where we do bioethics upstream from the clinic to the places where marginalized persons and communities have been pushed. Here we encounter not only the symptoms of social injustices that manifest in our hospitals as morbidity, mortality, and ethical quandaries, we encounter the root causes. From this location, we begin to gain first-hand knowledge of the complexities present in our clinical realities that allow us to see and understand patients and communities in new ways, opening up new avenues for action. A Catholic bioethics informed by the Catholic social tradition will begin with the myriad points of pain that cry out for justice experienced by the poor and marginalized in communities constrained by structural violence.

Part I, "Accompanying Vulnerable Communities," shifts our gaze to the fluid interface between the clinical setting and the communities that surround our hospitals. These chapters explore how the structural inequalities present in society bleed through the doors of our emergency departments, manifesting themselves in acute and chronic illnesses. The epidemic of gun violence, the invisible problem of trafficked labor, the lack of services for the mentally ill, and inadequate access to basic necessities (food, education, work) all have deleterious effects on health. The response of the health care system, while understandable, cannot be that of the nurse in the first chapter—"Just get used to it!" On the contrary, when confronted again and again with victims of structural violence, we should feel called to action. However, often we do not know where to start, overwhelmed with the complexities of the issues. What is more, while clinical care for these patients presents its own unique challenges, greater obstacles emerge when trying to discharge these patients back into the very environment that resulted in their hospitalization in the first place.

The social responsibility of Catholic health care institutions features prominently in the first part of the *Ethical and Religious Directives for Catholic Health Care Services* (ERDs) and proclaims the biblical mandate to care for all these persons and more. The clarion words of directive 3 are always worth highlighting:

> In accord with its mission, Catholic health care should distinguish itself by service to and advocacy for those people whose social condition puts them at the margins of our society and makes them particularly vulnerable to discrimination: the poor; the uninsured and the underinsured; children and the unborn; single parents; the elderly; those with incurable diseases and chemical dependencies; racial minorities; immigrants and refugees. In particular, the person with mental or physical disabilities, regardless of the cause or severity, must be treated as a unique person of incomparable worth, with the same right to life and to adequate health care as all other persons.[1]

Yet what does it mean concretely for Catholic health care to *distinguish* itself with regard to these members of our communities? On this point, Catholic bioethics is largely silent. This book takes a first step in redressing this silence.

In chapter 1, "Health Care Providers on the Frontline: Responding to the Gun Violence Epidemic," Michelle Byrne, Virginia McCarthy, Abigail Silva, and Sharon Homan boldly offer one suggestion. Noting that gun violence in the US has reached epidemic proportions, they draw on Catholic social thought to outline a series of methodological and practical steps that move us beyond the ethical dilemmas presented in the emergency department (ED) and the moral distress of

---

[1] United States Conference of Catholic Bishops (USCCB), *Ethical and Religious Directives for Catholic Health Care Services*, 6th ed. (Washington DC: USCCB, 2018).

caring for victims. They reframe the central concept of bioethics—that of personhood—to focus not solely on the personhood of the patient but to see bioethics as a shared act of personhood between bioethicist and patient/community. They then articulate a new array of principles affirmed in recent magisterial witness on gun violence—forgiveness, reconciliation, nonviolence, belonging, connectedness, solidarity, trust, mercy, hope, and dignity—that expands beyond the traditional bioethical framework. Their framework enables ethicists to envisage an array of responses—community-based intervention strategies, community-building relationships, basic research, and legislative advocacy—that enable a fitting and distinctively *Catholic* response to the problem.

In chapter 2, "Catholic Bioethics and Invisible Problems: Human Trafficking, Clinical Care, and Social Strategy," Alan Sanders, Kelly R. Herron, and Carly Mesnick focus on the global scourge of human trafficking and its intersection with health care, particularly the instances in which victims present in emergency departments. They likewise highlight interconnectedness—this time between health care associates, institutions, and trafficked persons—as the foundational ethical reality. While the ERDs do not specifically address victims of human trafficking, CST takes a clear stance on the social challenges that promote trafficking to take place. Forced labor, commodification of human beings, and unjust immigration policies all empower traffickers to continue seeking victims. Sanders, et al., introduce into our conversation a key concept that has, to date, largely eluded Catholic bioethics, namely, structural sin. Traditional Catholic bioethics, informed by the manualist tradition of Catholic moral theology, has long been concerned with individual sin, but has failed to tackle the role of structural sin. Empowered with this key tool of Catholic social thought, they argue that health care professionals need to be cognizant of warning signs for victims of human trafficking and highlight interdisciplinary programs that engage local nonprofits, law enforcement, and advocacy groups to support victims when they are ready.

The role of structural sin in fostering morbidity and mortality is clear in some instances; in others, its role is more subterranean. Pastoral theologian and counselor Bruce Rogers-Vaughn's masterful book *Caring for Souls in a Neoliberal Age* makes a compelling case role of economic inequality and the dynamics of neoliberal economics in fueling the epidemic rise in mental health issues since 1980.[2] These persons increasingly present in the emergency room with acute medical problems. In chapter 3, "Far from Disadvantaged: Encountering Persons with Mental Illness," Abraham M. Nussbaum, MD, a physician-psychiatrist takes up this issue. He recounts the story of Liêm, a patient that presents to the emergency room after an attempt to remove his own eye. His chapter takes Catholic health care to task for failing to provide sufficient access to behavioral health services for patients in need and critiques the biomedical model of mental illness that informs and limits bioethical engagement with these patients. He asks, "What does it mean to include persons with mental illness in familial, civil, and ecclesial societies of human happiness?" He challenges Catholic health care to return to its roots as exemplified in a series of activists and witnesses: Fr. Joan-Gilabert Jofré who founded the first psychiatric hospital, or the community of Geel, Belgium, which developed a system of foster care for mentally ill adults based around the relics of Saint Dymphna and today remains a paradigm for providing long-term care while integrating the mentally ill into the larger community. Nussbaum recommends a series of concrete steps designed to attend to the structural determinants that especially disadvantage patients with mental illness, including the bold suggestion of developing partnerships between Catholic health systems and Catholic parishes as agents of solidarity.

Such partnerships are neither simply theoretical nor impossible. In the final chapter of this section, "Integral Ecology in Catholic Health Care: A Case Study for Health Care and Community to Accelerate Equity," Cory D. Mitchell, Armand Andreoni, and Lena Hatchett ask: how do we develop a community-engaged approach to address the social inequalities—particularly around lack of access to food, education, and employment—that result in patients using the emergency room as their primary form of treatment? They draw on the example of Proviso Partners for Health (PP4H) to challenge bioethics to consider how the lack of resources available in the community perpetuates the inequalities faced by food insecure patients.

---

[2] Bruce Rogers-Vaughn, *Caring for Souls in a Neoliberal Age* (New York: Palgrave MacMillan, 2016).

They find in Pope Francis's notion of "integral ecology," articulated in *Laudato Si'*, a framework for working against the health disparities that affect disproportionately Black communities. The concept of integral ecology, paired with practices of reconciliation made real through the Rite of Penance, enables Catholic bioethicists—as well as leaders in Catholic health care institutions—to begin to address the systemic inequalities by engaging in a corporate examination of conscience, by accompanying patients within vulnerable communities, and by taking seriously their role as a resource for the community's health grounded in community relationships and collaborative partnerships.

Chapter 1

Health Care Providers on the Frontline: Responding to the Gun Violence Epidemic

Michelle Byrne, MD, MPH, Virginia McCarthy, Abigail Silva, and Sharon Homan

It is Friday evening during a holiday weekend. Seventeen-year-old Terrance was unloading a drum set from a van, preparing for a church choir rehearsal. A man walks up and opens fire on him and his bandmates. Terrance was rushed by ambulance to a nearby hospital—his elbow shattered, arm mangled, and his intestines and liver severely damaged. Terrance was the sixth gunshot victim the emergency team had seen that week. That night they went on to treat four more gunshot victims. Terrance was the only one who survived. One doctor vented her frustration saying, "Even if I can save this child, I have to send him right back into that violent neighborhood. When is this going to stop?" Feeling distressed, a new night shift nurse asked his manager how to cope. Though realizing she might sound insensitive, the nurse manager admitted the reality that trauma workers "just get used to it."

After two weeks in the hospital, Terrance completed five months of physical therapy to regain his day-to-day functions and eighteen months of psychiatric treatment to help manage symptoms of post-traumatic stress disorder. Since the shooting, he, his mother, and eight-year-old sister continue to live in fear of getting shot in their neighborhood. They have withdrawn from community and church activities and are stressed about the unpaid hospital and rehabilitation bills stacking up on their kitchen table.

Meanwhile, each week, gun violence victims flow steadily into the hospital. During the hospital's annual strategic-planning meeting, the chief medical officer noted, "this past year gunshot victims took up one-third of the orthopedic beds and consumed 20 to 30 percent of hospital resources. Because 51 percent of gunshot victims were uninsured, the hospital had lost $6 million in costs. How can we as a hospital and community address these injustices?"

❖   ❖   ❖   ❖   ❖

Terrance's story raises important questions at the intersection of health care and societal injustices arising from gun violence. Gun violence continues to plague communities across the United States. In the Chicago area, over 4,300 people were shot in the year 2016 alone.[1] Every day health care providers pronounce some victims dead and care for those who are wounded, all while keenly aware that emergency interventions play a very small role in stemming the tide of patients that flood their hospitals due to the gun violence crisis. The media broadcasts mass shootings such as those in Parkland, Florida, at Sandy Hook Elementary School, the Pulse Nightclub, and Las Vegas, but these deaths make up only a small percentage of the total lives lost to gun violence. Homicide, suicide, domestic violence, accidental incidents, and police shootings all contribute to the suffering endured across the country every day due to the gun violence epidemic.

Gun violence rips apart lives, families, and communities. Daily, the trauma of gun violence is witnessed and treated by those at hospitals across the country. At Loyola University Medical Center, a level-one trauma center located in the Western suburbs of Chicago, gun violence victims present to the hospital an average of three times a week. Families and victims share stories of grief and anger—a mother burying her fourth child because of gun violence; a teenager missing weeks of school due to rehabilitation for his gunshot-caused paraplegia. The gun violence epidemic has stimulated increased

[1] Madison Park, "Chicago Police Count Fewer Murders in 2017, but Still 650 People Were Killed," *CNN*, January 1, 2018, https://www.cnn.com/2018/01/01/us/chicago-murders-2017-statistics/index.html.

advocacy for legislation and system-level change amongst leading professional organizations in medicine, public health, psychology, law, and other fields. The American Medical Association, American Academy of Family Physicians, American Academy of Pediatrics, American College of Obstetricians and Gynecologists, American College of Physicians, and American Psychiatric Association advocate for gun violence to be recognized as a public-health issue of epidemic proportion, calling for restrictions in gun ownership, sale, and use, as well as advocating for safe storage—in short, for sensible gun laws. While these organizations call persistently for an increase in gun violence research and funding through the Centers for Disease Control and Prevention (CDC), health care professionals are left to care for Terrance and other victims like him with little hope for immediate and lasting change. Health care providers, often on the front lines of these tragedies, provide only brief episodes of tertiary care before discharging patients back to the same difficult situations that led to their admission in the first place.

This chapter explores the complex problem of gun violence, recommends that the bioethics community take a proactive stance, and suggests practical ways that bioethicists can lead critical conversations and mobilize the use of evidence-informed approaches that health care communities and communities of faith have used successfully in the past. Bioethicists—whether secular or Catholic—have not traditionally addressed the problem of gun violence. This chapter argues that the Catholic social tradition (CST) provides tools for the bioethics community to begin bringing its wisdom and experience to this important public health issue which continues to ravage our neighborhoods, schools, and churches, hurting those who are already most vulnerable in our communities. A perspective developed from CST includes not only practical interventions, such as hospital violence intervention programs, but new methodological tools including shifting the starting point of bioethics from the hospital to the heart of local communities. Through this shift, new "principles" emerge—such as reconciliation, nonviolence, connectedness—that change both the conceptual and practical landscape of bioethics itself. Insofar as the stream of victims bleeds through the doors of our emergency departments (EDs) and challenges health care providers and institutions to ask: "What ought we do?" this is—or should be—a question for bioethics.

Gun Violence and Public Health

Firearms play a critical role in many forms of violence including suicide, homicide, domestic violence, accidental incidents, mass shootings, and police shootings. The CDC reported that firearm-related deaths in the US rose in both 2015 and 2016, with 38,000 gun-related deaths in 2016, up 4,000 deaths from 2015. Two thirds of these deaths—22,000—resulted from suicide.[2] Additionally, the US gun homicide rate is twenty-five times higher than that of comparable nations across the globe.[3]

In part, the high rates of gun-related homicides and suicides can be attributed to the general availability of guns in the US. Over 300 million guns reside in roughly 32 percent of US households; between 300,000 and 600,000 of these are stolen each year (including semi-automatic rifles) and sold on the street, often illegally. Gun violence disproportionately impacts vulnerable and socially disadvantaged people and neighborhoods, particularly communities of color experiencing high rates of unemployment and high school dropout rates.[4] Spikes in violence in major cities like Chicago are major contributors to the grim annual statistics.[5]

To understand the scope, as well as the possibilities, for a dramatic reconsideration of the crisis of gun violence, motor vehicle safety provides an instructive example. In November 2017, Nicholas Kristof penned an in-depth *New York Times* editorial entitled, "How to Reduce Shootings," in which he describes, through a series of graphs, the shift in motor vehicle regulation between 1950 and today as an analogy for talking about gun regulation. He notes that successfully implemented regulatory practices included: seatbelts, design standards, speed limits, child safety seats, airbags, and mandatory defect reporting amongst motor vehicle manufacturers (as well as rigorous vehicle licensing, registration, and mandatory driver education

---

[2] Maya Rhodan, "Gun Related Deaths in America Keep Going Up," *Time*, November 6, 2017, http://time.com/5011599/gun-deaths-rate-america-cdc-data/.

[3] Robert Preidt, "How US Gun Deaths Compare to Other Countries," *Health Day*, February 3, 2016, https://www.cbsnews.com/news/how-u-s-gun-deaths-compare-to-other-countries/.

[4] Wendy Cukier and Sarah Allen Eagen, "Gun Violence," *Current Opinion in Psychology* 19 (2018): 109–12.

[5] Rhodan, "Gun Related Deaths," 2017.

classes in most states). Kristof observes, "We don't ban cars, but we work hard to regulate them—and limit access to them—to reduce the death toll they cause. This has been spectacularly successful, reducing the death rate per 100 million miles driven by 95 percent since 1921."[6] In 2014, the Violence Policy Center reported that gun deaths had overtaken motor vehicle deaths in twenty-one states and the District of Columbia. Yet regulation of gun ownership and use continues to be slow and highly contested, in large part due to the constitutional right for gun ownership which is defended fiercely by the National Rifle Association and other lobby groups.

Despite the lack of legislative efforts, the rash of gun violence deaths and mass shootings has catalyzed the medical and public health communities to begin reframing the problem as a public health issue. The field of public health is concerned with protecting the health of populations where they live, learn, work, and play.[7] As such, public-health practitioners focus not only on the individual patient in front of them, but equally on the social context and environment in which the patient exists. For example, while a cardiologist may focus on which specific medications a patient with coronary artery disease needs to prevent a heart attack, a public-health practitioner may be concerned with issues such as the patient's access to a grocery store with fresh produce, whether it is safe for the patient to exercise in his neighborhood, and whether the patient has insurance in order to afford the medications he needs. By considering these "big picture" problems, public-health experts address health care at a population level and seek to make systemic changes that affect individual patients, as well as entire groups of patients. Gun violence poses harm to individuals, their families, and communities and as such, it requires a comprehensive public-health response and solution.

A growing body of evidence suggests that gun violence affects primarily young men of color and often can be traced within social networks that are much smaller than the urban areas in which victims live. Though many people are fearful of random shootings in major

---

[6] Nicholas Kristof, "How to Reduce Shootings," *New York Times*, February 20, 2018, updated May 18, 2018, https://www.nytimes.com/interactive/2017/11/06/opinion/how-to-reduce-shootings.html.

[7] American Public Health Association, "What is Public Health?" https://www.apha.org/what-is-public-health.

cities, evidence shows that gun violence tends to occur between known contacts in predictable ways.[8] A study of a Boston neighborhood in 2012, for example, demonstrated that 85 percent of gunshot injuries occurred within a network of 763 people (less than 2 percent of the community's population).[9]

Gun violence spreads like an infectious disease. Violent acts tend to occur in clusters, spread from place to place, and mutate from one type to another—this is similar to the infectious disease model, in which an agent or vector initiates a specific biological pathway leading to symptoms of disease and infectivity.[10] Researchers have labeled this phenomena "social contagion," and it has been demonstrated in a variety of aspects of society from consumer behavior, to rule breaking, and to other health problems such as smoking and obesity.[11] With the issue of gun violence, perpetrators and victims are often connected within small groups, and incidents "spread" through the group leading to more and more shootings. While both secular and Catholic bioethicists have been quick to respond to potential threats of infectious epidemics—Ebola, Zika, SARS, and more— they have remained largely silent on the spread of gun violence that has reached epidemic proportions in the US. What accounts for this silence?

Gun Violence and Bioethics:
An Overlooked Epidemic

Secular bioethics applies general ethical principles, especially those of utility and autonomy, to the field of medicine and health care, ordinarily asking relevant questions to guide clinically based con-

---

[8] Andrew V. Papachristos, Christopher Wildeman, and Elizabeth Roberto, "Tragic, but not Random: The Social Contagion of Nonfatal Gunshot Injuries," *Social Science and Medicine* 125 (2015): 139–50.

[9] Andrew V. Papachristos, Anthony A. Braga, and David M. Hureau, "Social Networks and the Risk of Gunshot Injury," *Journal of Urban Health* 89, no. 6 (2012): 992–1003.

[10] Gary Slutkin, "Violence is a Contagious Disease," in *Contagion of Violence: Workshop Summary*, Institute of Medicine and National Research Council (Washington, DC: National Academy Press, 2012), 94–111.

[11] Paul Mardsen, "Memetics and Social Contagion: Two Sides of the Same Coin?" *The Journal of Memetics: Evolutionary Models of Information Transmission* 2 (1998): 68–86.

versation rather than providing sure and certain answers.[12] It places primary emphasis on the rights and well-being of autonomous individuals, focusing on decisions that individuals make regarding their health care. As such, the bioethics community has historically functioned largely outside the discipline of public health. From a traditional perspective, gun violence and gunshot wounds ask nothing more of bioethics than any other patient, family, health team, and institutional encounter. Either the patient is near death and relying upon surgical intervention to preserve life, or the injury has created a complex situation for treatment or discharge, and these circumstances draw the bioethicist into the conversation. Here the goals and scope of the encounter are narrow, focused on the provision of comprehensive care for one individual patient. The medical institution prioritizes the care of this patient, and the function of bioethics within the institution ensures that the care for this individual patient is as compassionate and comprehensive as possible. Bioethics interfaces traditionally with individuals, their support networks, clinical teams, and institutions—all within the confines of the hospital walls.

Catholic bioethics, like its secular counterpart, has yet to address questions of gun violence beyond the typical clinical questions. Yet while Catholic bioethics shares much in common with the secular framework, it grounds autonomy in a fuller understanding of what it means to be a human person. Being human means reflecting on what we ought to do to ourselves, others, society, and our physical world. Human personhood does not exist in isolation. Intrinsic to personhood is, in the words of John Kavanaugh, the "mutuality of being known and knowing, of being loved and loving."[13] This mutuality of knowing roots bioethics in a shared act of personhood, inviting the ethicist to consider most fully the broader context of the individual patient's condition, a perspective with which the public-health community is quite familiar. Thus, the Catholic tradition pushes bioethics to expand its purview beyond individuals and the roles and responsibilities of health care providers to questions of

[12] Center for Practical Bioethics, "What Is Bioethics?" https://www.practical bioethics.org/what-is-bioethics.

[13] John F. Kavanaugh, *Who Counts as Persons? Human Identity and the Ethics of Killing* (Washington, DC: Georgetown University Press, 2001), 15.

organizational context and considerations of social justice. The epidemic of gun violence calls bioethics to transform the conversation, look beyond patient encounters that take place in our medical institutions, and begin to address the issue in a holistic way.

Beyond Personhood:
Gun Violence and Catholic Social Thought

As Terrance's case illustrates, the trauma of gun violence cases weighs heavy on the families and clinical staff involved. No one ever really "just gets used to it." Kavanaugh charges that bioethics draws upon the fullness of the humanity of the *bioethicist herself*. But this shared act of personhood cannot be merely conceptual. The Catholic social tradition—informed by the insights of liberation theology—makes it clear that the essential knowledge needed to understand this issue can be found only by immersing oneself in communities. It calls bioethicists to alter their social locations, to locate themselves not only within the confines of the hospital but to sit in the midst of the communities that have experienced gun violence in order to delve deeper into the lived realities of patients who have suffered a gunshot wound. In this regard CST illuminates a new path forward for Catholic bioethics. Not only do the principles of CST affirm the dignity and essentially social nature of the human person as discussed above; they also proclaim that human dignity and the capacity to grow in community are directly affected by economics, politics, law, and policy. Only by immersion in community (solidarity) can bioethics gain the knowledge necessary to understand the issue, identify pressing ethical questions, and begin to envisage fitting courses of action. What is more, CST brings new principles to the table—including mercy, peacebuilding, solidarity, human dignity, rights and responsibilities, and the preferential option for the poor—that provide new conceptual tools to inform and shape a population-level paradigm for a person-centered and community-conscious bioethics.

Communities in which gun violence takes hold are laden with experiences of social injustice, striking at the very life and dignity of persons, disproportionately stigmatizing and affecting communities already wrought with economic and social stress, particularly communities of color. Those on the margins—namely, Black Americans, women in abusive relationships, children, and persons with mental health challenges—are the ones who suffer most. The gun violence epidemic weaves further violence into the very fabric of our culture: it perpetuates abuse, destroys love, and degrades hope in our homes, schools, and streets. These lived realities are fundamental to the patients we meet in the emergency department—their housing, family dynamics, race, mental health history, employment status, and education are key to their well-being. These realities are known to public-health experts as the social determinants of health. It is well established in the literature that despite being nonmedical factors, social determinants greatly influence who suffers from a variety of conditions and the outcomes they experience. For this reason, social determinants can be key practical tools upon which clinical teams build comprehensive patient-centered care plans.

This patient-centered approach, incorporating and adjusting for the lived reality of the patient, finds new language for hope and healing through principles of CST. The framing of the response of the United States Conference of Catholic Bishops (USCCB) to the "pervasive culture of violence" is grounded in mercy and peacebuilding, an approach that the Catholic Church has long espoused. Pope John XXIII addressed the Cuban Missile Crisis and the threat of nuclear war in his 1963 papal encyclical, *Pacem in Terris*. He called for a recognition of "Rights and Responsibilities" at the national level in a conversation focused on international peace. In 1994, the US Bishops issued a pastoral message, *Confronting a Culture of Violence: A Catholic Framework for Action*, in which they encouraged a culture of nonviolence, stating that violence destroys lives, families, and communities and stands in stark contrast to respect for the dignity of persons. The USCCB supported the Assault Weapons Ban (1994–2004) and continues to advocate for restricted sale of firearms and regulation of handguns.[14] The Catholic Church has been vocal against domestic abuse and violence against women, acknowledging, too, the toll that domestic violence takes on children. And most recently, in the months

---

[14] United States Conference of Catholic Bishops, "Assault Weapons Backgrounder," February 2005, http://www.usccb.org/issues-and-action/human-life-and-dignity/criminal-justice-restorative-justice/assault-weapons-background.cfm.

and years following mass shootings, the USCCB continues to speak out against gun violence and urges specific action around gun violence prevention.[15]

This message of gun violence prevention has been echoed and championed particularly by Cardinal Blase Cupich, Archbishop of Chicago. Cardinal Cupich advocates for peace and prevention, for an end to gun violence, via the practice of solidarity. During a Good Friday peace march in one of Chicago's neighborhoods most affected by gun violence, he spoke and marched alongside mothers who have lost children to shootings.[16] He has advocated at the Illinois State Capitol to urge legislators to support the Gun Dealer Licensing Act, which would require regular background checks and training for gun shop owners and employees.[17] The Cardinal has also shown his support for local hospital initiatives advocating for resources to support frontline health care providers, and urged our city and nation to stand together against gun violence and share the responsibility for prevention and healing.[18] At the institutional level, the Archdiocese of Chicago has developed an Institute for Violence Prevention to address this problem and streamline prevention initiatives with the goal of ending abject suffering introduced into lives of individuals and communities through gun violence.[19]

The suffering caused by gun violence not only affects the health of the individual involved but affects the health of our communities,

[15] United States Conference of Catholic Bishops, "Bishop Conference President Reaction to Shooting at Florida High School," February 14, 2018, http://www.usccb .org/news/2018/18-037.cfm.

[16] Michael J. O'Loughlin, "Cardinal Cupich Praises Activities Against Gun Violence at Good Friday Procession," *America*, March 30, 2018, https://www.americamagazine. org/faith/2018/03/30/cardinal-cupich-praises-activists-against-gun-violence-good -friday-procession.

[17] John Keilman, "Cardinal Cupich Calls on State Lawmakers to Display 'Moral Courage' and Override Gun Law Vet," *Chicago Tribune*, April 17, 2018, http://www .chicagotribune.com/news/local/breaking/ct-met-cardinal-cupich-gun-dealer-bill -20180417-story.html.

[18] "Remarks for Cardinal Blase J. Cupich at Loyola Medical Center in Maywood, Ill., on Gun Dealer Licensing Bill (Senate Bill 1657)," Archdiocese of Chicago, https://www .archchicago.org/en/cardinal-cupich-s-statement/-/article/2018/04/17/remarks -for-cardinal-blase-j-cupich-at-loyola-medical-center-in-maywood-ill-on-gun-dealer -licensing-bill-senate-bill-1657-.

[19] Archdiocese of Chicago, "Violence Prevention Initiatives," https://www.arch chicago.org/offices-and-ministries/violence-prevention.

striking at the life and dignity of the human family. The principles of CST call us to consider first those who are affected most by this issue, namely, communities of color, women in caught in domestic violence, and children. When looking at the problem of gun violence, it is important to note that both the shooters and those who are wounded suffer. While we know that most communities are caught in cycles of violence resulting from a lack of resources and opportunities for those who live there, there are limited possibilities for engaging in targeted research that studies the effects of gun violence within these communities.

For years, even funding for research on gun violence has been restricted due to lobbying efforts that prevented the conduction of federally funded, comprehensive research. In 1996, the Dickey Amendment was passed. The amendment states that "none of the funds made available for injury prevention and control at the CDC may be used to advocate or promote gun control."[20] Simultaneously, the CDC received a budget cut that delivered the message clearly. However, 2018 government spending bills timed soon after the Parkland, Florida, shooting, gave clarification on Capitol Hill that the Dickey Amendment did not specifically prohibit research into the causes of gun violence. While experts differ on their interpretation of whether this clarification will provide the needed impetus for an increase in gun violence research, advocacy for the dedication of CDC funding to the topic must certainly remain a priority.

The CST principle of rights and responsibilities is relevant here, calling us to consider the ways that the right to gun ownership comes into conflict with a number of other rights. Parents feel that they have the right to send their children to school without fear of a mass shooting. Neighbors feel that they have a right to safe streets. People of color feel they should have the right to walk and drive without being shot by police. Currently, policies and laws favor the right of gun ownership, leaving communities devastated by gun violence in many forms. Attempts to introduce regulatory policies are met frequently

---

[20] Nell Greenfieldboyce, "Spending Bill Lets CDC Study Gun Violence; But Researchers Are Skeptical It Will Help," *NPR*, March 2018, https://www.npr.org /sections/health-shots/2018/03/23/596413510/proposed-budget-allows-cdc-to -study-gun-violence-researchers-skeptical.

with gun owners protesting that policymakers and activists "stay away from their guns" or offering similar demands.

CST urges us to find another way forward—to balance rights and responsibilities in a way that protects the dignity of the human person and interrupts the unjust violence that devastates many of our communities. It is in navigating this space that the bioethics community can offer great help. Bioethicists are experienced in addressing nuanced conversations—ones where there is no clear answer on how to hold the autonomy of some individuals (in this case those who wish to own and sell guns) with the right to life and dignity of others in society (in this case those who are suffering from gun violence). Beyond autonomy and conflict of rights, however, bioethicists might broker conversations on reconciliation between shooter and victims, use peacemaking as a tool of community building, and help foster practices within community that promote belonging, a sense of connectedness, trust, and hope. They might also surface new issues traditionally not addressed by bioethics—that curbing the epidemic of gun violence will require improved health care access and treatment for those with addiction and mental health needs, mitigation of domestic violence, suicide prevention efforts, employment opportunities for young people, and creative approaches to criminal justice particularly regarding gang-involved incidents.

Practical Recommendations

Though the epidemic of gun violence continues to plague our communities, many efforts to decrease shootings have been successful across the country. For example, health care providers have been effective at decreasing shootings in communities through hospital violence intervention programs (HVIP).[21] These programs seek to combine brief in-hospital interventions with intensive community-based management after hospital discharge to reduce risk factors for

---

[21] "Lessons Learned: Evaluating Community- and Hospital-Based Models and Initiatives," in *Roundtable on Population Health Improvement. Community Violence as a Population Health Issue: Proceedings of a Workshop*, National Academies of Sciences, Engineering, and Medicine; Health and Medicine Division; Board on Population Health and Public Health Practice (Washington, DC: National Academies Press, 2017), https://www.nap.edu/read/23661/chapter/6.

re-injury and cultivate protective factors against it. HVIPs signifi-cantly impact the lives of gun violence victims: program participants have reduced misdemeanor offenses, decreased feelings of aggres-sion, and improved self-efficacy. Additionally, HVIPs successfully decrease both injury and criminal justice recidivism and save costs. These programs rely on practices of forgiveness, reconciliation, and nonviolence—central principles of CST. While HVIPs have demon-strated success and incorporate key aspects of CST, other programs can likewise draw on CST in an effort to interrupt the epidemic of gun violence.

Health care systems can help promote mental health and well-being in communities as a way to fight multiple forms of violence, including suicide. Ensuring accessible, high quality, and culturally competent mental health treatment is one component. However, promoting activities that allow community members to experience belonging/connectedness, control of destiny, dignity, hope/aspira-tion, safety and trust can build resilience.[22] Strategies may include rebuilding social relationships and networks, reclaiming and improv-ing public spaces, promoting community healing, and fostering eco-nomic stability and prosperity.[23]

Health care institutions can also leverage their academic affiliation or partner with academic institutions to support gun violence re-search. For example, electronic medical record data offer opportuni-ties to understand and subsequently improve the health of the populations that they serve.[24] Leveraging these data along with geo-graphic information systems can help identify geographic areas and targets where prevention efforts can take place.[25]

[22] Prevention Institute, *Back to Our Roots: Catalyzing Community Action for Mental Health and Wellbeing* (Oakland, CA: Prevention Institute, 2017).

[23] Howard Pinderhughes, R. Davis, and Myesha Williams, *Adverse Community Experiences and Resilience: A Framework for Addressing and Preventing Community Trauma* (Oakland, CA: Prevention Institute, 2015).

[24] Daniel J. Friedman, R. Gibson Parrish, and David A. Ross, "Electronic Health Records and US Public Health: Current Realities and Future Promise," *American Journal of Public Health* 103, no. 9 (2013): 1560–67.

[25] C. H. Lasecki, F. C. Mujica, S. Stutsman, A. Y. Williams, L. Ding, J. D. Simmons, and S. B. Brevard, "Geospatial Mapping Can be Used to Identify Geographic Areas and Social Factors Associated with Intentional Injury as Targets for Prevention Efforts Distinct to a Given Community," *Journal of Trauma and Acute Care Surgery* 84, no. 1 (2018): 70–74.

The Patient Protection and Affordable Care Act requires nonprofit hospitals to assess the health needs of the people in the communities they serve and to take steps toward addressing those needs.[26] These efforts are called Community Health Needs Assessments and they can provide an opportunity and mechanism by which gun violence can be identified as a health need that must be addressed. As such, prevention efforts can be implemented.

Beyond extending broader access to clinical services, Catholic health systems, informed by their bioethicists, can play a role in advancing legislation on restorative justice and the regulation of gun use in our communities. The role that health care institutions can play in advocacy efforts cannot be underestimated.[27] The issues that cause and maintain the epidemic levels of gun violence are multifactorial. Lobbying for gun violence research and stricter gun control measures, as well as against policies that threaten the social safety nets and break apart communities (e.g., school closings, anti-immigration laws) is in keeping with and supported deeply by CST.

Conclusion: Public Health and Bioethics

Bioethicists can be the yeast that leavens needed critical conversations about the social responsibility of Catholic health care to address gun violence. They can elevate the relevance and compatibility of CST with our national gun violence prevention guidelines *and* mobilize use of evidence-informed practices and policies to address gun violence. They can draw on the work of public-health researchers that understand questions of justice as fundamental aspects of creating healthy communities.

When considering whether the issue of gun violence fits into the purview of bioethics, some may counter that it is instead a social problem, fit to be addressed through policy change and the criminal

---

[26] Lindsey Wahowiak, "Community Needs Assessments Leading to Better Outcomes: ACA Requirement Fortifying Health," *The Nation's Health*, http://thenations health.aphapublications.org/content/47/4/1.4.

[27] For example, Catholic Health Initiatives successfully lobbied Sturm Ruger shareholders to direct the company to enact gun safety measure. "Investors Call for Meaningful Corporate Action to Address Gun Violence," Interfaith Center for Corporate Responsibility, March 29, 2018, https://www.iccr.org/investors-call-meaningful -corporate-action-address-gun-violence.

justice system. Yet if human dignity and personhood are truly realized in community with others, Catholic bioethics provides a starting
point for addressing gun violence in a way that extends beyond the
initial patient encounter. What is more, bioethicists are adept at wrestling with the perplexity of what constitutes the "good" of "health"
and why health matters for human well-being. CST offers Catholic
bioethics a panoply of principles and practices—forgiveness, reconciliation, nonviolence, belonging, connectedness, control of destiny,
dignity, hope/aspiration, safety, trust, and more—that create a vibrant
framework for more adequately addressing the texture of this vexing
health care problem.

The etiology and sequelae of Terrance's shattered intestines lie not
in a specific pathogen or genetic mutation but in a nexus of specific
social factors. These factors are indeed complex. The work of medical
and public health communities would benefit from the contributions
of bioethicists who bring skill and insight in navigating this complexity. With the collaboration of bioethics experts, those working for
healing in communities plagued by gun violence will be more effective. Bioethicists can offer a needed perspective and a skill set worth
sharing to a problem that continues to spread through our streets
and plague people already on the margins of society. As public health
professionals continue to address gun violence from a multitude of
angles, we invite bioethicists to join us as integral partners in the
reduction of gun violence in our communities.

Chapter 2

Catholic Bioethics and Invisible Problems: Human Trafficking, Clinical Care, and Social Strategy

Alan Sanders, Kelly R. Herron, and Carly Mesnick

Trisha, an eighteen-year-old African-American female, comes into the emergency department (ED) with an older male companion. She has presented to the ED before, and is exhibiting symptoms she has presented in the past—dizziness, severe headaches, and malnourishment. She does not have any identification cards, and when she is asked for information during the admission process, her male companion answers all of the questions for her. She looks withdrawn and keeps her head and eyes down during the conversation.

After admission, Trisha and her companion take seats next to each other in the waiting room and the male companion never leaves her side. He looks around every once in a while, glances at the TV at times, and looks at his phone. Trisha, on the other hand, keeps her head and eyes down and avoids any eye contact or pleasantries with others sitting or walking nearby. She has no belongings other than what she is wearing; she has no purse and no phone.

When the two are invited back into the examining room, her male companion follows close behind her with a hand on her arm to control her direction and interactions with staff. When the nurse comes in to examine Trisha, she immediately suspects some sort of abuse and neglect but when she asks Trisha about her condition, the companion again answers all questions for her. The nurse probes into the reasons for her conditions; the companion becomes defensive and asks that she just be treated so that they can leave. The nurse then asks for privacy so that she can examine Trisha more closely, but the companion refuses to leave.

Briefly leaving the exam room, the nurse returns with a physician who explains that she must have privacy to properly examine, diagnose, and treat Trisha's symptoms. The companion very reluctantly agrees but stays close by. Upon examination, the physician clearly sees signs of rape and sexually transmitted disease (STD), but even with privacy, Trisha is very reluctant to answer questions. She exhibits signs of trauma, such as hypervigilance, elevated anxiety, hopelessness, and symptoms of post-traumatic stress disorder (PTSD) including being easily startled, avoidance, trouble sleeping, irritability, and reports intrusive thoughts and memories of past traumatic events.

The physician tells Trisha that she shows signs of an STD and she responds, "I know, they told me that last time I was here." The physician also tells Trisha that she shows signs of rape and asks, "Have you been raped?" She only looks down with some tears forming in her eyes. The physician asks, "Is your companion outside responsible for any of this?" Again, Trisha does not respond as tears begin to drip down her cheeks. The physician then says, "Trisha, I want to help you. Can you tell me anything about your living situation or how this happened?" Finally, Trisha responds, "You don't understand. If I tell you anything I will be hurt more, and I might put others in danger."

❖   ❖   ❖   ❖   ❖

Trisha is a victim of global human trafficking, a form of modern-day slavery that exploits women, children, and men for sex or labor purposes. Any person can be a victim, but traffickers prey particularly on vulnerabilities, people with psychological, emotional, economic, and even socio-political challenges. Victims are often lured with promises of a better life, such as good employment, education, stability, or the promises of loving relationships.[1] Traffickers use violence,

---

[1] Catholic Health Initiatives, "Human Trafficking: How You Can Help," http://www.catholichealthinitiatives.org/human-trafficking-how-you-can-help.

threats, deception, debt bondage, and other manipulative tactics to get people to act against their will.

Until recently, few laws protected victims of human trafficking. In 2000, the United States passed the Trafficking Victims Protection Act (TVPA).[2] Prior to the TVPA, no comprehensive US federal law existed to protect victims of trafficking or to prosecute their traffickers. If victims were identified at all, they were identified only in terms of domestic abuse. Since then, the US Department of State has produced an annual *Trafficking in Persons (TIP) Report* that outlines progress made to eradicate trafficking in the United States and around the world.[3] The report includes victims' stories and assigns tiers or ratings to governments based on their efforts, or lack thereof, in prosecuting traffickers, protecting victims, and preventing trafficking cells.[4] These legislative efforts have shed light on the predatory actions of traffickers and their often hidden victims.

Like Trisha, victims of human trafficking are often reluctant to come forward out of fear—for their own safety or the safety of those closest to them. While human trafficking has been discussed frequently as a human rights problem, it has been rarely considered a problem of bioethics or health care. However, 88 percent of victims report having had some contact with a health care professional while being trafficked in the US.[5] Contact with a health care provider may be the only time a trafficked person is alone and in a safe space with a member of the public, making the clinical encounter vital to identifying victims and offering resources. However, traditional approaches to bioethics are ill-equipped to engage the complex social questions that enter the clinical setting with trafficked persons. While similarities exist between the care provided for victims of domestic violence, the social circumstances of trafficked persons present unique

[2] For federal legislative efforts regarding human trafficking, see United States Department of State, "U.S. Laws on Trafficking in Persons," https://www.state.gov/j/tip/laws/.

[3] United States Department of State, "Diplomacy in Action," https://www.state.gov/j/tip/rls/tiprpt/.

[4] "2014 State Ratings on Human Trafficking Laws," February 2015, https://polarisproject.org/resources/2014-state-ratings-human-trafficking-laws.

[5] L. M. Hachey and J. C. Phillippi, "Identification and Management of Human Trafficking Victims in the Emergency Department," *Advanced Emergency Nursing Journal* 39, no. 1 (2017): 31–51.

challenges. This essay outlines what constitutes human trafficking, details how health care professionals and organizations can support victims, and offers practical recommendations for advocating on behalf of victims and creating collaborative partnerships within the community.

Human Trafficking: An Invisible Problem

Human trafficking is a hidden social problem, especially in developed countries such as the US. The International Labour Organization estimates that there are 20.9 million victims of human trafficking globally; 68 percent are trapped in forced labor, 26 percent are children, and 55 percent are women and girls.[6] There is no official estimate of the total number of victims in the US, but Polaris—an organization that fights modern-day slavery—estimates that the total number of victims is in the hundreds of thousands. Yet only 31,000 cases were reported to the Polaris national hotline between 2010 and 2017.[7] This under-reporting suggests that victims do not feel that the process for reporting ensures them of better or safer alternatives.

Most people link "human trafficking" to sex trafficking, such as forced or coerced prostitution. Yet the majority of trafficked victims are used for labor-related jobs. For every woman or child enslaved in commercial sex there are at least fifteen men, women, and children enslaved in agricultural and domestic slave labor.[8] Unfortunately, trafficked labor is cheap, producing great returns and fueling the problem. The growing gap between the rich and poor created by globalization exacerbates the problem as more and more persons desperately seek ways out of generational or systemic poverty. Traffickers capitalize on this desperation by promising a better life in return for cooperation, and victims find out only too late that they have inadvertently given up their identity and freedoms completely to their traffickers. Victims of agricultural and domestic labor are

[6] Polaris Project, "The Facts," October 26, 2017, https://polarisproject.org/human-trafficking/facts.

[7] Polaris Project, "2016 Hotline Statistics," https://polarisproject.org/resources/2016-hotline-statistics.

[8] E. Benjamin Skinner, *A Crime So Monstrous: Face-to-Face with Modern-day Slavery* (New York: Free Press, 2008).

harder to recognize, especially if they have relatively adequate nutrition and living conditions or if they are not subject to direct physical abuse. While Trisha's story may be the one most closely associated with trafficking victims, it is important to consider that "Men, women, and children are trafficked for various purposes, including domestic servitude, agricultural and plantation work, commercial fishing, textiles, factory labor, construction, mining, and forced sex work as well as bride trafficking and petty crime."[9] Thus, the awareness of human trafficking needs to expand beyond sex trafficked individuals, to identify and support those have been victimized by traffickers in a global economic system that relies unjustly on low wage (or no wage) labor.

Increased awareness of how to identify and support victims of human trafficking begins by recognizing their vulnerability. Certain factors make this difficult to do. Historically, trafficked persons have often been criminalized based on their "work" and because of that have not come forward. In 2015, National Human Trafficking chronicled the story of "Daniel" who reported that he and several other agricultural workers who came to the US on a work visa had their passports confiscated, suffered verbal and physical abuse, and sustained injuries and low-wages, yet despite the fear of reporting their trafficker, they wanted support.[10] They cited their immigration status as a key factor in delayed reporting. In 2016, the National Institute of Justice cited immigration status as a powerful way to control domestic workers who have been brought but overstayed a visa.[11] In Daniel's case, however, he overstayed through no fault of his own because his trafficker had denied his freedom to leave and withheld his passport. Yet his fear of prosecution by the US government for "unlawful entry to the US" is real, despite being smuggled in by a US businessman.

---

[9] C. Zimmerman and L. Kiss, "Human Trafficking and Exploitation: A Global Health Concern," *PLoS Medicine* 14, no. 11 (2017): e1002437.

[10] Human Trafficking Hotline, "Labor Trafficking Story: Daniel," https://human traffickinghotline.org/resources/labor-trafficking-story-agriculture-daniel.

[11] National Institute of Justice, "How Does Labor Trafficking Occur in U.S. Communities and What Becomes of the Victims?," September 2016, https://www.nij .gov/topics/crime/human-trafficking/Pages/how-does-labor-trafficking-occur.aspx.

To treat victims of human trafficking as criminals furthers their abuse and neglect. While trafficking has long been considered a legal challenge and one that relies on law enforcement as the primary intermediaries, others have made the case that human trafficking is a public health challenge. As a public health issue, health care professionals and the wider public can play an important role in identifying and redressing the inequalities faced by victims of all forms of human trafficking. Given Catholic health care's commitment to justice and marginalized communities, room must be made in Catholic bioethics to more deeply understand and inform others about the many challenges faced by these communities.

Catholic Bioethics and Human Trafficking

Like gun violence, human trafficking has been overlooked within Catholic bioethics due to its almost exclusive focus on clinical questions. For Catholic health care, many of the more complex moral questions center around individual or personal decisions regarding treatments such as artificial nutrition and hydration and sterilization. In fact, the word "bioethics" is often conflated with "medical ethics," meaning, that the primary ethical framework is the provider-patient relationship and the nature of informed consent, such as referenced in Part III of the *Ethical and Religious Directives for Catholic Health Care Services* (ERDs).[12] A victim of human trafficking does not fit very well into this individualized moral-technical context.

The picture changes, however, if one considers the first part of the ERDs. Part I of the ERDs—aptly named "The Social Responsibility of Catholic Health Care Services"—pays significant attention to the unique role Catholic health care plays in caring for those vulnerable within society. It demands that health care institutions attempt to understand the larger perspective of a victim's plight in order to be better informed about how to care for vulnerable populations. What is more, it calls for "social responsibility," specified as "service to and advocacy for those people whose social condition puts them at the margins of our society and makes them particularly vulnerable."[13]

---

[12] United States Conference of Catholic Bishops (USCCB), *Ethical and Religious Directives for Catholic Health Care Services*, 5th ed. (Washington DC: USCCB, 2009).

[13] Ibid., directive 3.

The challenge in the clinical setting is how to recognize and address the vulnerabilities of trafficked persons and meet their overall health needs.

Human Trafficking, the Catholic Social Tradition, and Structures of Sin

Building on the ERDs, the CST provides a more comprehensive approach for attending to victims of human trafficking. Not only has attention to labor been at the heart of the CST from its inception; the CST also provides language for understanding the heart of the problem—namely social sin—as well as its remedy, solidarity. These tools have equipped the church to become an international voice against human trafficking.

Attention to the plight of workers has been part of the CST since its beginning and has resounded through the modern encyclicals. Pope Leo XII's 1891 *Rerum Novarum*—known by its English title as "On the Condition of Labor"—is a key reference point for today's victims of human trafficking.[14] Modern human trafficking is a result of changes in the nature of work and the treatment of human beings due to the rise of industrialization and globalization. Trafficked individuals come to be seen as another commodity, violating the very core of their human dignity. This reality echoes what Pope Francis has spoken consistently about as endemic to what he describes as a throw away culture, which "advances by silencing, ignoring and throwing out everything that does not serve its interests."[15] He notes that this culture permits individuals to be used until they are discarded as "useless." He addresses specifically the reality of human trafficking as modern day slavery: "slavery for work, sexual slavery, slavery for profit."[16] While recognizing the vulnerability of individuals is an

---

[14] This attention to labor continues throughout almost all of the magisterial documents, with particular focus in John Paul II's *Laborem Exercens* (On Human Work), 1981.

[15] Pope Francis, "Meeting with the Population: Greeting of The Holy Father, Jorge Basadre Institute (Puerto Maldonado)," January 19, 2018, https://w2.vatican.va/content/francesco/en/speeches/2018/january/documents/papa-francesco_20180119_peru-puertomaldonado-popolazione.html.

[16] Ibid.

important first step, greater strides need to be made in creating just structures and legislative action that challenge the throw-away culture, especially for migrant victims of trafficking.

Theologian Tisha Rajendra argues that the tenuous status of migrants makes them vulnerable because they are insufficently protected under current legislation. Rajendra describes what she sees as CST's emphasis on a "cosmopolitan principle" that draws on solidarity and humanity's interconnectedness as a way of framing the obligation of Catholic institutions to respect the dignity of all persons from all cultures.[17] The tradition, she notes, foregrounds a commitment to human dignity centered on human persons as the image and likeness of God, an image that is relational and interdependent, modeled on the Trinity. Yet we often do not see ourselves as connected to those who are exploited—whether they be migrants or trafficked persons or others on the margin. Thus, "the first step in turning [pathological] interdependence based on exploition [exemplified in human trafficking] to interdependence based on solidarity is to become aware of the relationships that connect us to the most vulnerable members of society."[18]

CST also highlights another concept crucial for understanding a reality as pervasive and destructive as human trafficking, namely, social or structural sin. Structural sin, first identified by liberation theologians and then integrated into CST by John Paul II in his encyclical *Sollicitudo Rei Socialis* (On Social Concern), "are categories which are seldom applied to the situation of the contemporary world. However, one cannot easily gain a profound understanding of the reality that confronts us unless we give a name to the root of the evils which afflict us."[19] Problems rooted in structural or social sin give the impression of being insoluble or insurmountable. While rooted in personal sin and always connected to the concrete acts of individuals, at the heart of structural sin lies what John Paul II identifies as twin "idolatries": "the all-consuming desire for profit, and . . . the thirst for power, with the intention of imposing one's will upon

---

[17] Tisha M. Rajendra, "Migration in Catholic Social Thought," *Concilium* (2011): 3, 37.

[18] Ibid., 38.

[19] Pope John Paul II, *Sollicitudo Rei Socialis* 36.

others."[20] As such, social sin is woven into the fabric of society, not necessarily through direct intent but rather through collective and systematic biases and corruption.

The concept of social or structural sin is crucial for understanding human trafficking. It challenges an individualistic understanding of moral culpability. In a homily given in memory of the twenty thousand African immigrants who have died in the past twenty-five years trying to reach Europe, Pope Francis asked, "Who is responsible for the blood of these brothers and sisters of ours? All of us respond: 'It wasn't me. I have nothing to do with it. It was others, certainly not me.'"[21] Pope Francis, not blaming any specific individual, points to a collective moral responsibility. Human traffickers are certainly immoral actors who should be prosecuted for their crimes, but looking only at individual moral actors misses the bigger picture of the economic and social structures that entrap persons, enabling traffickers to prey on victims in the first place. Social justice is the larger perspective and process of eliminating these evil structures.

Concerns about the structural sin of human trafficking have been raised by the church since the beginning of the new millennium. In a 2002 letter on the occasion of an international conference on "Twenty-First Century Slavery—The Human Rights Dimension to Trafficking in Human Beings," Pope John Paul II stated that "the trade in human persons constitutes a shocking offense against human dignity and a grave violation of fundamental human rights."[22] In 2007, the Pontifical Council for the Pastoral Care of Migrants and Itinerant People published a statement on human trafficking calling for the US federal government, in cooperation with state and local governments, to increase educational efforts so that all Americans become aware of the problem, place an emphasis on the recovery and care of victims, and provide victims with legal protections and

---

[20] Ibid. 37.

[21] Cindy Wooden, "Pope Calls for Repentance over Treatment of Migrants," *Catholic News Service*, July 8, 2013, http://www.catholicnews.com/services/englishnews/2013/pope-calls-for-repentance-over-treatment-of-migrants.cfm.

[22] "Letter of John Paul II to Archbishop Jean-Louis Tauran on the Occasion of the International Conference 'Twenty-First Century Slavery—The Human Rights Dimension to Trafficking in Human Beings,'" May 15, 2002, http://w2.vatican.va/content/john-paul-ii/en/letters/2002/documents/hf_jp-ii_let_20020515_tauran.html.

social services as soon as possible.[23] The 2002 letter, the 2007 statement, and several additional interventions made by Pope Francis denounce human trafficking and encourage local and national efforts to increase awareness of this grave social sin. What might it mean for bioethicists and health care providers to likewise denounce and give increased awareness to trafficking victims who appear in our EDs?

Structural Sin and Catholic Bioethics

The concept of structural sin, undergirded by Catholic teaching on trafficking and a deep commitment to the interconnectedness between health care providers and vulnerable patients, enables Catholic bioethicists to approach Trisha's situation in new and different ways. The immediate focus in her story as narrated earlier was on her immediate health presentation, as it should have been. However, as the complexity around her situation began to emerge, it became important for the health care team to gather as much information about her history as possible. What forms of social support, if any, does she have? What about her family history? After exploring these routine clinical questions, however, more outreach and collaborative efforts need to develop that link health care institutions with advocacy and support services. It is the interdisciplinary nature of structural injustices, which make them complex and difficult to break down.

When asking the routine clinical questions over time, the staff at the ED learned Trisha is the oldest of three siblings, all of whom experienced domestic abuse. Both parents struggled with alcohol and drug addiction along with other mental health concerns, and eventually all of them were sent to live with their grandmother. However, the grandmother was frail and had many chronic conditions and relied primarily on Trisha to act as the parent. During this time Trisha met Jerry, her eventual trafficker. Jerry started coming to her grandmother's home, telling Trisha he loved her and that he would take

---

[23] Pontifical Council for the Pastoral Care of Migrants and Itinerant People, "People on the Move: Statement on Human Trafficking, no. 105," December 2007, http://www.vatican.va/roman_curia/pontifical_councils/migrants/pom2007-105/rc_pc_migrants_pom105_statement-human-barnes.html.

care of her and her family. He bought them groceries, took Trisha to get her hair and nails done, and assumed a caretaking role for Trisha and her siblings. However, Jerry also began posting pictures of Trisha online and got her addicted to heroin, telling her it would help relieve her stress. Over time, he convinced her to live with him and began selling her for sex to those who responded to his online posts. If Trisha refused, he would lock her in a room for days with no food, no water, and no toilet.

If a person like Trisha is simply freed from the grips of their trafficker(s), the chance that they will flourish on their own are slim to none. They suffer from trauma, both the trauma of being trafficked and the trauma of the circumstances that enabled their trafficking to occur in the first place. Without a more comprehensive approach, such as adequate housing, education, and counseling, victims have little chance of truly escaping their circumstances. Ultimately, human trafficking is more than a law enforcement or domestic violence issue; it is a public health issue, deeply informed by social determinants of health, including where victims and potential victims live, work, recreate, and learn. Insofar as it erupts within clinical settings, trafficking highlights how these distinctions—between public health or social ethics—are false distinctions. It is a place where public health and social ethics meet bioethics, calling all three areas to adapt and transform.

Yet supporting patients like Trisha beyond the clinical walls is complicated but necessary for addressing her well-being. As such, it will require multidisciplinary teams across many human service organizations working together to end human trafficking and support survivors. A social approach to human trafficking involves defining scope; identifying risk and protective factors of victimization, perpetration, resilience; investigating health care screening and response protocols; and implementing prevention strategies. When viewed through this lens, the solution shifts from only enforcing laws or treating presenting health issues to including a whole community and fostering systemic change.[24]

---

[24] Emily F. Rothman, et al., "Public Health Research Priorities to Address US Human Trafficking," *American Journal of Public Health* 107, no. 7 (July 1, 2017): 1045–47.

Accompanying Victims, Dismantling the Structures of Sin: Practical Recommendations

None of the documents of CST address the role of health care in connection to human trafficking. Nevertheless, health care has a role to play in the development of a social strategy to holistically address the needs of the victims of human trafficking. Victims of human trafficking can be assisted, if they wish, in multiple ways through their interactions in the health care system and with health care professionals. In order to meet the needs of this unique and vulnerable population, Catholic bioethicists should lead a multifaceted approach that focuses on emphasizing education, interdisciplinary care in the clinical setting, a broader understanding and utilization of community-based resources, and advocacy both for and with victims.[25]

First, caring for vulnerable persons creates challenges in the clinical setting when elements of abuse are present. In these instances, there is a greater need to expand efforts to raise awareness of challenges victims face and provide guidance for physicians, nurses, social workers, and chaplains on how to identify, interact with, and treat suspected victims and keep them safe.[26] Many counties in the US offer certification for training in recognizing the signs and symptoms of human trafficking. A director of an emergency department (ED) can become a certified trainer in human trafficking and provide training to all staff members in the ED. Over time the education and training can expand to other areas of the hospital. Health systems as a whole can raise awareness and provide training through a variety of mechanisms, such as newsletters and online learning certified for the continuing education of busy health care professionals.

Drawing on Pope Francis's framing of the church and its ministries as a field hospital, treating victims means treating their wounds but

---

[25] For resources developed by Dignity Health, see "Taking a Stand Against Human Trafficking," https://www.dignityhealth.org/hello-humankindness/human-trafficking.

[26] For resources on how to identify victims of human trafficking in the clinical setting, see National Human Trafficking Resource Center, "Identifying Victims of Human Trafficking: What to Look for in a Healthcare Setting" and National Human Trafficking Resource Center, "Framework for a Human Trafficking Protocol in Healthcare Settings."

may not mean solving all of their problems comprehensively in the clinical encounter.[27] One phrase that is helpful in assisting victims of human trafficking is to "treat, but not rescue." Although this may seem counterintuitive, treating and not rescuing is important given the danger victims face. For victims of human trafficking, the goal is to create a relationship of trust, relying on experts (particularly the skills of crisis nurses, chaplains, and social workers) to offer resources, support, and to create options for victims who may feel like they have none. Probing questions should be asked very tentatively, if at all. After interacting with someone suspected of being a victim, health care providers should contact the Polaris National Human Trafficking Hotline as follow-up rather than to attempt to free an individual immediately.[28]

According to the US Department of Health and Human Services Substance Abuse and Mental Health Services Administration (SAMHSA), the trauma-informed approach is the best-practice model for those who encounter trafficked persons and others who have been affected by traumatic events. Trauma-informed care assumes that the provider realizes the widespread impact of trauma, recognizes the signs and symptoms of trauma, responds by fully integrating knowledge about trauma into policies, procedures, and practices, and the provider seeks to actively resist retraumatization.[29]

While the clinical setting provides an initial point of contact in which victims can be cared for, other organizations such as immigration, law enforcement, local health-clinics, local advocacy alliances, and other social service agencies can provide valuable resources for victims and serve as collaborative partners for health care institutions to work proactively to serve the needs of trafficked persons in a holistic manner. Collaborating with law enforcement creates an opportunity to identify that victims of trafficking are in the area. One option would

---

[27] Interview with Pope Francis by Fr. Antonio Spadaro, https://w2.vatican.va/content/francesco/en/speeches/2013/september/documents/papa-francesco_20130921_intervista-spadaro.html.

[28] Polaris National Human Trafficking Hotline, https://polarisproject.org/get-assistance/national-human-trafficking-hotline.

[29] W. L. Macias-Konstantopoulos, "Caring for the Trafficked Patient: Ethical Challenges and Recommendations for Health Care Professionalism," *The AMA Journal of Ethics* 19, no. 1 (2017): 85.

be to develop a community taskforce: "members of this proposed joint task force would include one or two human trafficking resource officers, front line health care providers, and members of the local human trafficking law enforcement task force."[30] This alliance would create immediate connection to additional resources to train hospital staff and provide a structure by which a patient could choose to leave their victimizer under the protection of law enforcement. However, if a patient does choose to leave, additional services would be needed. The alliance may consider expanding its community-based collaborations beyond law enforcement to build wrap-around services such as housing, education, and counseling to help freed victims recover from their trauma and begin building a new life for themselves.

One example that demonstrates the practical application of collaborating and working in solidarity with victims is to explore beginning a Crime and Trauma Assistance Program (CTAP) through a federal grant provided through the Victims of Crime Act (VOCA) or related entity. CTAP can grow services that provide counseling and therapy for persons experiencing trauma from a variety of injustices. CTAP staff may be comprised of clinical social workers, clinical counselors, and marriage and family therapists, among others, who provide a variety of therapy modalities such as EMDR (Eye Movement Desensitization Reprocessing), TF-CBT (Trauma Focused-Cognitive Behavioral Treatment), and Traumatic Incident Reduction. CTAP also provides training, education, and consultation opportunities for the local hospital's or health system's employees, local agencies, and organizations that provide other assistance, advocacy, and supplemental treatments to those affected by traumatic events. With regard to human trafficking, CTAP can train SANE nurses (Sexual Assault Nurse Examiners), the hospitals' nursing staff, case management, social workers, and emergency department on the signs and symptoms of human trafficking and how to make referrals to the CTAP program. The CTAP site can be located near the main hospital but should be in a discreet location so that victims do not feel labeled

---

[30] Megan Helton, "Human Trafficking: How a Joint Task Force Between Health Care Providers and Law Enforcement Can Assist with Identifying Victims and Prosecuting Traffickers," *Health Matrix* 26, no. 1 (2016): 456.

by entering the doors; the program serves victims for years, if not indefinitely.

Finally, local efforts both in the clinical and community setting create an opportunity for intentional advocacy work on the behalf of victims. Advocacy professionals within the health system can examine state laws to see where improvements can be made, such as effectively prosecuting traffickers, removing punitive measures for identified victims in cases of prostitution or immigration violations, and improving state-wide education efforts for providers. It is pointless to prosecute a victim for prostitution or immigration, for example, when the victim did not have a choice in his or her services. Often the focus of many advocacy efforts is sex- trafficking victims; however, victims of trafficking likewise include child-labor and other non-sex forms of labor. Thus, advocacy work connected to the antiquated immigration laws within the US is sorely needed.

Conclusion

In Trisha's case, training in trauma-informed care provides the clinician with a lens for safely and tentatively probing beyond her current medical conditions and immediate concerns of abuse and neglect into a wider social history that might shed light on her complete entrapment by others that has taken away her freedoms and violated her human dignity. It also provides other staff with training on how to recognize signs and symptoms of this wider history, and when and how to communicate with each other about red flags and alerts that need to be made to local authorities and/or national hotlines. Trisha's case presents the challenge of how health care can engage structural injustices.

For Catholic health care, creating structures to support these victims and patients is a part of our social responsibility. Rajendra points to the cosmopolitan principle of CST that breaks down barriers to identifying commonly held dignity and the importance of practicing solidarity. Papal letters, encyclicals, and addresses have focused consistently on the challenges posed by structures of violence. Rather than ignore the victims of these structures, Catholic health care needs to find a way to develop trust with patients and partnerships with the community to truly treat the whole person.

Chapter 3

Far From Disadvantaged: Encountering Persons with Mental Illness

Abraham M. Nussbaum, MD

Illness incapacitates a person; each illness incapacitates in its own fashion. Congestive heart failure incapacitates a person's cardiac output, acute renal failure incapacitates a person's glomerular filtration, and mental illness incapacitates a person's agency. A person experiencing depression has an incapacitated volition to make a choice, while a person experiencing psychosis has an incapacitated ability to distinguish between real and perceived choices.

A person whose mental illness impedes their ability to act in the world often falls out of the world's familial, civil, and ecclesial societies. Persons with mental illness are less likely than their peers to ever marry and more likely to divorce, even if they desire family.[1] Persons with mental illness are less likely than their peers to be employed and more likely to be disabled, even if they desire work.[2] Persons

[1] J. Breslau, E. Miller, R. Jin, N. A. Sampson, J. Alonso, L. H. Andrade, E. J. Bromet, G. de Girolamo, K. Demyttenaere, J. Fayyad, A. Fukoa, M. Gălăon, O. Gureje, Y. He, H. R. Hinkov, C. Hu, V. Kovess-Masfety, H. Matschinger, M. E. Medina-Mora, J. Ormel, J. Posada-Villa, R. Sagar, K. M. Scott, and R. C. Kessler, "A Multinational Study of Mental Disorders, Marriage, and Divorce," *Acta Psychiatrica Scandinavica* 124, no. 6 (2011): 474–86.

[2] Y. B. Suijkerbuijk, F. G. Schaafsma, J. C. van Mechelen, A. Ojajarvi, M. Corbiere, and J. R. Anema, "Interventions for Obtaining and Maintaining Employment in Adults

with mental illness are less likely than their peers to experience accommodation and more likely to experience stigma in religious communities, even if they desire faith.[3]

Within the Catholic social tradition (CST), all people are created to participate in these three interdependent societies—family, work, and faith. In the encyclicals, the popes describe the human person as a social creature constituted by social engagement. John XXIII wrote in *Pacem in Terris*, "any human society, if it is to be well-ordered and productive, must lay down as a foundation this principle, namely, that every human being is a person, that is, his nature is endowed with intelligence and free will."[4] CST declares that to be a person is to be a social creature endowed with intelligence and will, but leaves unsaid how to include a person whose intelligence or will is so incapacitated by mental illness that they stand alone.

When contemporary bioethicists consider what it means to include a person with mental illness in a human society, they focus upon the inclusion of such a person in the society of biomedicine. Bioethicists discuss the ethical implications of culture within psychiatric care,[5] the professional ethics of psychiatric practice,[6] and the ethics of conducting research on psychiatric subjects.[7] Bioethicists often leave unsaid how to include a person whose free will is incapacitated by mental illness in the human societies beyond medicine, to speak about persons with mental illness as something more than patients.

Persons with mental illness are sometimes patients participating in biomedical treatment. They are sometimes also companions and cousins in families, candidates and citizens in civic life, and choristers

---

with Severe Mental Illness: A Network Meta-analysis," *Cochrane Database of Systematic Reviews* 9 (2017): Cd011867.

[3] A. Smolak, R. E Gearing, D. Alonzo, S. Baldwin, S. Harmon, and K. McHugh, "Social Support and Religion: Mental Health Service Use and Treatment of Schizophrenia," *Community Mental Health Journal* 49, no. 4 (2013): 444–50.

[4] John XXIII, *Pacem in Terris* 9.

[5] See, for example, Ahmad Ukashah, J. Arboleda-Florez, and N. Sartorius, *Ethics, Culture, and Psychiatry: International Perspectives* (Washington, DC: American Psychiatric Press, 2000).

[6] See Laura Weiss Roberts, *A Clinical Guide to Psychiatric Ethics* (Arlington, VA: American Psychiatric Association Publishing, 2016).

[7] See James M. DuBois, *Ethics in Mental Health Research: Principles, Guidance, and Cases* (Oxford: Oxford University Press, 2008).

and communicants in ecclesial life. To account for the range of experiences of a person with mental illness, the questions bioethicists ask—especially Catholic bioethicists—should be expanded by CST, which implicitly asks what it means to include persons with mental illness in the familial, civil, and ecclesial societies foundational for human happiness. To extend the CST vision of engagement in these foundational societies, Catholic parishes should explicitly consider their responsibility to persons with mental illness and Catholic health systems should extend psychiatric services, especially for the estranged and indigent.

Encountering Liêm, Alone

Liêm and I met on the adult inpatient psychiatry service of the academic safety-net hospital at which I work. The hospital is a governmental authority with a social mission to care for vulnerable persons. Many of the patients have public insurance. Many of the patients have been turned away from other hospitals. Many of the patients have delayed care until they accepted care at our facility.

Liêm accepted our care against his will. His family initially brought him to a large Catholic hospital in the area that provides technical services which generate profit margins—cardiology, oncology, and orthopedic services—but no psychiatric services. So Liêm was transported by deputies, in handcuffs, to our public hospital.

When our nurses unshackled Liêm, they found his wrists encircled by friction burns. Those red circular abrasions echoed the darker, deeper, linear abrasions on his face. Around his right eye were hurried marks of violence that signified Liêm's determination to cast out the offending eye. Liêm tried to claw his right eye out with his fingers because he believed Matthew 5:29—"If your right eye causes you to sin, tear it out and throw it away"—was written for him alone. Liêm likely would have fulfilled the command, but his older brother discovered Liêm in the act. The brother saved Liêm's eye long enough for physicians to look at it.

The eye was infected, so we prescribed antibiotics to fight the likely pathogens. Liêm refused antibiotics, preferring infection. The eye was damaged, so we consulted ophthalmologists who recommended extraction of his irreversibly compromised orbit. Liêm refused surgery, preferring self-extraction.

Liêm suffered from schizophrenia, an oft-disabling and progressive mental illness that erodes neurocognitive function, impairs reality perception, and sometimes distorts agency to the point that a young man will autoenucleate his own eye.[8] Liêm declined biomedical treatments, so we asked our hospital ethics service which treatments Liêm could refuse and which he could be compelled to accept. The bioethicists met the medical team and reviewed Liêm's records. They found that Liêm's illness so impaired his autonomy that he was no longer able to make decisions for himself. They advised that an alternative "decision-maker" be identified to substitute their agency for Liêm's own.

Autonomy, Bioethics, and the Person as Decision-Maker

Clinical bioethicists, like those who evaluated Liêm, encourage and assess the ability to govern one's self. Bioethicists typically assess individual autonomy, identifying the minimal conditions at which a person can exercise his or her own authority through interviews and reviews of available records. In doing so bioethicists determine if a person is the power behind the reasoning that results in a person's behavior. The bioethicists who evaluated Liêm determined that psychosis was the power behind his behavior, so Liêm lacked autonomy. He lacked the minimal power of self-government to be the "decision-maker" in his care.

In their assessment the clinical bioethicists did not employ a relational account of autonomy, an understanding of the way Liêm made decisions in the context of social relationships. They did not ask how he came to read Matthew in so literal a fashion that he would sacrifice his sight. They did not even ask why he was named Liêm, a name which revealed his relationships.

Liêm's parents named him after Saint Vincent Liêm, the first martyr of the Vietnamese church. Liêm's parents fled persecution in Vietnam and raised Liêm to revere the saint's heroism. Of their six children, Liêm was the only unmarried one, the only one to drop out of school, and the only one who had been escorted out of Mass for interrupting

---

[8] M. Shah, L. Sun, S. Elmann, I. Vrcek, R. Mancini, H. J. Kim, J. Carrasco, and R. Shinder, "Self-inflicted Enucleations: Clinical Features of Seven Cases," *Orbit* 36, no. 3 (2017): 154–58.

the priest. Liêm fell out of his family's plans for marriage, an educated future, and out of their parish life. Alone, Liêm took to reading Scripture and concluded that Matthew 5:29 spoke to his sins. He was refusing antibiotics, corrective surgery, and psychiatric medications as a large act of penance and a small act of martyrdom.

If a clinical bioethicist wanted to understand Liêm's actions in a relational fashion without asking relational questions like why he was named Liêm, they would meet obstacles. If a bioethicist sought counsel from the biomedical literature, they would find a culturally specific account of autoenucleation that pathologizes Liêm's faith by characterizing autoenucleation as a sequelae of Christian beliefs.[9] If a bioethicist sought a culturally specific care setting, they would find that while the first institutions for care of persons with mental illness in the United States were developed by Protestant communities, very few were developed by Catholics.[10] If a bioethicist sought a specifically Catholic guild of psychiatrists to mediate between psychiatry and Liêm's faith, they would find that while such a guild existed in the twentieth century, none exists today.[11] Finally, if a bioethicist turned to the Catholic bioethics literature, they would find very limited discussions of what it means to care for persons with mental illness.

The Missing Persons of Catholic Bioethics

In magisterial documents, the care of persons with mental illness is discussed either as an illustration of other concerns or in brief papal missives.[12] There is no mention of the care of persons with mental illness in magisterial bioethics texts like *Donum Vitae* and *Dignitas*

---

[9] See R. S. Shiwach, "Autoenucleation—A Culture-Specific Phenomenon: A Case Series and Review," *Comprehensive Psychiatry* 39, no. 5 (1998): 318–22.

[10] Heather H. Vacek, *Madness: American Protestant Responses to Mental Illness* (Waco, TX: Baylor University Press, 2015). Catholics have not typically built mental health institutions but have relied upon the state to do so; see also B. D. Kelly, "Hearing Voices: Lessons from the History of Psychiatry in Ireland," *Irish Medical Journal* 110, no. 3 (2017): 537.

[11] A. M. Nussbaum, "Profession and Faith: The National Guild of Catholic Psychiatrists," *Catholic Historical Review* 93, no. 4 (2007): 845–65.

[12] See John Paul II, "Address to Participants in the International Congress on the Human Mind," *Acta Apostolicae Sedis* 83, no. 8 (1991): 66–672; Benedict XVI, "Effective Help Needed for those with Mental Illness," *L'osservatore Romano* 1926 (2006): 2.

Personae. Perhaps as a result, the only mention within the United States Conference of Catholic Bishops' *Ethical and Religious Directives for Catholic Health Care Services* is that "the person with mental or physical disabilities, regardless of the cause or severity, must be treated as a unique person of incomparable worth, with the same right to life and to adequate health care as all other persons."[13] In the Directives, persons with mental illness are recognized as persons with rights but grouped among the disabled, even though many persons with mental illness are not disabled, and mental illnesses incapacitate a person differently than other illnesses.

While persons with mental illness go missing in magisterial documents and ethical directives, they are readily found in the human societies identified by the encyclicals. According to the World Health Organization, a single class of mental illnesses, depressive disorders, is the leading cause of non-fatal disability worldwide.[14] According to the United States Substance Abuse and Mental Health Services Administration, approximately one in five American adolescents and adults had a diagnosable mental illness in the past year, and approximately one in twenty-five American adults is seriously impaired by a mental illness.[15] And when a Catholic health system recently surveyed the residents of their underserved community, respondents identified poor mental health as their most pressing concern.[16]

When persons with mental illness appear in Catholic health care literature, authors typically propose ways to better include persons with mental illness in the society of medical care. In the pages of

[13] United States Conference of Catholic Bishops, *Ethical and Religious Directives for Catholic Health Care Services*, 5th ed. (Washington, DC: USCCB, 2009), 11–12.

[14] World Health Organization, *Depression and Other Common Mental Disorders: Global Health Estimates* (Geneva: World Health Organization, 2017), license CC BY-NC-SA 3.0 IGO, http://apps.who.int/iris/bitstream/10665/254610/1/WHO-MSD-MER-2017.2-eng.pdf.

[15] Substance Abuse and Mental Health Services Administration, "*Key Substance Use and Mental Health Indicators in the United States: Results from the 2016 National Survey on Drug Use and Health* (HHS Publication No. SMA 17-5044, NSDUH Series H-52)" (Rockville, MD: Center for Behavioral Health Statistics and Quality, Substance Abuse and Mental Health Services Administration, 2017), https://www.samhsa.gov/data/.

[16] A. Carrillo and C. L. O'Grady, "Responding to Chicago Communities: Residents List Mental Health Care as Top Need," *Health Progress* (Jan–Feb 2018): 29–33.

Health Progress, the journal of the Catholic Health Association, readers can find articles about integrating mental health services into primary care clinics,[17] using telepsychiatry to provide access to psychiatric services in rural communities,[18] and imagining the success of the quality improvement movement within medicine as a model for transforming the care of persons with mental illness.[19] These initiatives, many with profound merit, are adopted from secular psychiatric practice rather than birthed from Catholic models of care.

Liêm was sent away from a Catholic hospital which offered no psychiatric services even though such services were first developed by Catholic communities.

Forgotten Witnesses from the Tradition

Liêm needed psychiatric hospitalization; Father Joan-Gilabert Jofré founded the first psychiatric hospital in Western society. In 1409, Jofré observed a group of children in Valencia, Spain, mocking and striking a disturbed man, crying out "The madman, the madman, here comes the madman."[20] Jofré stopped the children and sheltered the man in a local convent. Two days later Jofré delivered a sermon calling his parishioners to action. He said their city lacked

> a hospital house where the innocent and frenzied would be drawn together . . . it would be a very holy thing and work for Valencia to build a hostel or hospital where such insane or innocent persons could be housed so that they would not be wandering through the city and could not hurt nor be hurt.[21]

---

[17] J. Brunelle and R. Porter, "Integrating Care Helps Reduce Stigma," *Health Progress* (Mar–Apr 2013): 26–29.

[18] S. Linquist and B. Erickson, "A Network Touches the Hard-to-Reach: Expanding Access to Mental Health Services through Telehealth," *Health Progress* (Jan–Feb 2018): 23–27.

[19] R. Hochman, "The Substance Abuse and Mental Health Epidemic: It is Time to Ignite a Transformational Campaign," *Health Progress* (Jan–Feb 2018): 19–22.

[20] Ruben D. Rumbaut, "The First Psychiatric Hospital of the Western World," *American Journal of Psychiatry* 128, no. 10 (1972): 125–29.

[21] J. J. López-Ibor, "The Founding of the First Psychiatric Hospital in the World in Valenica," *Actas Espanolas De Psiquiatria* 36, no. 1 (2008): 6.

Soon after, his congregants built the Hospital of Santa María of the Holy Martyr Innocents. They named their hospital after the children Herod slaughtered, who are acclaimed as saints despite dying before they had reached the age of reason. The company of saints makes room for those without reason; Jofré and his congregants similarly found room in their communal life for persons with mental illness, figuratively turning "madmen" into "holy innocents" deserving of humane care. Their hospital admitted local and foreign patients, provided the full range of contemporary treatments, pioneered a humane form of inpatient treatment, and inspired mental hospitals throughout the Iberian Peninsula as well as in Cuba, Guatemala, and Mexico.

Liêm also needed supportive housing; Saint Dymphna, the seventh-century martyr, inspired a tradition of psychiatric foster care. According to legend, Dymphna was born to an unbelieving Celtic king and his Catholic wife. When Dymphna's mother died, the king insisted that Dymphna become his bride. Dymphna refused her father, fled across the North Sea, and founded an oratory near Amsterdam. Dymphna's father, literally mad with rage, sought her relentlessly and when he found her, martyred Dymphna and her three companions. In the ensuing centuries, Geel, the Belgian town where Dymphna was killed, became a favorite pilgrimage site for the deranged, depressed, and disturbed. In recognition of cures attributed to Dymphna, the church canonized her in 1247 as a virgin martyr who resisted irrational madness. Canonization increased Dymphna's pilgrims, and Geel made room by constructing a hospital for pilgrims in 1286. The number of pilgrims grew even further, and the community increased its services, consecrating a church dedicated to her cult in 1349, adding an infirmary in 1480, and in the fifteenth century, a system for lodging Dymphna's pilgrims in the homes of villagers. Many pilgrims never left the hospitable homes of Geel, and a system of foster care for mentally ill adults developed around the relics of Saint Dymphna. Today, the adult foster care for the mentally ill in Geel remains a paradigm for providing long-term care while integrating the mentally ill into the larger community.[22]

[22] Jackie L. Goldstein and M. M. Godemont, "The Legend and Lessons of Geel, Belgium: A 1500-year-old Legend, a 21st Century Model," *Community Mental Health Journal* 39, no. 5 (October 2003): 441–58.

The ongoing example of Geel poses a question to contemporary psychiatry—why can it not similarly integrate persons with mental illness into community settings? It also puts a question to Catholic parishes and health systems—where are today's Dymphna-inspired hospitality rooms or Holy Innocent-inspired hospitals for persons with mental illness?

Seeking Liêm, Social, in the Encyclicals

If we seek rationale for building these kinds of services, we find it, at least implicitly, in CST. Explicitly, the encyclicals make little mention of persons with mental illness. However, the tradition was inaugurated by Leo XIII when he declared, "There naturally exist among [humankind] manifold differences of the most important kind; people differ in capacity, skill, health, strength; and unequal fortune is a necessary result of unequal condition. Such unequality is far from being disadvantageous either to individuals or to the community."[23] Leo XIII was writing about the condition of workers, but by acknowledging the reality of "unequal fortune" and insisting that "unequality" is far from a disadvantage, Leo XIII prepared fertile ground for renewing psychiatric services.

In a biomedical model, unequal fortune is accounted individually as pathology to be corrected, so Liêm was assessed individually against standards of mental health. He fell short because his mental illness incapacitated his agency, so he was involuntarily committed to treatment. Hospitalized on our unit, Liêm was isolated from his family, his culture, and his faith. His meals were prepared for him, his days were scheduled for him, and his physical movement was restricted to a locked unit. The very treatments we prescribed, despite our intentions, decreased Liêm's agency. On the unit we encountered Liêm, as in the words of *Octogesima Adveniens*, in a

> world dominated by scientific and technological change [where] methodological necessity and ideological presuppositions too often lead the human sciences to isolate . . . certain aspects of man, and yet to give these an explanation which claims to be

[23] Leo XIII, *Rerum Novarum* (Vatican City: Libreria Editrice Vaticana, 1891) 17.

complete or at least an interpretation which is meant to be all-embracing from a purely quantitative or phenomenological point of view.[24]

We privileged a scientific way of understanding Liêm which isolated his pathology and autonomy from a relational understanding, making "it impossible to understand [Liêm] in his totality."[25]

By contrast, the encyclicals teach that unequal fortune is a reality borne through engagement in human societies. The family is the first society, the society of origin, so Paul VI wrote that a person "finds his true identity only in his social milieu, where the family plays a fundamental role," growing in wisdom, and learning to harmonize individual rights with communal living.[26] It is in the family that a person like Liêm learns to live in solidarity with others. Liêm was angry at his brother for interrupting his autoenucleation, but his family visited daily, easing Liêm's estrangement.

The civic life is the second society, the society where a person has the agency to exercise their rights and duties. CST describes a person as naturally social and meant to live with others and to work for one another's welfare. A well-ordered human society requires that each person contribute generously to the establishment of a civic order in which rights and duties are acknowledged and fulfilled. Acting in civic life a person has both a right to work and a duty to work. A person's labor is not just a commodity to be exchanged, John XXIII wrote, but "a specifically human activity," whose remuneration "must be determined by the laws of justice and equity."[27] The state exists to pursue justice and equity—the common good—and to reduce unequal fortune by protecting its most vulnerable citizens. The state provides necessary social services; John XXIII named health care as a necessity of life and affirmed that "systems of social insurance and social security can . . . be instrumental in reducing imbalances between the different classes of citizens."[28] The job of the state, John XXIII wrote, is to provide necessary social services at the lowest

[24] Paul VI, *Octogesima Adveniens* (Vatican City: Libreria Editrice Vaticana, 1971) 38.
[25] Ibid. 36.
[26] Paul VI, *Populorum Progressio* (Vatican City: Libreria Editrice Vaticana, 1967).
[27] John XXIII, *Mater et Magistra* (Vatican City: Libreria Editrice Vaticana, 1961) 18.
[28] Ibid. 136.

or least centralized competent authority, and to offer these services without "depriving the individual citizen of his freedom of action. It must rather augment [one's] freedom while effectively guaranteeing the protection of his essential personal rights."[29] The state must provide services, on the basis of subsidiarity, that augment the freedom to act in the world. Today, persons with mental illness often receive services so focused on public safety that they decrease the agency of an individual person, as when Liêm's family sought care for his eye only to see Liêm's hands shackled.

Encountering Liêm, Far From Disadvantaged

Liêm's agency was incapacitated by schizophrenia and its treatments, increasing his isolation from society. If we had evaluated Liêm from a perspective informed by CST, or seen him in a facility which embodied CST, we could have simultaneously acknowledged Liêm's unequal fortune in developing schizophrenia, prescribed the best available treatments, and seen Liêm as far from disadvantaged. Liêm had relationships, however strained, to which he could be restored; Catholic bioethicists and health systems similarly have relationships to CST, however strained, which can be restored through practicable ways.

First, biomedical care is a means to becoming fully human, rather than an end in itself. The biomedical model trains practitioners to diagnose and treat pathophysiological dysfunction. It also trains people outside the health professions to look at their bodies and assess them functionally. The encyclicals implicitly rebuke functional accounts of person by situating biomedical care as a means. John XXIII wrote that every person has the right "to the means which are suitable for the proper development of life; these are primarily food, clothing, shelter, rest, medical care, and finally the necessary social services."[30] Medical care serves the human good, but health is not the good itself.

Second, Catholic health systems could include other means suitable for human development in psychiatric treatment plans. In a

[29] Ibid. 155.
[30] John XXIII, *Pacem in Terris* (Vatican City: Libreria Editrice Vaticana, 1963) 11.

biomedical model, our obligation to an ill person like Liêm is complete when his symptoms remit, or at least no longer impair his behavior. The encyclicals encourage a broader assessment of whether or not Liêm has access to the material conditions—food, shelter, and rest—he needs to be fully human. Reducing food insecurity, providing housing, and ensuring rest are both salutary, which is the concern of biomedicine, and humanizing, which is the concern of the Catholic social tradition.

Third, Catholic health systems can encourage vocational rehabilitation and supported employment. The encyclicals conceive of work as an activity constituent of being fully human. John XXIII wrote that "work, which is the immediate expression of a human personality, must always be rated higher than the possession of external goods which of their very nature are merely instrumental."[31] People work not just to obtain goods but to become themselves.[32] A person with mental illness needs a form of work that allows expression of their human personality.

Fourth, Catholic bioethicists could define and assess "mental illness" relationally. In medicine, mental illness is a dysfunction delimited to the individual, which neglects the ways mental illness is socially determined.[33] It also neglects the ways mental health is social engagement. In CST people are intrinsically social, so a single person is never an independent unit of analysis. People, no matter how ill, are related to other people and responsible to other people, so psychiatric treatment plans should include relational accounts of persons with mental illness.

Fifth, all Catholics can advance the agency of persons with mental illness in civic society. Persons with mental illness are excluded from civic society in multiple ways. Literally, persons with serious mental

---

[31] Ibid. 107.

[32] This vision of work is bolstered by findings in the biomedical literature, where a large clinical trial of persons with schizophrenia found that the best clinical outcomes were experienced by persons who are employed. R. Rosenheck, D. Leslie, R. Keefe, J. McEvoy, M. Swartz, D. Perkins, S. Stroup, J. K. Hsiao, J. Lieberman, and CATIE Study Investigators Group, "Barriers to Employment for People with Schizophrenia," *American Journal of Psychiatry* 163, no 3 (2006): 411–17.

[33] Michael T. Compton and Ruth S. Shim, eds., *The Social Determinants of Mental Health* (Washington, DC: American Psychiatric Publishing, 2015).

illness die roughly ten years before their peers.[34] While living, persons with serious mental illness are often imprisoned or jailed, a removal from civic life which often forecloses future involvement in civic life. Exclusion from civic life limits the action of persons with mental illness. Encouraging and enabling a person with mental illness to participate in civic life—by volunteering, voting, running for office, organizing direct action, and engaging in civil disobedience—builds agency, so they are themselves a treatment for mental illness.

Sixth, Catholic health professionals could encourage membership in familial society. Persons with mental illness are often estranged from their families for many reasons. Families are often perplexed by the thoughts or behaviors of a person with mental illness. Families are often exhausted by the demands of caring for a person with mental illness. Families often simply no longer exist in the ways assumed by the social teaching encyclicals. And yet CST insists that the family is the first society, reminding us that we become ourselves through these fundamental interpersonal relationships. In psychiatric services we should support and encourage membership in families, ideally families of origin, but also found families which can endure trials and differences.

Seventh, church leaders should enable membership in the found family that is the church. The sociologist Robert Orsi recently observed that "Any honest description of very many religious spaces in contemporary America would have to include some reference to the presence there of strange, disturbed, possibly psychotic people loudly sharing their distress with the worshippers."[35] Orsi was wondering why people with mental illness are edited out of sociological accounts of worship. We might similarly ask: why are the ordinary experiences of people with mental illness often ignored in parish life? Instead of excluding persons with mental illness, a parish could welcome and value people with mental illness by hosting peer support groups, a devotion to Saint Dymphna, organizing support ministries,

---

[34] E. R. Walker, R. E. McGee, and B. G. Druss, "Mortality in Mental Disorders and Global Disease Burden Implications: A Systematic Review and Meta-Analysis," *JAMA Psychiatry* 72, no. 4 (2015): 334–41.

[35] Robert Orsi, *Between Heaven and Earth: The Religious Worlds People Make and the Scholars who Study Them* (Princeton, NJ: Princeton University Press, 2005), 165.

advocating for justice for persons with mental illness, and helping Catholic health systems offer high quality, low-cost care for persons with mental illness by turning their homes into Geel-inspired foster homes. Parishes can, in short, encourage solidarity between persons with and without mental illness, while advocating for treatments characterized by subsidiarity.

The Catholic social tradition insists that a person is fully human only when in relationships with other people. Surely this includes relationships with persons with mental illness like Liêm. Persons without mental illness can become more human by visiting a person with mental illness in their home, the hospital, or at Mass. Persons with mental illness, persons like Liêm, are readily found in all these places. In relationship with Liêm, perhaps he could have read Matthew 5:29 in conversation with others instead of, to considerable harm, reading the parable alone.

Chapter 4

Integral Ecology in Catholic Health Care: A Case Study for Health Care and Community to Accelerate Equity

Cory D. Mitchell, Armand Andreoni, and Lena Hatchett

The Proviso Partners for Health (PP4H) initiative benefits low-income African American and Hispanic individuals in four target communities of Maywood, Bellwood, Broadview, and Melrose Park in the Proviso Township in the western suburbs of Cook County, Illinois.[1] With a total population of 98,822 (2015 Census estimates), this service area is characterized by consistently high unemployment and poverty rates. The latest unemployment figures show Maywood with the highest rate among these communities at 11.7 percent, almost twice the state unemployment rate of 6 percent, followed by Bellwood (9.7 percent) and Broadview (7.7 percent). All of these rank among the highest in the Chicago metropolitan area. The reality of high rates of unemployment and underemployment were reflected in the community health needs assessment (CHNA) which showed that between 21.8 percent and 45.6 percent of the population falls under the federal poverty level.[2]

CHNAs are required of every nonprofit hospital under the Affordable Care Act (ACA) and often reveal important information about

[1] For a complete overview of PP4H, see https://www.provisopartners.com.
[2] Alliance for Health Equity: Hospitals and Communities Improving Health Across Chicago and Cook County, healthimpactcc.org.

key factors that contribute to the health of individuals within a particular community. In addition to the poverty levels, the assessment revealed a high level of food insecurity and high rates of chronic disease. A study on food access found this area to have the greatest percentage of residents living in a food desert.[3] Mortality rates in suburban Cook County show west suburban Cook having the highest rates for heart disease, cancer, and stroke. Additionally, Behavioral Risk Factor Surveillance System data in the CHNA show 59 percent of respondents being overweight or obese, while 16 percent reported being current smokers and 15 percent were binge drinkers.[4] This community suffers from a variety of health risk factors, but perhaps the most significant is the lack of access to quality food and a safe environment to live, work, and play.

To address these issues, PP4H seeks to establish a sustainable local food policy, systems and environmental change to promote community health and well-being in terms of affordable and accessible fruits and vegetables throughout Proviso Township. Benefits from this effort will appeal to other distressed areas and encourage them to participate to achieve the same goals. Likewise, surrounding sponsors will hopefully consider lending the same opportunity to other residents in their areas as well. Insofar as the local built environment lacks affordable and accessible opportunities for physical activity, PP4H seeks to capacitate community residents and municipalities to improve access to affordable options for physical activity to reduce obesity and enhance community well-being.

The PP4H model partners community and academic facilitators using the REAL framework for equity: (1) resilience, (2) economics, (3) accountability, and (4) love. Within this partnership, members leverage resources and support one another to accomplish the common goals of health and economic opportunity. The partnership has thirty-one active organizational partners and reaches a list of over 150 individuals and organizations in Proviso, including Loyola Uni-

---

[3] D. Block, et al., "Food Access in Suburban Cook County," in *Oak Forest (IL): Cook County Department of Public Health* (2012).

[4] Health Impact Collaborative of Cook County, "Community Health Needs Assessment Central Region," June 2016, http://allhealthequity.org/wp-content/uploads/2018/08/POST-Central-Report.pdf.

versity Health System (a member of Trinity Health) and Loyola University Chicago Stritch School of Medicine and Marcella Niehoff School of Nursing. Currently, fifty-five individuals are working on thirty equitable policy initiatives including food justice, community capacity building, active recess, school wellness policy, and tobacco.

The partnership has a collaborative structure that involves five hubs: (1) elementary school wellness, (2) high school wellness, (3) food justice, (4) built environment (community safety), and (5) tobacco-free living. Each hub is co-led by one person representing the community and one person representing an organization. Each hub works in teams to identify equitable goals, strategies, and action steps for the community action plan. The entire design, planning, implementation, evaluation, and dissemination process is guided by community improvement advisors and academic partners who are formally coached in the art of community of solutions skills from the Robert Wood Johnson foundation 100 Million Healthier Lives SCALE initiative.[5]

❖ ❖ ❖ ❖ ❖

PP4H is one example of community partnerships that can develop between a hospital and the local community to address community health needs, especially around food. The focus on equitable food access is a social, health care, and moral challenge in America. Roughly 13 percent of Americans have insecure access to food on a regular basis.[6] But as with most vital goods, services, and resources in the United States, inequities plague how food is accessed. While 13 percent of the US population is food insecure, nearly 23 percent of African Americans and almost 19 percent of Hispanics struggle with food access.[7] Much of this inequitable access to food is both racialized and spatialized such that African Americans and Hispanics have fewer supermarkets and more poor quality foods in their often

---

[5] S. Stout, *Overview of Scale and a Community of Solutions: Scale 1.0 Synthesis Reports* (Cambridge, MA: Institute for Healthcare Improvement, 2017).

[6] Elena David, *Food Insecurity in America: Putting Dignity and Respect at the Forefront of Food Aid* (Samuel Centre for Social Connectedness, 2017).

[7] Ibid.

low-income segregated neighborhoods compared to White neighborhoods.[8] These social dynamics are a painful reminder that food insecurity is not a simple economic problem of individuals but is systematically structured; like education and employment, devalued groups disproportionately bear the brunt of insufficiency and its sequelae.[9, 10]

Likewise, the consequences of food insecurity are many and varied. The risk of high blood pressure, which can lead to cardiovascular disease (CVD) and stroke, is increased by approximately 21 percent for people experiencing food insecurity.[11] Additionally, the risk of diabetes is increased by about 50 percent.[12] Smoking and alcohol consumption are also associated with food insecurity.[13] Even mental health and employability can be damaged by the lack of equitable access to food.[14] Moreover, food insecurity can lead to both internalizing and externalizing behaviors among youth; educational outcomes can suffer as a result.[15] To be sure, American inequality almost ensures that the relationships between food insecurity and poor outcomes are bi-directional due to a lack of a robust social safety net for the most disadvantaged. Poor physical and mental health, as well as unemployment and low-wage work can lead to greater food insecurity, which can in turn exacerbate poor health and employment outcomes.[16] Food injustice is a vicious cycle indeed.

---

[8] Renee E. Walker, Christopher R. Keane, and Jessica G. Burke, "Disparities and Access to Healthy Food in the United States: A Review of Food Deserts Literature," *Health and Place* 16, no. 5 (2010): 876–84.

[9] Douglas S. Massey and Nancy Denton, *American Apartheid: Segregation and the Making of the Underclass* (Cambridge, MA.: Harvard University Press, 1993).

[10] David R. Williams and Chiquita Collins, "Racial Residential Segregation: A Fundamental Cause of Racial Disparities in Health," *Public Health Reports (1974–)* 116, no. 5 (2001).

[11] Ibid.: 404–16.

[12] Ibid.

[13] Jin E. Kim and Janice Tsoh, "Cigarette Smoking and Food Insecurity in Socioeconomically Disadvantaged Young Adults," *Drug and Alcohol Dependence* 156 (2015): e110–e111.

[14] Elena David, "Food Insecurity in America: Putting Dignity and Respect at the Forefront of Food Aid," Samuel Centre for Social Connectedness (2017).

[15] Christian King, "Food Insecurity and Child Behavior Problems in Fragile Families," *Economics & Human Biology* 28 (2018): 14–22.

[16] "What Are the Connections between Food Insecurity and Health?" *Feeding America: Hunger and Health*, https://hungerandhealth.feedingamerica.org/understand-food-insecurity/hunger-health-101/.

Food insecurity is not just a social or health care issue, it is a moral dilemma. How can we have localities of lack in the land of plenty? What is the appropriate social and/or institutional response to food injustice in a country that has been historically inept at addressing domestic market failure related to the provision of vital goods and services for people of color? If the *Ethical and Religious Directives for Catholic Health Care Services* (ERDs) remind Catholic health care to pay particular attention to the poor and disenfranchised, do Catholic health systems have unique obligations for addressing fragmented and inequitable market-based systems that may have deleterious effects on patient populations? This chapter seeks to provide a creative and concrete case study that demonstrates how one health system in partnership with a community movement addresses these questions and challenges using Pope Francis's framework of integral ecology. PP4H re-envisions equitable structures and policies in the Trinity Health System's Transforming Communities Initiative. We conclude with recommendations that can be spread and scaled to health system and community partnerships to improve food justice, community health, and well-being.

Why Is Food Justice Overlooked?

As previously stated, when the market (and society in general) fails to meet the needs of people of color, those in power usually pay scant attention. In fact, throughout much of American history, policymakers have passed implicitly and explicitly racist policies and laws, which in turn led to implicitly and explicitly biased institutional and individual practices.[17] National narratives also help to undermine social concern for the marginalized. These narratives include the myth of meritocracy and rugged individualism. Such narratives function to magnify the virtue of individual effort. Any person who cannot pull themselves up by their own "boot straps" is thought of as deviant, lazy, and/or undeserving.[18] Our national policies and narratives obscure how privilege and opportunity are structured through

---

[17] Ibram X. Kendi, *Stamped from the Beginning: The Definitive History of Racist Ideas in America* (New York: Nation Books, 2016).

[18] Ibid.

time and space to create and maintain a society of haves and have nots.[19, 20, 21] This focus on individual effort also calls our attention away from unjust systems in order to put the onus for perceived deviance squarely on the shoulders of marginalized populations.

The only obligation(s) explicated by society is the obligation for each person to make the right choices in what is often believed (by the haves) to be an unbiased society in which one can move from "rags to riches" with grit and determination.[22] To date, American society including Catholic health care professionals, have no real substantive language or framework to help think through and address the intersection of food insecurity and oppression. We are stuck seeing food access as an individual or family economic issue and, as a result, miss how social capital, social support, and social cohesion are just as important (if not more so) for food justice as economics.[23] The PP4H is one example of how Catholic health care systems can create a just and sustainable integral ecology.

Catholic Bioethics and Food Justice

In a library search using the search terms, "Catholic bioethics food insecurity," we found no relevant articles. This lacuna is disheartening because Catholic self-understanding and the heart of Catholic sacramental life—Communion—is centered on eating a meal together.[24] Indeed we find our greater humanity in Communion with the Triune God, with each other, and often in eating together. Thus, food justice should be a critical concern for Catholic bioethicists, but it does not appear in the literature. Indeed, the issue of systematic in-

[19] Jeffrey Reiman, *The Rich Get Richer and the Poor Get Prison: Ideology, Class, and Criminal Justice*, 8th ed. (Boston, MA: Allyn and Bacon, 2007).

[20] Gregory D. Squires and Charis E. Kubrin, *Privileged Places: Race, Residence and the Structure of Opportunity* (London: Lynne Rienner, 2006).

[21] Kendi, *Stamped from the Beginning*.

[22] Linda Lutton, "The View from Room 105: Can Schools Make the American Dream Real for Poor Kids?," *WBEZ* 91.5 Chicago, January 16, 2017, https://www.revealnews.org/episodes/reveal-presents-the-view-from-room-205/.

[23] Christian King, "Informal Assistance to Urban Families and the Risk of Household Food Insecurity," *Social Science & Medicine* 189 (2017): 105–13.

[24] "The Eucharist," in *Catechism of the Catholic Church*, 2nd ed. (United States Catholic Conference—Libreria Editrice Vaticana, 1997), 1324.

justice receives scant attention from traditional bioethicists precisely because of the discipline's narrow focus on technologies, therapies, and procedures.

While such a reductionist approach aligns with traditional secular medical ethics and may have its roots is casuistry, it makes it difficult to bring macro-level and mezzo-level issues into view. This is akin to having procedural laws that tell lawyers what rules must be followed in order to litigate a case without having recourse to substantive law, which creates and defines the "why" of law. The only possible result is such a case would be disjointed piecemeal legislation with little rhyme or reason. The same is true of a reductionist Catholic bioethics; it only gets part of the picture at the risk of missing fundamental causal factors. As a result, Catholic bioethics attempts to salve symptoms without addressing problems at their root cause.

A reductionist Catholic bioethics will inevitably strain against the current of change as it seeks to articulate rational theo-technological arguments for or against procedures without broader concern for the inequalities and power dynamics that shape the way those technologies and procedures are allocated and (mis)used. Because Catholic health systems are part of community ecosystems, traditional Catholic bioethics is challenged to help guide health systems in making operational decisions that benefit the common good in a strategic and systematic way. Here, we find Catholic bioethics suffers from inadequate engagement with Catholic social teaching, which tends to be well reasoned and multilevel in nature, in that it addresses issues at the individual, family, institutional, and societal levels.[25] Food justice requires such an approach.

Integral Ecology in Catholic Social Teaching

PP4H is consistent with the concept of integral ecology explicated in Pope Francis's encyclical *Laudato Si'*. Ecology is all about relationships, and an integral ecology amplifies the focus on human relationships with each other and our (built and natural) environment. Integral ecology is fundamentally holistic, affirming that "everything

[25] Bernard V. Brady, *Essential Catholic Social Thought*, 2nd ed. (Maryknoll, NY: Orbis Books, 2017).

is closely related." An integral ecology sees all aspects of the world—human, social, and natural—as deeply intertwined, deeply interconnected. As a result, seemingly unrelated concepts—such as meaningful work, the environment, spirituality, culture, and more—are understood as part of an integrated whole. These interconnections encompass persons as well. After discussing the biblical narrative of Cain and Abel (which happens to have implications for sharing and food), Francis goes on to say: "These ancient stories, full of symbolism, bear witness to a conviction which we today share, that everything is interconnected, and that genuine care for our own lives and our relationships with nature is inseparable from fraternity, justice and faithfulness to others."[26] The pope also tells us to be indignant about the kind of inequality that views or treats one human or a group of humans as more worthy than others.

When we normally talk about ecology or *Laudato Si'*, many Catholic health care leaders will automatically jump to climate change and reducing facility-level carbon footprints.[27] However, humans require healthy social and economic systems as well as environmental systems if they are to be healthy. As the pope notes:

> We are convinced that "man (sic) is the source, the focus and the aim of all economic and social life." . . . We are faced not with two separate crises, one environmental and the other social, but rather with one complex crisis which is both social and environmental. Strategies for a solution demand an integrated approach to combating poverty, restoring dignity to the excluded, and at the same time protecting nature.[28]

PP4H collaborates to deliver such an integrated approach for its four targeted communities.

Within a framework of integral ecology, we see other principles of CST at play. Integral ecology is made possible for Proviso because it relies on solidarity *through* subsidiarity to enhance the common good. In concrete terms, this means that PP4H collaborates with community

---

[26] Pope Francis, *Laudato Si'* 70.

[27] See *Health Care Ethics USA* (Summer 2015). See also Ron Hamel's chapter in this volume (chap. 13).

[28] Pope Francis, *Laudato Si'* 127, 139.

members so that leadership and learning are shared. Residents are valued as experts in their own lives who have just as much to teach us as we have to teach them.[29] They are valued as human beings with innate dignity, and they help guide PP4H in decision-making and solution-finding. The whole process is organic and accords with Francis's articulation of integral ecology.

In our collective experience, we know that connections between the built environment, the natural environment, employment, and social relations are important levers for food justice and health. In fact, green space can significantly reduce blood pressure upon exposure.[30, 31] "Neighborhoods, even those recently built, are congested, chaotic and lacking in sufficient green space. We were not meant to be inundated by cement, asphalt, glass and metal, and deprived of physical contact with nature."[32] However, as previously stated, social relationships and meaningful employment are important too. Integral ecology helps us to use systems thinking to address systematic inequalities with the Proviso communities.[33]

Applied Integral Ecology: Shifting the Paradigm

As a way to address food insecurity, Catholic ministries have been avid supporters of food banks and charitable food. While charitable food systems are a necessity for short term needs, food justice advocates demand sustainable food systems that can explore combined long-term solutions for enhancing food systems. Researchers in Europe and Canada have asked the moral question of whether food

---

[29] Mark S. Homan, *Promoting Community Change: Making It Happen in the Real World*, 4th ed. (Belmont, CA: Thomson Brooks/Cole, 2008).

[30] Michael J. Duncan, et al., "The Effect of Green Exercise on Blood Pressure, Heart Rate and Mood State in Primary School Children," *International Journal of Environmental Research and Public Health* 11, no. 4 (2014): 3678–88.

[31] Eugenia C. South, et al., "Neighborhood Blight, Stress, and Health: A Walking Trial of Urban Greening and Ambulatory Heart Rate," *American Journal of Public Health* 105, no. 5 (2015): 909–13.

[32] Pope Francis, *Laudato Si'* 44.

[33] Leah Frerichs, et al., "Integrating Systems Science and Community-Based Participatory Research to Achieve Health Equity," *American Journal of Public Health* 106, no. 2 (2016): 215–22.

charity undermines sustainable food solutions.[34, 35] A multilayered approach that combines short-term emergency food with workforce development and long-term career training in the food industry can build sustainability in low-income communities of color. Three Chicago-based organizations, including PP4H, have workforce development opportunities to address food justice and reflect integral ecology (Windy City Harvest, Cook County Green Corps, Greater Food depository).[36, 37, 38] Each of these organizations works with African American and Hispanic men who are underemployed, formerly incarcerated, and/or have struggled to train for and maintain meaningful employment.

PP4H was founded upon a spirit for working together before it was an actual growing partnership. In 2006, Maywood experienced high rates of obesity among African American women; at the same time, fresh food outlets were declining.[39] Because healthy food access is associated with better cardiovascular health, the standard thinking was that "food deserts" could be thwarted only by building new food outlets and bringing food stores back.[40] In practice, the local food economy in Maywood hit rock bottom in 2012 when a new mid-range grocery store closed after eighteen months. The local food economy was failing because of social, historic, and cultural racism and segregation.

---

[34] M. Caraher and A. Cavicchi, "Old Crises on New Plates or Old Plates for a New Crises? Food Banks and Food Insecuity," *British Food Journal* 116, no. 9 (2014), https://doi.org/10.1108/BFJ-08-2014-0285.

[35] Tiina Silvasti and Graham Riches, "Hunger and Food Charity in Rich Societies: What Hope for the Right to Food?" in *First World Hunger Revisited: Food Charity or the Right to Food?*, ed. Graham Riches and Tiina Silvasti (London: Palgrave Macmillan UK, 2014): 191–208.

[36] Lena Hatchett, et al., "'Something Good Can Grow Here': Chicago Urban Agriculture Food Projects," *Journal of Prevention & Intervention in the Community* 43, no. 2 (2015).

[37] Lena Hatchett, et al., "Cook County Green Corps African American Trainee Experience in a Green Job Training Program," *Journal of Sustainability Education* (September 2014).

[38] Greater Chicago Food Repository, "Chicago's Food Bank," https://www.chicagosfoodbank.org/.

[39] Amy H Luke, et al., "Leptin and Body Composition of Nigerians, Jamaicans, and US Blacks," *The American Journal of Clinical Nutrition* 67, no. 3 (1998): 391–96.

[40] Jeffrey J. Wing, et al., "Change in Neighborhood Characteristics and Change in Coronary Artery Calcium: A Longitudinal Investigation in the Mesa (Multi-Ethnic Study of Atherosclerosis) Cohort," *Circulation* 134, no. 7 (2016): 504–13.

Throughout the country, less than ten supermarkets are owned by African Americans, and African American neighborhoods have roughly 50 percent fewer chain supermarkets than White neighborhoods.[41, 42] Unlike traditional approaches, PP4H uses a value(s)-based solution for increasing economic and food justice opportunities. The urban farm grows and cultivates relationships with residents, trains youth, and distributes local food to support African American and Hispanic owned growers and sellers, who in turn distribute food to schools and health clinics.

PP4H learned from community members to re-envision power, goods, and resources in the form of value(s)-based employment. Trinity Health System Transforming Community Initiatives supports the sustainable effort with a grant and low-interest investment loans.[43] Traditionally, coalitions operate with staff and volunteers that represent public health researchers or hospital staff supervising community volunteers. To redesign for equity and value-based employment, PP4H practices shared learning and leadership in the PP4H Community Leadership Academy.[44, 45, 46, 47] Community members and multi-sector stakeholders generate real-world policy, systems, and environmental solutions for injustice from person, place, and policy perspectives.[48] To date we have coached thirty adults and youth as

---

[41] Tom Perkins, "Why Are There So Few Black-Owned Grocery Stores?" *Civil Eats* (2018), https://civileats.com/2018/01/08/why-are-there-so-few-black-owned-grocery-stores/.

[42] Lisa M. Powell, et al., "Food Store Availability and Neighborhood Characteristics in the United States," *Preventive Medicine* 44, no. 3 (2007): 189–95.

[43] Betsy Taylor, "Trinity Health Grant Initiative Seeks Community Transformations," *Catholic Health World* (March 15, 2016).

[44] Byrd K. Coleman, J. Scaccia, S. Stout, M. Schall, S. Callender, J. Anderson, N. Behrman, A. Budnik, D. Smith, L. Brown, W. Douglas, R. Bussey, E. McDermott, E. Munene, F. Mullin, L. Hatchett, J. Pohorelsky, T. VanLanen, B. Pairolero, and Z. Mann, *Engaging Community Members with Lived Experience: Scale 1.0 Synthesis Reports* (Cambridge, MA: Institute for Healthcare Improvement, 2017).

[45] Jonathan P. Scaccia, et al., "Community Health Improvement and the Community Psychology Competencies," *Global Journal of Community Psychology Practice* 8, no. 1 (2017).

[46] Stout, *Overview of Scale*.

[47] "100 Million Healthier Lives," https://www.100mlives.org/initiatives/.

[48] Rachel Davis, Danice Cook, and Larry Cohen, "A Community Resilience Approach to Reducing Ethnic and Racial Disparities in Health," *American Journal of Public Health* 95, no. 12 (2005): 2168–73.

Community Improvement Advisors and change agents to collaboratively design, implement, evaluate, and disseminate equitable solutions. While training community members is not a novel approach in health care, outsourcing Community Improvement Advisors as consultants and change agents who are paid at the same levels as health professionals is a welcomed violation of systemic racism, classism, and the current inequitable power structures.[49, 50] The PP4H Community Leadership Academy is the *start* of a journey into leadership that results in community members tailoring their unique perspectives of justice, knowledge, skills, and experience to become community change agents. To date, over $300,000 has been invested into the process and we have gained innovative health and economic solutions from emerging leaders who were formerly incarcerated, out-of-work, and underemployed.

PP4H is on track to coach sixty people to promote the community of solutions skills locally and nationally in the next two years and to leverage resources and assets worth three million dollars.[51] Our shared power and leadership approach to capacity building creates a pathway for people who live with injustice to coach health care professionals about equity and human centered design, systems thinking, implementation, and evaluation for community health. This collaboration space generates innovative policy, systems, and environmental change strategies that work for sustainable social change. This approach is one way we live out our values and simultaneously value our partners while enhancing our local integral ecology.

Incarnating Integral Ecology: Where to Start

Many health care professionals may be interested in rolling out their own integral ecology intervention or PP4H model and wonder

---

[49] Bita Arbab Kash, Marlynn Lee May, and Ming Tai-Seale, "Community Health Worker Learning and Certification Programs in the United States: Findings from a National Survey," *Health Policy* 80, no. 1 (2007): 32–42.

[50] A. Witmer, et al., "Community Health Workers: Integral Members of the Health Care Work Force," *American Journal of Public Health* 85, no. 8_Pt_1 (1995): 1055–58.

[51] Stout, *Overview of Scale*.

where to start. We recommend that corporate discernment conversations and processes must first search out the breaches of equitable interconnectedness inside the organization, as well as with the communities it serves. Earlier we referred to this type of discernment as an equity audit or examination of corporate conscience.[52] This examination should review hiring practices, workforce diversity (including executive staff), board membership, supplier location and diversity (including hiring practices), billing practices, implicit bias in clinical care (clinician panel data can be used to obtain this information) within the organization, in addition to surfacing the community health disparities identified by the CHNA. Leave no stone unturned. Making community rounds is also crucial. Since many executives and staff members do not live in the communities they serve, walking tours around the neighborhood(s) help providers see how residents actually live while potentially surfacing unmet need(s) and building goodwill. We build relationships and insights based on such contextualized encounters with the other. This is where integral ecology starts.

Like Catholic social teaching, the PP4H framework for equity is grounded in human dignity.[53] As human beings, we are more than just "rugged individuals." We are social beings who are interconnected with each other and creation. Interconnectedness is virtually an unmapped concept in bioethics. Traditional Catholic and even secular bioethics often promotes the primacy of autonomy at the expense of other human dimensions such as the need for interpersonal relationships.[54] However, "the dignity of the human as an individual is to be understood in the context of community. The freedom of each individual is itself a thoroughly social reality."[55] We find our humanity in humanity.

---

[52] See, for example, Linda Skrla, James Joseph Scheurich, Juanita Garcia, and Glenn Nolly, "Equity Audits: A Practical Leadership Tool for Developing Equitable and Excellent Schools," *Educational Administration Quarterly* 40, no. 1 (2004/02/01 2004): 133–61.

[53] Stout, *Overview of Scale*, 30.

[54] Tom Beauchamp and James Childress, *Principles of Biomedical Ethics*, 7th ed. (New York: Oxford University Press, 2013).

[55] John Sachs, *The Christian Vision of Humanity: Basic Christian Anthropology* (Collegeville, MN: Liturgical Press, 1991), 35–36.

An implicit but critical ingredient to building the sort of sustainable interconnectedness that integral ecology calls for is reconciliation. Few currently see reconciliation as related to Catholic bioethics,[56] but a bioethics shaped by integral ecology and the CST will integrate this principle as more fundamental than autonomy.[57] The work of St. Thomas Aquinas underpins early CST as a Thomistic *personalism* is grounded in human dignity, not in the primacy of the individual as totally autonomous over and above interconnectedness.[58] In a broken and sinful world, radical interconnectedness can succumb to ruptures that require reconciliation. Reconciliation is what ministry is about (2 Cor 5:18). It is how Christ healed and should be the essence of Catholic health care.

A good place to start this critical, integral, ecological work of reconciliation is the format of the Rite of Penance. For most Catholic health systems, there must first be a recognition that something is amiss. The status quo is not sustainable or in accordance with a truly Christian worldview. Corporately reflecting on Scripture passages such as the narrative about the sheep and goats in Matthew 25:31-46 or the nature of love, reconciliation, and hope in 1 John 3:11-24, tailored for non-Christian staff as well, might be a next step. Organizations can then confess their shortcomings with community stakeholders after their examination of corporate conscience in light of Scripture. Then a *metanoia* (change of ways) is required. This change can be in the form of truly equitable collaboration like the partnerships demonstrated by PP4H. Finally, a form of institutional absolution is implicitly granted to the health system when the community agrees to collaborate because love covers a multitude of sins (1 Peter 4:8).

In order to achieve an integral ecology, charity cannot be separated from justice. Traditional community benefit practices, such as charity

---

[56] One ethicist who counters this trend is M. Therese Lysaught. See her "Love your Enemies: Toward a Christoform Bioethic," in *Gathered for the Journey: Moral Theology in Catholic Perspective*, ed. David Matzko McCarthy and M. Therese Lysaught (Grand Rapids, MI: Eerdmans, 2007), 307–28.

[57] For more on the centrality of reconciliation and peacemaking to Catholic social thought, see Byrnes, et al., in chapter 1.

[58] D. Thomas Williams, *Who Is My Neighbor? Personalism and the Foundations of Human Rights* (Washington, DC: The Catholic University of America Press, 2005), 139.

care, are necessary but insufficient. PP4H demonstrates how solidarity working through subsidiarity can build true community, which is superior to approaches solely based on charity because it advances equity and the common good rather than rely on inequitable power dynamics and disparate access to resources. Recall that we started our initiative with a CHNA, which nonprofit hospitals must conduct at least once every three years under the Affordable Care Act.[59] Once community needs and assets are identified, a hospital can partner with community members using the principles of participatory action research.[60] Engaging in participatory action research helps to ensure that solidarity operates through subsidiarity so that those most affected by decisions have the most impact on those decisions.

[59] https://www.nlm.nih.gov/hsrinfo/community_benefit.html.
[60] Mark S. Homan, *Promoting Community Change: Making It Happen in the Real World*, 4th ed. (Belmont, CA: Thomson Brooks/Cole, 2008).

PART TWO

Countering Injustice in the Patient-Physician Encounter

In part I, we stood at the door of the emergency department, watching as the pain of our communities crossed that threshold and finding ourselves called back out into our local communities in response. In part II, we move further into our institutions—into the quiet encounters in the office of an ob-gyn, a pediatrician, a geriatrician, and the more frantic context of the ICU. Here the tools of Catholic social thought raise new issues that are largely invisible in Catholic health care: caring for gender non-conforming children, emphasizing racial dynamics in prenatal care, or highlighting new dimensions of issues that seem well-mapped like ecological or racial dynamics in end-of-life care. Not only do social injustices mutely walk into the physician's office, these patients can encounter further marginalization and unjust treatment from physicians, nurses, and other health care providers— sometimes unwittingly, sometimes intentionally.

Marginalization in health care can take place in a variety of ways— race, education level, economics, gender. These factors can pose barriers to receiving equitable care. For many of the patients highlighted in this section, the effects of meeting injustice in the health care setting can be devastating. Each of these chapters emphasizes the importance of accompaniment, narrative, access to health care, as well as understanding how values influence patient choices and the care that they receive. While each chapter takes a different approach to addressing these challenges, what remains fundamental is the necessity of listening to the patient's story and responding from where she is, not where the health care team thinks she ought to be. By listening to patient stories and responding to their needs, health care professionals and institutions are compelled to expand the services offered to these vulnerable patients, thereby gaining trust within these communities that have been historically marginalized within health care.

In chapter 5, "Neglected Voices at the Beginning of Life: Prenatal Genetics and Reproductive Justice," Aana Marie Vigen uses the narrative of Flora to highlight the racial and ethnic disparities in US maternal and birth outcomes. Her ethnographic approach evinces the subtle and myriad ways that these disparities pervade how women of color, and in particular Black women, are treated in US health care. To address these disparities, she asks how social analysis might provide a broader understanding of prenatal care and prenatal genetics. She challenges ethicists and mission leaders to expand the notion of what constitutes justice in prenatal care by exploring the longstanding racial inequalities suffered by Black women and infants in the US. Moving beyond limits of the standard pro-life/pro-choice binary toward a framework of reproductive justice, her chapter takes more of a public health approach that emphasizes the inherent interdependent nature of human beings. With Paul Farmer, she avers that "if disease and ill health make a preferential option for the poor, then providers ought to do so as well." Doing so highlights the importance of attending to the social locations of both patients and providers.

Women of color are not the only patients who meet injustice in the clinic. In chapter 6, "Bewildering Accompaniment: The Ethics of Caring for Gender Non-Conforming Children and Adolescents," Michael McCarthy challenges Catholic hospitals to expand how we think of accompanying gender non-conforming (GNC) patients, particularly children and adolescents. With regard to GNC patients, Catholic bioethics focuses almost exclusively on the question of surgical interventions. However, the decision for gender affirming surgery is made much later in life, usually after an uneven experience within the health care setting that leads GNC persons to feel isolated and rejected by the health care system itself. Experiencing such rejection earlier in life has devastating consequences for a GNC pediatric or adolescent patient, resulting in significantly higher suicide rates when compared to the cisgender population. McCarthy foregrounds the practice of accompaniment—a version of solidarity—to propose a framework for attending to GNC patients in their pediatric and adolescent years. The practice of accompaniment not only enables Catholic health care to reframe the ethics of caring for GNC patients; it also challenges it to take the lead by expanding access to health care services beyond the thirty-five centers for pediatric and adolescent GNC patients that currently exist.

While end-of-life care has received much attention in Catholic bioethics, the ways in which a variety of injustices inflect such care has not. In chapter 7, "Greening the End of Life: Refracting Clinical Ethics through an Ecological Prism," Cristina Richie offers a proposal for enhancing ethical decision-making at the end of life by incorporating environmental concerns. While the intersection of clinical ethics and end-of-life care making tends to focus on immediate clinical decisions, Richie seeks to promote greater awareness around the environmental effects of health care interventions. She notes how the *Ethical and Religious Directives* specifically incorporate ecological concerns raised within Catholic social thought. However, this ecological framing rarely enters end-of-life conversations or advanced care planning prior to acute end-of-life decisions. By raising the question of environmental ethics at the end of life, Richie applies Green Bioethics to advanced care planning, providing a model for how it might function with regard to other instances of informed consent and patient decision-making.

While Aana Marie Vigen encourages a deeper consideration of racial disparities at the beginning of life, Sheri Bartlett Browne and Christian Cintron raise similar concerns at the end of life. Their chapter, "Racial Disparities at the End of Life and the Catholic Social Tradition," reflects on the death of an infant, highlighting concerns of mistrust, dignity, faith, and the sin of racism that have historically plagued health care institutions. They make clear how the standard framework of secular bioethics, adopted by Catholic bioethics, is deeply informed from a White and Western perspective. They are critical of how hospitals function as "White spaces," and how even Catholic theological anthropology disadvantages how Black patients are perceived and treated. By drawing on the Catholic social tradition, they aim to offer a liberating paradigm that challenges health care institutions to more intentionally cultivate relationships with Black patients by focusing on better education of health care staff through community partnerships that collaborate with local Black churches. They close by emphasizing that a key area of justice rests with diversifying the face of health care, a field that remains disproportionately White.

Chapter 5

Neglected Voices at the Beginning of Life: Prenatal Genetics and Reproductive Justice

Aana Marie Vigen

"Flora" is an insightful person.[1] Along with being a mother to twins, she identifies as a Black[2] woman and as a student. She hopes to become a life coach for people in rehab from addiction. She gave birth in March 2017. At the time, she was seventeen. She saw both an ob-gyn at one clinic and maternal fetal health physicians at a different high-risk clinic. She had some genetic screening via blood work along with checks for congenital anomalies via ultrasounds. She reports that some procedures and results were not well explained to her. Moreover, while pregnant Flora had several things on her mind: school; insurance (her Medicaid coverage was stopped for a time due to a change in her mother's employment); she needed car seats and a breast pump. Additionally, many days Flora had significant back pain due to the twins' positioning. She remembers loving her ob-gyn but feeling less comfortable at times with the way she was treated at the high-risk clinic.

---

[1] "Flora" is a pseudonym. Interview with the author, February 22, 2018.

[2] I capitalize Black, Latina, and Hispanic as a way to decenter white identity as the (un)conscious, generalized norm or standard so often operative in western bioethics and society. I do not alter capitalizations when quoting other sources.

A couple years before meeting Flora, I had begun reflecting on the uncomfortable paradox of my personal experience of excellent prenatal care alongside overwhelming data on persistent racial-ethnic disparities in US maternal and birth outcomes. I sought to explore two basic questions: first, what medical policies or practices would most improve the health and well-being of US women and children—especially those who are often at risk of being poorly or underserved? Second, what approaches to prenatal care and prenatal genetics will empower women to be as healthy as possible and to experience good birth outcomes? I then began to do qualitative interviews with health care providers (genetic counselors, physicians) and with Black and/or Latina new moms so that I might hear how they think about these questions in their own contexts.

❖ ❖ ❖ ❖ ❖

"Prenatal genetics" elicits a variety of responses—from blank stares to appreciative interest to worried brows. Some regard genetic testing as crucial to improving birth outcomes; others see it as inextricably tethered to abortion and/or eugenics. I think both postures fail to see the limits inherent in their respective stances. Moreover, both positions often attend insufficiently to social context.

This chapter offers an alternate way of thinking about prenatal care and genetics that I hope might lead eventually to more astute, commonsensical approaches and practices. Rather than ask about the ethics of prenatal genetics in a vacuum, it starts with social analysis. Understanding social dynamics is integral to understanding how prenatal genetics plays out differently in different women's lives depending on a number of socio-economic and racial-ethnic factors.

Specifically, I follow Loretta Ross and other founders of Sister-Song.[3] They, along with scholars such as Dorothy Roberts, foreground reproductive justice—rather than choice or life—as the primary normative moral framework. Loretta Ross and Rickie Solinger explain:

[3] SisterSong: Women of Color Reproductive Justice Collective, https://sistersong .nationbuilder.com/.

At the heart of reproductive justice is this claim: all fertile persons and persons who reproduce and become parents require a safe and dignified context for these most fundamental human experiences. Achieving this goal depends on access to specific, community-based resources including high-quality health care, housing and education, a living wage, a healthy environment, and a safety net for times when these resources fail. Safe and dignified fertility management, childbirth, and parenting are impossible without these resources.[4]

Rather than ask abstractly "is prenatal genetics ethical or not?" a reproductive justice framework helps us situate the topic within the larger social, racial, and economic context of US medical care for women. And in so doing, it presses us to give focused and sustained attention to longstanding, unjust inequities.

Vital Context:
US Maternal Mortality and Birth Outcomes

Maternal Mortality

The US has the highest rate of maternal mortality among industrialized peers, and the number of maternal deaths is rising even as it declines elsewhere. Annually, 700 to 900 women die from "pregnancy or childbirth-related causes, and some 65,000 nearly die." Sixty percent of these deaths are preventable.[5] Numerous reasons fuel this unacceptable trend:

> New mothers are older than they used to be, with more complex medical histories. Half of pregnancies in the U.S. are unplanned, so many women don't address chronic health issues beforehand. Greater prevalence of C-sections leads to more life-threatening

[4] Loretta J. Ross and Rickie Solinger, *Reproductive Justice* (Oakland, CA: University of California Press, 2017), 9.

[5] Nina Martin and Renee Montagne, "The Last Person You'd Expect to Die in Childbirth," *ProPublica* and *NPR*, May 12, 2017, https://www.propublica.org/article/die-in-childbirth-maternal-death-rate-health-care-system. In terms of mothers' near deaths, see Katherine Ellison and Nina Martin, "Nearly Dying in Childbirth: Why Preventable Complications are Growing in the U.S.," *NPR*, December 22, 2017, https://www.npr.org/2017/12/22/572298802/nearly-dying-in-childbirth-why-preventable-complications-are-growing-in-u-s.

complications. The fragmented health system makes it harder for new mothers, especially those without good insurance, to get the care they need. Confusion about how to recognize worrisome symptoms and treat obstetric emergencies makes caregivers more prone to error.[6]

Investigative journalists Nina Martin and Renee Montagne note that while more research is needed, it is reasonable to say that the US has prioritized infant health—including reducing preterm births and improving birth outcomes—while few postnatal efforts have focused on risks and needs of new mothers.

Moreover, racism is a fundamental factor that we must stop ignoring and denying.[7] ProPublica and NPR collected over 200 stories from Black mothers in 2017. A recurring theme is how unconscious bias affects their care and makes them feel disrespected by medical providers:

> The young Florida mother-to-be whose breathing problems were blamed on obesity when in fact her lungs were filling with fluid and her heart was failing. The Arizona mother whose anesthesiologist assumed she smoked marijuana because of the way she did her hair. The Chicago-area businesswoman with a high-risk pregnancy who was so upset at her doctor's attitude that she changed OB-GYNs in her seventh month, only to suffer a fatal postpartum stroke. Over and over, black women told of medical providers who equated being African American with being poor, uneducated, noncompliant and unworthy.[8]

Regardless of fame (e.g., Serena Williams)[9], education attained, socioeconomic class, or profession, Black women are too often not believed or heard at key moments in their health care.

---

[6] Martin and Montagne, "The Last Person You'd Expect to Die in Childbirth."

[7] See P. R. Lockhart, "What Serena Williams's Scary Childbirth Story Says About Medical Treatment of Black Women," *Vox*, January 11, 2018, https://www.vox.com/identities/2018/1/11/16879984/serena-williams-childbirth-scare-black-women.

[8] Nina Martin and Renee Montagne, "Nothing Prevents Black Women from Dying in Pregnancy and Childbirth," *ProPublica*, December 7, 2017, https://www.propublica.org/article/nothing-protects-black-women-from-dying-in-pregnancy-and-childbirth.

[9] Serena Williams recounts her birth and postpartum story in a February 2018 issue of *Vogue* magazine, https://www.vogue.com/article/serena-williams-vogue-cover-interview-february-2018.

For her part, Flora recounts feeling respected by her regular ob-gyn (a Latina female) who asked Flora important questions and for her input. Her OB reassured her when her insurance was temporarily discontinued, explaining that they would work it out and not to worry. She also made sure that Flora was able to get a breast pump and connected her with an advocate who helped her prepare for the babies. Flora felt that this doctor gave her information and options *and also asked* Flora for her thoughts. Given the frequency of their appointments *and because of how* this doctor engaged her, Flora trusted her and felt comfortable in her care.

In contrast, while Flora appreciated that the doctors and staff at the high-risk clinic were paying close attention to the twins' development, she also felt they talked less with her than her OB:

> At the high-risk clinic . . . they just felt like I didn't know any-thing. . . . I had done research on things that I should and should not do, should and should not eat. . . . I got myself well educated. So for them to treat me like I didn't really know any-thing, and I wasn't trying as hard to follow directions. I didn't appreciate that.[10]

She also commented, "It's as if they are talking around you in a different language, and you just have to sit there and listen."

While Flora herself did not have complications, the racial-ethnic disparity among the 700 to 900 maternal deaths in the US is startling: Black women are three to four times more likely to die as a result of complications related to pregnancy and/or childbirth than white women.[11] "Put another way, a black woman is 22 percent more likely to die from heart disease than a white woman, 71 percent more likely to perish from cervical cancer, but 243 percent more likely to die from pregnancy- or childbirth-related causes."[12] Being pregnant is quite literally life-threatening for Black women.

---

[10] Interview with the author. Note: She saw several different doctors at the high-risk clinic, one of whom was a Black male physician.

[11] Per the Centers for Disease Control and Prevention (CDC), the pregnancy-related morality rate for Black women was 43.5 vs. 12.7 for white women from 2011–2013. See CDC, "Reproductive Health: Pregnancy Mortality Surveillance System," https://www.cdc.gov/reproductivehealth/maternalinfanthealth/pmss.html.

[12] Martin and Montagne, "Nothing Prevents Black Women from Dying in Pregnancy and Childbirth."

Infant Mortality and Birth Defects

The picture for infants has improved somewhat in recent years, yet worrisome trends persist. The US infant mortality rate[13] is still nearly twice as high as peer industrialized nations.[14] In 2015, out of nearly 4 million annual live births over 23,000 infants died before their first birthday.[15] In 2015, the infant mortality rate for non-Hispanic white infants was 4.82, 5.20 for infants identified as Hispanic, and a shocking 11.73 for Black, non-Hispanic infants—over twice as high as the rate for non-Hispanic whites.[16] Every year over twice as many Black infants die before their first birthday than white infants. Thankfully, after a month in the NICU, Flora's twins went home and are doing well. They celebrated their first birthday in March 2018.

Why do infants die in these early months? Per the CDC, the top five causes of infant death in 2015 were (in order of frequency): "1. Birth defects, 2. Preterm birth and low birthweight, 3. Sudden infant death syndrome; 4. Maternal pregnancy complications 5. Injuries."[17] Thus, birth defects,[18] many with associated genetic markers, are a signifi-

---

[13] The infant mortality rate is the number of deaths per 1000 live births before a first birthday. It is one of the baseline measurements that gauges not only maternal and child health but the overall health of a society.

[14] "In 2010, there were 6.1 deaths for every 1,000 live births in the United States, which was higher than the rates of 25 other countries in the [CDC] report, including Hungary, Poland, the United Kingdom, and Australia. In the top-ranked countries of Finland and Japan, the infant mortality rate was 2.3 deaths per 1,000 live births." Rachael Rettner, "US Ranks Behind 25 Other Countries in Infant Mortality," *LiveScience*, September 24, 2014, https://www.livescience. com/47980-us-infant -mortality-full-term-babies.html.

[15] Per the CDC, "Infant Mortality," https://www.cdc.gov/reproductivehealth /maternalinfanthealth/infantmortality.htm.

[16] See Sherry L. Murphy, Jiaquan Xu, Kenneth D. Kochanek, Sally C. Curtin, and Elizabeth Arias, "Deaths: Final Data for 2015," *National Vital Statistics Reports* 66, no. 6 (November 27, 2017): 14, https://www.cdc.gov/nchs/data/nvsr/nvsr66/nvsr66 _06.pdf.

[17] CDC, "Infant Mortality."

[18] While the CDC uses the term "birth defect," some object to this terminology. The CDC discusses birth defects in this way: "Birth defects are structural changes present at birth that can affect almost any part or parts of the body (e.g., heart, brain, foot). They may affect how the body looks, works, or both. Birth defects can vary from mild to severe. The well-being of each child affected with a birth defect depends mostly on which organ or body part is involved and how much it is affected. Depending on

cant concern, "accounting for 20 percent of all infant deaths."[19] To be sure, genetics is not the only important root cause and not all birth defects lead to death. Many individuals born with congenital anomalies live comparably as long and as fulfilled as other adults.

Given the complexity and frequency, let us explore congenital anomalies further. According to the CDC, every year, approximately 3 percent, or 1 out of every 33, of babies are born with a birth defect. In other words, out of nearly four million live births, approximately 120,000 infants each year are affected by a congenital anomaly. With respect to race-ethnicity, the CDC notes that for select birth defects (e.g., cleft lip, trisomy 18, encephalocele) Native Americans, Alaska Natives, non-Hispanic Blacks, and Hispanics experience a much higher rate than their non-Hispanic white counterparts. For a few select birth defects, Hispanics and non-Hispanic Blacks, experience a much lower rate than their non-Hispanic white counterparts.[20]

While Down syndrome (trisomy 21) is the most common of the twenty-one major birth defects noted by the CDC (one out of 691 births per year),[21] many other conditions populate the radar of health care providers. Congenital heart defects and neural tube defects (both of which often have associated genetic markers) are also a significant concern. Some congenital anomalies are relatively easy to detect

---

the severity of the defect and what body part is affected, the expected lifespan of a person with a birth defect may or may not be affected." CDC, "Birth Defects: Facts About Birth Defects," https://www.cdc.gov/ncbddd/birthdefects/facts.html.

I use the term to signify not only a difference or variation but a problem in the structural functioning of a human organ or system. Yet I recognize this distinction is open to interpretation and to debate, as many who are deaf and also those who identify as GLBTQAI rightfully make clear.

[19] T. J. Mathews, Marian F. MacDorman, and Marie E. Thoma, "Infant Mortality Statistics from the 2013 Period: Linked Birth/Infant Death Data Set," *National Vital Statistics Reports* 64, no. 9 (August 6, 2015), https://www.cdc.gov/nchs/data/nvsr/nvsr64/nvsr64_09.pdf.

[20] See CDC, "Key Findings: Racial and Ethnic Differences in the Occurrence of Major Birth Defects," https://www.cdc.gov/ncbddd/birthdefects/features/racialethnicdifferences.html; see also Mark A. Canfield, Cara T. Mai, Ying Wang, et al., "The Association Between Race/Ethnicity and Major Birth Defects in the United States, 1999–2007," *American Journal of Public Health* (September 2014), http://ajph.aphapublications.org/doi/full/10.2105/AJPH. 2014.302098.

[21] CDC, "Birth Defects: Data and Statistics," https://www.cdc.gov/ncbddd/birthdefects/data.html.

prenatally while others are far more vexing. In all, many layers of complexity merit attention.

First, it is important to emphasize that these anomalies range from severe and life-threatening to very mild in their expression. In fact, there are ranges of severity experienced *within* several conditions, for example, Down syndrome and osteogenesis imperfecta (also known as brittle bone disease). Similarly, one person may have a rather mild (or relatively treatable) form of spina bifida or heart defect while another's health is much more significantly and chronically constrained.

Second, while some congenital disorders are clearly caused by one factor (e.g., a defective gene on chromosome 15 that causes Tay-Sachs or heavy alcohol consumption during pregnancy causing fetal alcohol syndrome), others are caused by a complex mix of factors or an unknown cause.[22] Overall, congenital anomalies are correlated with a web of several influential—and often interrelated—factors, such as inherited genetics; a lack of folic acid in one's diet; environment (chronic exposure to toxins, pollutions, stress, etc.); lack of access to early prenatal care; medical history/diagnoses prior or during pregnancy; smoking or drinking alcohol during pregnancy; and advanced maternal age. Thus, genetic anomalies constitute one important piece of a larger puzzle.

Third, for some women, genetic family histories constitute a particularly significant part of their health profile—for example, women who have themselves or who have biological family member(s) with diseases that are known to be directly linked to genetic factors (e.g. Tay-Sachs, phenylketonuria, trisomies 13, 18, 21, sickle cell disease, osteogenesis imperfecta, cystic fibrosis, Huntington's disease, breast cancer with genetic mutations BRCA 1 or 2). Some individuals with such family histories want to learn everything they can about their genetic profiles during pregnancy while others want less or no information.

---

[22] The CDC: "For most birth defects, we think they are caused by a complex mix of factors. These factors include our genes (information inherited from our parents), our behaviors, and things in the environment. But, we don't fully understand how these factors might work together to cause birth defects." CDC, "Birth Defects: Facts About Birth Defects."

Catholic Bioethics and Prenatal Genetics

As a Lutheran, I aim for modesty in describing Catholic bioethics. In that spirit, I think it is fair to identify two common but contrasting themes found in both official Catholic teaching and mindsets. On the one hand, the Catholic tradition emphasizes the intrinsic value of all human life, leveraging respect, human dignity, and *imago Dei* as the most authoritative ethical guides. In medical ethics, these norms are often applied in a deontological use (universal, duty-based) of natural law, as seen in *Humane Vitae* and *Dignitas Personae*. In assessing the morality of prenatal genetics, this view holds that genetic testing is never ethical if used to justify abortion. On the other hand, the tradition also expresses a more contextual form of natural law as seen in *Pacem in Terris*, which prioritizes the role of human conscience and experience. Prenatal genetic screening can help inform that conscience. Furthermore, while official Catholic teaching is unambiguous when it comes to using genetic testing to decide whether or not to have an abortion, it is *not* against testing if used to help prepare for the birth of a child. *Dignitas Personae* and *Donum Vitae* are crystal clear on both points.

Moreover, and regardless of actual ethical positions taken on prenatal genetics, in most traditional arguments autonomy is the central norm. Either it is leveraged to prioritize the autonomy of the pregnant woman *or* the fetus's inherent dignity that demands guarding its future autonomy. Either way, individual autonomy is commonly understood as a (if not *the*) critical issue at stake. In short, whatever one thinks about the ethics of prenatal genetics, it is likely conceptualized primarily in individualist terms—for example, what a person should/should not do or what information to which a person or family has an inherent right. This hyper-focus on individual autonomy and dignity often sidelines other moral norms—the common good, solidarity, and the preferential option, while questions regarding the larger social context are almost never raised.

Insights from the Catholic Social Tradition

Catholic ethics are textured, and the Catholic social tradition (CST) in particular contributes vibrant social, economic, and cultural analysis to a range of topics from labor and poverty (*Rerum Novarum*,

Laborem Exercens) to the multi-headed lethal beast of climate change (*Laudato Si'*). Michael Rozier, SJ, underscores how CST fits well with the core values of public health because of shared emphases on the well-being (common good) of all and on balancing individual rights and responsibilities with those that are social and structural in nature.[23] For example, the church consistently calls society to provide social, economic, educational, childcare, and health care supports needed to welcome children across the spectrum of health and ability.

CST also connects the common good to intrinsic human dignity in order to emphasize that we are inherently interdependent creatures—born into relationship with others just as God is inextricably in relation to creation. Thus, being made in God's image means not only that we are beloved; it also means that we *are accountable to one another*. Everyone needs care, love, and help of various kinds; no one is wholly self-sufficient. Our well-being—as individuals and as a society—is bound up with others. This lens of human interdependence then, in addition to that of autonomy, ought to inform prenatal care.

And also because of our interdependence, we ought to align ourselves—our priorities—with those in greatest need, making a preferential option for those suffering most from present structural inequities. The preferential option, rooted in Latin American liberation theology, does not mean that God loves those impoverished or marginalized in society more than those who are not. Rather, it points to the fact that while God loves all people (and all creation), God in Christ starts with the hurts and needs of those most likely to feel unloved, ignored, and suffering—and calls us to do likewise—to embody this love and justice in the world as we are able. It is a kind of "theo-ethical triage." To paraphrase Paul Farmer, if disease and ill health make a preferential option for the poor, then providers of care had better do so as well.[24]

---

[23] See Michael Rozier, "Religion and Public Health: Moral Tradition as Both Problem and Solution," *Journal of Religion and Health* (2017) 35: 1059.

[24] See Paul Farmer, *Pathologies of Power* (Berkeley, CA: University of California Press, 2005), 140. See also Michael Griffin and Jennie Weiss Block, eds., *In the Company of the Poor: Conversations with Dr. Paul Farmer and Fr. Gustavo Gutierrez* (Maryknoll, NY: Orbis, 2013).

Finally, CST urges us to practice what we pray and espouse. Offering lip service to ideals of equality and justice do very little lasting good. Instead, CST asks people to create concrete actions of creative moral resistance and transformation. Embodying solidarity with those at the margins of power structures means that those with relative power put their material resources and energies in service of pragmatic interventions—enacting specific changes to specific policies, laws, and practices—that benefit those with less. Solidarity also means listening deeply to—and following the lead of—those who know most intimately what it means to be dispossessed by systems of power.[25] Indeed, solidarity represents the opposite of a "savior" mentality. It is *not* about coming in and fixing things for others for whom we patronizingly express charity, and even worse, pity. Rather, solidarity requires those in power *to listen* to those who are too often silenced or ignored and *to be changed* by what they hear. It is only then that people can discern collaboratively how to transform present structures and practices so that they are more just and respectful.

Concrete Proposals

So how might pre- and postnatal care change if we genuinely value the lives of women and children? First, we who generally experience good birth outcomes and who can access excellent health care, especially those who identify as white, need to listen deeply to people who too often do not. Second, in light of what we hear, together as a society, we need to support mothers comprehensively, for example, by adequately funding new parent classes, affordable childcare, and other social safety nets. Just one example is paid parental leave.[26] Still in 2018, the US ranks last among its industrial peers. No federal law requires paid leaves.[27] As many in public and community health note,

---

[25] Tisha Rajendra, "Burdened Solidarity: The Virtue of Solidarity in Diaspora," *Journal of the Society of Christian Ethics* 39, no. 1 (2018).

[26] "Most European countries ensure paid parental leaves, publicly supported child care for preschool children, and cash grants to families with children." Lisa Sowle Cahill, *Theological Bioethics* (Washington, DC: Georgetown University Press, 2005), 180.

[27] The one federal law enacted, The Family Medical Leave Act, "offers only unpaid leave of up to 12 weeks a year to care for yourself, a child or a family member. It is restricted to workers in companies with more than 50 employees, who work full-time

economic policy *is* health policy, education policy *is* health policy. As Rozier observes, "socio-economic factors are twice as influential on our overall health as medical care. And . . . zip code is a stronger predictor of health than our genetic code."[28]

A caveat: calling for strong attention to social determinants of health does *not* mean that genetics does not matter or that there is no need for prenatal genetic testing and counseling. Rather, the point is that instead of narrowly focusing on prenatal genetics in the abstract ("is it ethical or not?"), we need to situate it within a larger context of prenatal (and pre-conception) medical care and women's health. Simply put, *both* a woman's genetic makeup *and* her social location (e.g., racial-ethnic, socio-economic class) hold vital information about her specific health risks. Putting these diverse factors into conversation can contribute to a fuller analysis of her health and needs. Even more, if more women and girls have access to high quality, comprehensive, attuned and caring health care and reproductive education *before* pregnancy, they may be more equipped to negotiate questions and options related to prenatal genetics when and if they become pregnant.

Third, we need to attend to the social locations of both patients *and* providers. The results from genetic testing confirming congenital anomalies can present particular challenges for some women. For example, Flora at 17 and living with socio-economic constraints, appreciated holistic care and social services. If one or both of the twins had been diagnosed with a congenital anomaly, she likely would have needed additional information and support. Certainly, more affluent women also benefit from these same resources. Yet it is important to acknowledge that because of entrenched racial and socio-economic inequities, some women may need more support

---

and have been with the firm for more than one year, and thus doesn't cover 40 percent of the U.S. workforce." Brigid Schulte, "The U.S. Ranks Last in Every Measure When It Comes to Family Policy, in 10 Charts," *The Washington Post*, June 23, 2014, https://www.washingtonpost.com/blogs/she-the-people/wp/2014/06/23/global-view-how-u-s-policies-to-help-working-families-rank-in-the-world/?utm_term=.92edafcec522. See also, Charlotte England, "Paid Maternity Leave: US is Still One of the Worst Countries in the World Despite Donald Trump's Family Leave Plan," *The Independent*, March 1, 2017, http://www.independent.co.uk/news/world/americas/paid-maternity-leave-us-worst-countres-world-donald-trump-family-leave-plan-women-republican-social-a7606036.html.

[28] Rozier, "Religion and Public Health," 1061.

than others. Reproductive justice demands that *all* women—across race and class lines—are empowered with the agency, support, and information needed to be captains of their own lives—make reproductive decisions and to parent children in safe and healthy environments.

Moreover, health care providers and bioethicists need to attend to our own social locations. In clinical ethics we focus too often on individualized understandings of patient-provider relationships. Yet, it is never just a patient and a doctor or nurse talking together in a room. Both always bring their "baggage" to the encounter—their respective worldviews and values rooted in particular social, racial, gender, sexual, religious, and economic identities. Whether or not health care providers are consciously aware of these filters makes a real difference. Too often, stereotypes and assumptions about which patients are "intelligent, responsible, who will be or are good parents," etc., poison doctor-patient relationships. Flora felt her OB truly knew her and respected her. However, she felt that the doctors and staff at the high-risk clinic gave her far less credit and made more assumptions about her given her age and possibly racial identity. She felt they primarily gave her instructions to follow, rather than actively involving her in her own care.[29]

Power dynamics matter. While everyone makes assumptions and can be guilty of stereotyping others, health care providers wield significant control in the clinical context—what topics are discussed, what options are presented, what referrals and recommendations are made. When providers (un)consciously make assumptions about

---

[29] Flora explained that her cervix was opening too early and they would continually remind her that she should not be walking much, "So they would be like, any appointment I came to, they were like, 'Your cervix is opening a little bit more. We need you to stop doing this.' Like keep reminding me as if I'm not following directions." Flora felt they assumed that she was not taking their directions seriously and that bothered her because she was trying hard not to do things that would cause her cervix to open further. She remarked, "Young parents doesn't mean they're irresponsible parents. That might mean that they have more access to more knowledge, and they might be trying to learn." In all, Flora felt less informed and less respected at the high-risk clinic than with her OB, even as she appreciated their expertise: "I think they enhanced [my prenatal care] in certain ways, and in certain ways I don't think that they helped. I think that going to a high-risk clinic when your pregnancy is high risk is very important because those are the people that can help you and have better technology to help you. But there are certain ways where they could overstep boundaries, and they need to be more willing to accept how you feel about your status."

their patients' intelligence, wishes, or values, they often misstep and fail to build solid communication, trust, and rapport with patients. We need to foster health care cultures that push providers to stop, reflect, and check assumptions so that they can truly see and hear the person before them.

To take Flora's cue, health care providers would do well to step back a bit from getting through the procedures to make sure they fully hear and respond to patients' priorities and questions by creating more space for conversation and collaboration and explaining topics with clarity and humility. Flora had wished that someone had given her written material, perhaps a handout naming and describing the various options as well as what the procedure entailed, what they would be screening for or diagnosing. In her case, she was aware that some genetic screening was being done but was not as clear on the names of the screens or their results. Women ought to have a more than a vague sense of the testing and procedures done to them. Current health care structures do not reward such time and attention. Certainly, many providers feel overwhelmed by the volume of their work. Yet discerning the most fitting and helpful kinds of prenatal genetic testing and counseling for particular patients is hard to achieve without first having a strong relationship and significant trust levels.

Conclusion

CST helps us to take a deep read of particular situations and people. It can help us move from abstract concepts to thinking more concretely about what good health care really looks and feels like to specific peoples. Rozier observes that "For health care organizations [and I would add bioethics], ethics is not just about arriving at a solution to the dilemma; *ethics is about choosing where to focus one's effort and why.* . . . In this way, the ethical concerns that these moral traditions help address is less about any specific ethical dilemmas and more about broadly informing one's life and the health of the community."[30] I would even go further: bioethics in the twenty-first century must doggedly raise critical questions about what is and is not

---

[30] Rozier, "Religion and Public Health," 1061 (emphasis mine).

on our collective radars and cultivate strong moral imagination for addressing complex problems even more than it applies general principles to case studies or cultivates virtue in individual professionals. Bioethics, more than ever, needs to immerse itself in the muck of structural suffering and social sin experienced every day by so many in the United States (and globally).

Central norms in CST can embolden those of us in relative positions of power in society to reflect on the ways that privilege and social (dis)advantage (profession, insurance, race, class, immigration status, gender, disability, sex, etc.) shape particular experiences of medical care. This exercise can then create an opening for health care providers to think about what it means to live in solidarity with those who must contend with the social sin of being at disproportionate risk of having poorer health and of receiving inadequate health care. There is no defensible excuse for why the United States cannot do much better in terms of racial-ethnic disparities in maternal and infant health.

With respect to prenatal genetics, when we rush too quickly to take a stand for or against it in the abstract, we miss important social context. Flora views the option to do genetic testing as important to prenatal care *and* she also thinks it is important that women be given choices about what kinds, if any, of testing or counseling services they wish to pursue.[31] Certainly many clinics, especially those with ample resources, offer detailed information and conversation. Yet, in Flora's experience, her providers could have done better at giving her specific information about testing options—what kinds of things they would be looking for and what kinds of results she wanted to know versus those she did not want to know. In particular, Flora wanted to know if there were any life-threatening issues for the twins, but she did not want to know if one or both had Down syndrome. While lines can blur, life-threatening vs. other kinds of impairments

---

[31] She commented, "I think that people should let people have choices. Maybe you want to know if your kid has Down syndrome or autism or anything. But sometimes that's more stressful during your pregnancy to know than not knowing. . . . I feel like they should have like a paper listing all the tests that they would do. And you might want to have a paper of all the tests that they need for their specific pregnancy and give them a choice to further explain it and let them decide if they want to know certain things, or if they feel like to them that they need to have."

were an important distinction to her. In short, for Flora, it was not a zero-sum issue. And again, while prenatal genetics was on her mind, so were many other things—back pain, preparing her home for the babies, and making sure her insurance was restarted. Her OB got this; the providers at the high-risk clinic less so. For Flora, prenatal genetics was one discrete part of a much larger matrix of tests, concerns, needs, and priorities.

Medical providers need to strive to better align care plans with patient's specific values, priorities, and needs and take them seriously as agents of their own lives. Flora did not want extensive genetic testing; however, other women do. Educating patients about options, risks, what results mean, etc., is vital. Yet, it is just as important is to check one's own presumptions about what pregnant women will (not) want or "what is best" for them. Flora took her pregnancy seriously and worked hard to educate herself about what to do, eat, and also avoid as soon as she learned she was pregnant. She wanted her health care providers to take her seriously as well.

Incorporating CST into bioethical analysis and practice will help shine a spotlight on injustice and envision steps to make meaningful changes to health care practices and institutional structures. We need to work on two fronts simultaneously: first, targeting racial-ethnic and socio-economic disparities in maternal and infant mortality and morbidity is urgent. In so doing, we—as providers of medical care and as a society—should understand that prenatal genetic testing, by itself, is not a "magic key" that will unlock the secret to ameliorating these disparities in outcomes. Second, we need to enact policies and practices that help providers to listen to patients and to reflect critically on the assumptions they often make. The more care providers fully hear—and collaborate with—their prenatal patients, especially those most at risk of being unseen and unheard, the more they will find ways to incorporate genetics into prenatal care in ways that are both fitting and just.

Chapter 6

Bewildering Accompaniment: The Ethics of Caring for Gender Non-Conforming Children and Adolescents

Michael McCarthy

Thia was born biologically male. Yet she never felt comfortable as a boy. Her parents say that from a very early age she would not tolerate being called a boy. She exclusively wore dresses, bright colors, and rejected outright all "boy things"—cars, trucks, sports, action figures, etc. When she visited her grandparents she always complained that they forced her to do "boy" things and refused to let her wear dresses or bring any "girl" toys.

At school she was required to dress as a boy; teachers would get mad when she wanted to be herself. She had difficulty making friends, and some local parents would not let her play with their kids. With a few close friends, the family was open about Thia's questions and her insistence that she was a girl. They all listened, supported, and loved Thia. Yet it was clear that they were all concerned. Her parents were at a loss for what to do.

In addition to Thia's questions, her family also had concerns. Should they try and stop behaviors such as crossdressing and promote a more "masculine" environment, even though she would reject it? Who could they to talk to? Various pediatricians either dismissed Thia's behavior as a phase or clearly felt uncomfortable with the topic. Through an online support group, they found answers to questions, but as adolescence began, things grew more complex. Thia suffered bouts of severe depression and anger. She now dressed as a boy. She hated her body. Her lament, which as a little boy was "Why didn't God make me a girl?!" was now "Why was I born at all?!" Her parents knew she was depressed and angry but had unhelpful experiences in the health care environment. When their concerns for their daughter's life became greater than guarding their family's secret, they visited a physician who affirmed that Thia was dressing as a boy but did not use her preferred pronouns of she and her. He referred them to a clinic that specialized in gender dysphoria that was three states and several hundred miles away.

❖   ❖   ❖   ❖   ❖

When questions of gender identity are raised in Catholic health care, they tend to focus on the role of health care professionals facilitating the process of physiological transition from one gender to another. While the ethical permissibility of gender affirmation surgery and hormone treatment in Catholic health care facilities continues to be debated, few discuss how to support gender nonconforming (GNC) children and their parents as they wrestle with identity questions, questions that can arise rather early in life. During those years, patients, accompanied by parents who may be confused, ashamed, frightened, or affirming, encounter the health care system at a variety of touchpoints—pediatric wellness visits, school immunizations, annual check-ups, sports physicals, and visits for illness—illnesses which at times arise from social stresses subsequent to challenging gender norms in a heteronormative society. Each touchpoint can be fractured by ethical failure and misrecognition.

How health care professionals interact with gender-questioning individuals and their families shapes their mental and physical well-being and raises a spectrum of ethical questions. Very little, however, has been written about what responsibilities Catholic health care has in caring for GNC children who are members of our patient communities. While sexual complementarity and gender ideology have a place in the larger discussion, this chapter focuses specifically on Catholic social teaching (CST) as a primary resource. CST enables us to ask much broader questions regarding individual well-being and the importance of accompanying GNC children and their parents as members of the Catholic health care community.

This chapter will first describe terminology used in the LGBTQ+ community and why positive interactions with health care professionals are a matter of life and death for many GNC pediatric patients. While we tend to rush to interventions, either encouraging heteronormative behavior or moving toward gender transition, a middle path consistent with treatment options and CST is a path of accompaniment. Secondly, this chapter critiques traditional gender normative approaches within Catholic moral theology that focus solely on the act of transitioning and limit the role Catholic health care can play, rather than accompanying individuals coming to understand themselves in relationship to the world. Third, given the complex medical concerns of GNC individuals, the chapter offers a broader perspective on how to approach gender identity from the CST. Finally, it offers examples of how Catholic health care can better welcome and address the needs of gender questioning children.

Encountering Discrimination in the Clinical Setting

For many, terminology swirling around gender identity can be confusing. Thus, a few initial clarifications are helpful. First, it is important to distinguish between sex and gender. Sex pertains strictly to biological distinction between male and female. Gender is associated with social characteristics typically associated with being male and female. Thus, sex is a biological category determined primarily by one's chromosomes, whereas gender functions as sociological category that typically is thought of within a gender binary.[1]

Most individuals would be referred to as cisgender; here natal sex and gender identity align. However, some individuals identify outside of traditional gender binaries of male and female. Gender minorities or GNC individuals understand themselves as somehow different than the gender of their natal sex. They may best be understood on a gender continuum. "People with nonconforming gender identities can identify with more than one gender (e.g., bigender), no gender

---

[1] For further discussion of gender, see Jana Marguerite Bennett's chapter in this volume (chap. 11).

(e.g., agender), or feel that their gender fluctuates or is undefinable by traditional terms (e.g., genderfluid)."[2] Some may understand themselves as transgender, "individuals for whom gender identity and assigned sex at birth are not fully concordant."[3] For these individuals, navigating health systems can present unique challenges.

Many GNC individuals lack broad access to patient-centered care that is nondiscriminatory. Negative interactions with health care professionals can begin early on in life. In a 2011 survey of over 6,000 transgender Americans, 19 percent of respondents reported being refused health care due to their transgender or GNC status. An additional 28 percent had postponed necessary healthcare when sick or injured, and 33 percent had delayed or not sought preventive care because of experiences of health care discrimination based on GNC or transgender status.[4] Reported experiences of discrimination include: refusing to treat, harsh or abusive language, health care professionals being rough during examination, verbal abuse, and being blamed for their health status.[5] A 2015 National Transgender Discrimination Survey (NTDS) found that nearly 33 percent of patients cited a negative experience with their health care provider within the last year.[6] Many reported having to educate their provider on what constituted appropriate care for transgender patients. While in some instances, health professionals may have been trying to understand the patient's perspective, in general patients felt that they were offering on the job health professional education.

While these experiences are unacceptable in caring for any patients, they have serious ramifications for the health and well-being of GNC patients and may therefore be even more damaging. A 2014 national

[2] Kristen L. Eckstrand, Henry Ng, Jennifer Potter, "Affirmative and Responsible Health Care for People with Nonconforming Gender Identities and Expressions," *AMA Journal of Ethics* 18, no.11 (2016): 1108.

[3] Jaime M Grant, Lisa A. Mottet, Justin Tanis, Jack Harrison, Jody L. Herman, and Mara Keisling, *Injustice at Every Turn: A Report of the National Transgender Discrimination Survey* (Washington, DC: National Center for Transgender Equality and National Gay and Lesbian Task Force, 2011), 4, http://www.thetaskforce.org/injustice-every -turn-report-national-transgender-discrimination-survey/.

[4] Grant, et al., *Injustice at Every Turn*, 76.

[5] Ibid.

[6] S. E. James, J. L. Herman, S. Rankin, M. Keisling, L. Mottet, and M. Ana, *The Report of the 2015 U.S. Transgender Survey* (Washington, DC: National Center for Transgender Equality 2016), 97.

survey on transgender discrimination reports that experiencing rejection from health care professionals correlates with a 60 percent increase in prevalence of suicide attempts, roughly the same as being rejected by their family.[7] While the rate of attempted suicides amongst the national cisgender population hovers around 4.6 percent, for transgender persons it is 41 percent. "Analysis of demographic variables found prevalence of suicide attempts was highest among those who are younger (18–24: 45 percent); multiracial (54 percent); and American Indian or Alaska Native (56 percent)."[8] These individuals indicated a lower educational attainment (high school or less: 48–49 percent) and a lower annual household income (less than $10,000). These findings point to a lack of social capital, the ability to find access to necessary resources in the community and to leverage those resources to their benefit. As with so many other health care disparities, persons from marginalized communities like GNC are further marginalized by race, education, and socio-economic status—limited resources further isolate individuals.

Health Care Resources for Gender Questioning Patients

In health care, accompaniment means that we are typically focused on treatment, but good treatment is based on good data. Unfortunately, only limited data exists regarding "which gender-affirming services—social, psychological, medical, or legal—are desired by GNC people," fueling a general lack of understanding.[9] Data is limited as GNC or transgendered individuals are reluctant to face compounded discrimination within the broader community. However, suicide data suggests that GNC and transgendered persons lack mental health support—something pediatric patients need long before surgical or

---

[7] Ann P. Haas, Philip L. Rodgers, and Jody L. Herman, "Suicide Attempts among Transgender and Gender Non-Conforming Adults" (Los Angeles, CA: Williams Institute, 2014), 12, https://williamsinstitute.law.ucla.edu/wp-content/uploads/AFSP-Williams-Suicide-Report-Final.pdf. While health care is an important indicator, these statistics indicate that guidance, accompaniment, and conversation with those closest to GNC persons is important. Like family members, these individuals are also coming to understand who they are and what their gender identity means for their own self-understanding and place in the world.

[8] Haas, et al., "Suicide Attempts," 2.

[9] Eckstrand, et al., "Affirmative and Responsible Health Care," 1110.

hormonal interventions. Catholic health care's external focus on medical transitions, rather than a broader range of support or counseling services, further marginalizes an already maligned population.

Clinics specializing in caring for GNC children and adolescents are few and far between. As of 2014, there were thirty-five clinical care programs in the US offering support specifically for GNC children.[10] Of the thirty-five programs, thirteen are in the Northeast, eight in the Midwest, six in the Southwest, seven on the West Coast (five in California), and one in the southwest (Dallas, Texas). Unfortunately for children like Thia, these thirty-five programs are operational in only eighteen states. All of them are located in urban areas, and none are affiliated with Catholic health care.

Services in these clinics vary, but most are not directed specifically toward transition and instead focus on helping children articulate who they are, particularly if they are manifesting symptoms of gender dysphoria.[11] The most common approach when caring for GNC children is nondirective treatment. Nondirective treatment seeks

---

[10] Sam Hsieh and Jennifer Leininger, "Resource List: Clinical Care Programs for Gender-Nonconforming Children and Adolescents," *Pediatric Annals* 43, no. 6 (2016): 238–44.

[11] *The Diagnostic and Statistical Manual of Mental Disorders* (DSM-5) lists several criteria for diagnosing gender dysphoria that differ between adults and adolescents. In adolescents and adults, gender dysphoria diagnosis involves a difference between one's experienced/expressed gender and assigned gender, and significant distress or problems functioning. It lasts at least six months and is shown by at least two of the following with a marked incongruence between one's experienced/expressed gender and primary and/or secondary sex characteristics: (1) a strong desire to be rid of one's primary and/or secondary sex characteristics; (2) a strong desire for primary and/or secondary sex characteristics of the other gender; (3) a strong desire to be of the other gender; (4) a strong desire to be treated as the other gender; and (5) a strong conviction that one has typical feelings and reactions of the other gender. In children, gender dysphoria diagnosis involves at least six of the following and an associated significant distress or impairment in function lasting at least six months: (1) a strong desire to be of the other gender or an insistence that one is the other gender; (2) a strong preference for wearing clothes typical of the opposite gender; (3) a strong preference for cross-gender roles in make-believe play or fantasy play; (4) a strong preference for toys, games, or activities stereotypically used or engaged in by the other gender; (5) a strong preference for playmates of the other gender; (6) a strong rejection of toys, games, and activities typical of one's assigned gender; (7) a strong dislike of one's sexual anatomy; and (8) a strong desire for physical sex characteristics that match one's experienced gender.

"to remain neutral with respect to gender identity and to have no therapeutic target with respect to gender identity outcome. The goal is to allow the developmental trajectory of gender identity to unfold naturally without pursuing or encouraging a specific outcome."[12] What is distinctive about this approach is its central emphasis on child, parent, and community-based interventions aimed at supporting the child and enhancing self-esteem. Contacts are made to reach out to family, friends, and schools to describe what is best needed to support GNC children. Given increased awareness around gender identity, expanding available resources becomes an urgent question of justice. Focusing on questions of identity, self-esteem, and self-understanding, combined with the health risks that emerge absent these critical developmental conversations, should shift the ethical framing beyond the discussion of gender ideology that guides the Catholic bioethical imagination.

Gender Ideology and the Catholic Moral Tradition

Traditional approaches to GNC patients in Catholic bioethics focus exclusively on medical interventions and the pervasiveness of "gender ideology." While there is no official Catholic teaching on questions of transgender status, clearer teachings surround surgical interventions or hormonal therapies that render patients sterile.[13]

---

[12] W. Byne, et al., "Report of the American Psychiatric Association Task Force on Treatment of Gender Identity Disorder," *Archives of Sexual Behavior* 41, no. 4 (2012): 759. Much of the data suggests that that approximately 80 percent of GNC children will "desist" rather than "persist" in their dysphoria. This data, however, was primarily generated under the previous DSM-4 classification of gender identity disorder. Under the DSM-4 classification, the American Psychiatric Association (APA) identified three modes of treatment: decreasing gender expansive behavior, nondirective intervention, and encouraging interaction. The first approach is most similar to the pediatric professions' categories one and two. While the focus is not on "conversion or reparative therapy," it does attempt to assist the child to live the gender aligned with their biological sex and reduce activities associated with the opposite gender. In the second approach, the goal is to remain neutral and let the child lead. The presumption here is that allowing the child to engage in gender expansive activities and to create an environment that does not judge or interfere with the activity has a greater potential to enhance the self-esteem of the child. The final category encourages transition and affirms the identification with the child's non-natal sex.

[13] United States Conference for Catholic Bishops, *Ethical and Religious Directives for Catholic Health Care Services*, 6th ed. (Washington, DC: USCCB, 2018).

These teachings are directly connected to magisterial teaching on sexuality. Thus, the inferred matrix for viewing GNC pediatric and adolescent patients is the sexual theology grounded in the unitive and procreative nature of marital sex.

Recently, the *National Catholic Bioethics Quarterly* published multiple essays chronicling concerns around hormonal therapy and gender affirmation surgery. John DiCamillo argues that human desires and the medical feasibility of facilitating gender transitions must be understood through the union of the body and soul. For DiCamillo, biological sex establishes an individual's sexual and gender identity.[14] Thus, he poses that while gender dysphoria may be a real condition, health care interventions should aim to realign gender identity with natal sex rather than to focus on transitioning. "Gender transitioning is intrinsically immoral and so cannot serve the good of the person, even if it provides certain short-term reported relief of dysphoric symptoms."[15] For DiCamillo, God's image is manifested in one's biological sex; attempts to disconnect sex and gender he names as gender ideology.

The phrase "gender ideology" first appears in John Paul II's encyclical *Evangelium Vitae* where it is described as an instance of the division between the culture of life and the culture of death. Gender ideology falls into the culture of death because it is a "freedom [that] negates and destroys itself, and becomes a factor leading to the destruction of others, when it no longer recognizes and respects its essential link with the truth."[16] The truth in this context is two-fold. First, gender transitions reject the truth of natal sex as reflecting God's image understood through a gender binary. Second, a choice against one's natal sex is "non-reproductive," a key characteristic of the culture of death.[17] Thus, any surgical intervention that misaligns a person with their natal sex violates church teaching while also harming the intended nature of the human person.

---

[14] John DiCamillo, "Gender Transitioning and Catholic Healthcare," *National Catholic Bioethics Quarterly* 17, no. 2 (2017): 217.

[15] Ibid., 221.

[16] John Paul II, *Evangelium Vitae* 19.

[17] Juan Vaggione, "Francis and 'Gender Ideology': Heritage, Displacement and Continuities," *Religion and Gender* 6, no. 2 (2017): 302–3.

In December 2017, various religious leaders continued raising concerns about gender ideology in a letter entitled "Created Male and Female." They argued, drawing on the longstanding principle of medical ethics, that medical institutions are obliged to

> "first, do no harm." Offering services that promote gender ideology harms individuals and societies by sowing confusion and self-doubt. Health care, and in particular Catholic health care itself, has a compelling interest, therefore, in maintaining policies that uphold the scientific fact of human biology and supporting the social institutions and norms that surround it.[18]

However, two problems plague their argument. First, what constitutes "harm" or what types of "harm" may be caused is unclear. Young GNC adults killing themselves is certainly a harm that may be mitigated by access to broader health care services. These medical problems will not be addressed by refusing to enter into dialogue with patients. Second, combating gender ideology does not seem to fall within the purview of health care that relies on patient-centered and evidenced based medicine. The scientific evidence does not demonstrate with the same certitude of "Created Male and Female" that a gender binary is a biological fact.

In a synthesis of over 150 articles addressing the biological origins of gender identity and orientation, Katherine O'Hanlon, et al., conclude that sexually dimorphic traits are "innate, immutable and innocent human features."[19] Their review of research exploring fetal development demonstrated important findings that posit gender identity and sexual orientation are conferred during the first half of pregnancy. While genitals develop during the first trimester, "the brain becomes imprinted in the latter half gestation, [making it] possible for fetal brain to be imprinted differently than the genitals."[20] These findings and other nascent areas of study such as genetics,

[18] "Created Male and Female: An Open Letter from Religious Leaders," http://www.usccb.org/issues-and-action/marriage-and-family/marriage/promotion-and-defense-of-marriage/created-male-and-female.cfm.

[19] Katherine A. O'Hanlon, Jennifer C. Gordon, and Mackenzie W. Sullivan, "Biological Origins of Sexual Orientation and Gender Identity: Impact on Health," *Gynecologic Oncology* 149, no. 1 (2018): 40.

[20] Ibid., 35.

epigenetics, neuroanatomy continue to reveal new insights into the genetic features of human development and sexual identity. Kevin Fitzgerald argues that these new insights call for an update to "our understanding of sexual characteristics and gender identification and the various ways in which both can be experienced and expressed in human beings."[21]

From a bioethics perspective, an appropriate rationale for making an ethical recommendation must be based on medical facts. If the new biological evidence is emerging because of information generated through a greater capacity for targeted research, then the theological framing informed by outdated science likewise needs to be reconsidered.

Reframing Gender Questions

Where traditional Catholic bioethics focuses on GNC persons' reproductive biology, Catholic social thought views them through a different lens. It understands GNC patients as persons in our culture who are vulnerable and marginalized. This lens changes not only what we see when we look at these patients; it changes how we understand the ethical dynamics of their lives. While Catholic sexual ethics focuses on surgical acts, CST asks about access, vulnerability, and responsibility. First, it highlights the lack of resources noted in Thia's story, where her social location limited her possibilities to meet her needs as both a GNC child and adolescent regarding clinical care and accompaniment. Second, it brings into view a different moral question: how do we support GNC children to safely ask and begin to answer the foundational question of the moral life, "Who am I?" For many GNC children, like Thia, it is difficult to even articulate this question or to answer it honestly. Many need help processing how to answer that question for themselves. Third, what is the responsibility of Catholic health care in accompanying children as they struggle to answer this question?

Creating more clinical spaces for children to explore the basic questions of moral action is vital to guarding against feelings of isolation and hopelessness. Theologian Craig Ford notes that "Sex and gender

---

[21] Kevin Fitzgerald, "Viewing the Transgender Issue from the Catholic and Personalized Health Care Perspective," *Health Care Ethics USA* 24, no. 2 (2016): 8.

identity are among the elements of one's self that one must explore not only introspectively in the sacred space of one's conscience, but also in community."[22] Isolation, rejection, or misrecognition—being told you are other than how you understand yourself to be recognized by God—within a community tasked to care for you, particularly the health care community, are actions that violate human dignity. Being immersed in such structural violence can impede a child's ability to answer the basic questions of the moral life: Who am I? Who am I called to be? Who am I becoming by my actions? These questions are not only the questions of virtue; they are foundational questions that GNC individuals begin to ask themselves as children. GNC children's inability to reconcile their identity or explore those questions openly and honestly leads to a profound vulnerability, as demonstrated in the rise in suicide rates. Catholic health care's ministry of continuing the healing ministry of Jesus Christ relies on a ministry of accompaniment and making people whole.

Yet accompaniment and wholeness is often what GNC children lack. Falling back on traditional sexual morality fails to answer questions that many children and parents are asking. While some argue that engaging in questions of gender identity and accompanying those children in a clinical setting capitulates to sexual ideology, "for many thoughtful Christians, the realization at play here has little to do with political correctness or accommodation to liberal culture; it is rather a question of love for persons, of psychological wholeness, and of theological integrity and development in new horizons of understanding."[23] Christopher Pramuk captures beautifully why GNC individuals seeking help in health care cannot be viewed solely via Catholic teaching on sexuality, but instead must be seen as fellow pilgrims seeking greater self-understanding and strangers whom Christians and their institutions are called to welcome.

Welcoming the stranger allows for greater possibilities of accompanying families who may be wrestling with challenges of having a GNC child and creates avenues for moving toward the child herself, rather than maintaining a categorical distance. Welcoming the family

---

[22] Craig Ford, "Transgender Bodies, Catholic Schools, and a Queer Natural Law Theology of Exploration," *Journal of Moral Theology* 7, no. 1 (2018): 94.

[23] Christopher Pramuk, "God Accompanies Persons: Thomas Merton and Pope Francis on Gender and Sexual Diversity," *Merton Annual* 28 (2015): 77–78.

and child requires an attitude of acceptance, a space for discerning and accompanying an individual and her family through understanding who one is and how one ought to act most authentically. It is precisely this quest for authenticity that calls Catholic health care to create spaces to walk with GNC patients and families.

Creating a Socially Constructive Space

By focusing specifically on offering appropriate care to GNC children and adolescents, Catholic health care could stem some of the negative experiences that GNC persons experience within health care at an earlier age. Given that childhood and adolescent care centers focus on accompaniment, support, and education, there is no reason Catholic institutions cannot explicitly expand services for this vulnerable population. By focusing on GNC pediatric patients, Catholic health care can improve health outcomes for GNC and transgender people simply by creating a more welcoming environment. Simple actions that embody gender-affirming care include: respecting patient's pronouns, identifying one's bias in caring for various patient groups or preferred treatment options, and developing strategies that assist children and parents to navigate health care systems.

In an effort to better educate staff, Catholic health systems would do well to turn to the World Professional Association for Transgender Health *Standards of Care*,[24] which states:

1. Directly assess gender dysphoria in children and adolescents.

2. Provide family counseling and supportive psychotherapy to assist children and adolescents with exploring their gender identity, alleviating distress related to their gender dysphoria, and ameliorating any other psychosocial difficulties.

3. Assess and treat any co-existing mental health concerns of children or adolescents (or refer to another mental health professional for treatment). Such concerns should be addressed as part of the overall treatment plan.

[24] World Professional Association for Transgender Health, *Standards of Care for the Health of Transsexual, Transgender, and Gender Nonconforming People* (2011), https://www.wpath.org/media/cms/Documents/Web%20Transfer/SOC/Standards%20of%20Care%20V7%20-%202011%20WPATH.pdf.

4. Refer adolescents for additional physical interventions (such as puberty suppressing hormones) to alleviate gender dysphoria. The referral should include documentation of an assessment of gender dysphoria and mental health, the adolescent's eligibility for physical interventions, the mental health professional's relevant expertise, and any other information pertinent to the youth's health and referral for specific treatments.

5. Educate and advocate on behalf of gender dysphoric children, adolescents, and their families in their community (e.g., day care centers, schools, camps, other organizations). This is particularly important in light of evidence that children and adolescents who do not conform to socially prescribed gender norms may experience harassment in school putting them at risk for social isolation, depression, and other negative sequelae.

6. Provide children, youth, and their families with information and referral for peer support, such as support groups for parents of gender nonconforming and transgender children.

While some discussion may need to be generated around recommendation four within Catholic institutions, these guidelines establish a higher standard of care for GNC children and can be made to work within the parameters of the ERDs, providing a clearer way to offer accompaniment to GNC children and their families.

Bewildering Accompaniment

In amplifying the anemic services available for GNC and transgender pediatric and adolescent patients, Catholic health care professionals should practice bewildering accompaniment as they support their patients in a process of self-recognition and discernment in light of their gender identity. James and Evelyn Whitehead argue that bewilderment is a value that fits the framework for entering into a caring relationship with GNC and transgender individuals. Scripturally, they note that bewilderment transforms into "a celebration of God's extravagance."[25] Jacob wrestling with the angel, the Israelites

---

[25] James Whitehead and Evelyn Whitehead, "Transgender Lives: From Bewilderment to God's Extravagance," *Pastoral Psychology* 63, no. 2 (2014): 172.

wandering in the desert, and Jesus' own forty days in the desert all communicate a restlessness, a dis-ease with the reality that confronts them. Yet, what emerges in this process of self-discovery is God's grace through the lives transformed by the individual's bewilderment.

Bewilderment experienced by GNC individuals, if met with welcoming, hospitality, and openness, can result in a process that can lead to a deeper sense of self-understanding, a place in which they can answer who am I. Yet, more frequently, GNC and transgendered individuals experience rejection, both from health care professionals and their families. Catholic health care is uniquely positioned to educate their own health professional staff and to accompany families in supporting and creating a loving place in which the child can experience God's love.

While Pope Francis's pontificate has not resulted in the official acceptance that many in the LGBTQ+ community have called for, his personal comments have engendered hope. In 2015, Francis met with a Spanish transgendered man, Diego Neria Lejarraga, who quoted the pope as saying, "God loves all his children, 'as they are.' He went on: 'You are a son of God and the Church loves you and accepts you as you are.' "[26] And in 2018, a Chilean gay man and survivor of the that country's sexual abuse crisis, Francis told him, "God made you like this and loves you like this and it doesn't matter to me. The pope loves you like this, you have to be happy with who you are."[27] If the pope has the freedom to accompany and create space within the Catholic community for those who have felt excluded and marginalized, then Catholic health care likewise has the responsibility to accompany and not judge those who are seeking care and accompaniment.

Even though official church teaching may restrict the surgical procedures that can be offered, it does not restrict opportunities to accompany families and children like Thia amidst their gendered

[26] Thomas Fox, "Report: Pope Francis Meets with, Hugs Transgender Man," *National Catholic Reporter,* January 30, 2015, https://www.ncronline.org/blogs/ncr-today/report-pope-francis-meets-hugs-transgender-man.

[27] Inés San Martín, "Abuse Victim Says Pope Francis Told Him 'Being Gay Doesn't Matter,' " *Crux,* May 21, 2018, https://cruxnow.com/vatican/2018/05/21/abuse-victim-says-pope-francis-told-him-being-gay-doesnt-matter/.

bewilderment. The dearth of pediatric institutes focusing on GNC and transgendered questions represents an opportunity to witness to CST's emphasis on caring for those on marginalized or stigmatized by society. Given that rejection by family and health care professionals occurs all too often with detrimental effects on the gender questioning population, Catholic health care ministries can become leaders in caring for children and families as they navigate a difficult, but potentially grace-filled journey of self-discovery. To welcome and accompany the stranger, perhaps one who appears as a stranger to herself is an opportunity to witness to the wisdom of the Catholic social tradition and Christ's healing ministry.

Chapter 7

Greening the End of Life: Refracting Clinical Ethics through an Ecological Prism

Cristina Richie

A fifty-six-year-old Hispanic man was admitted to University Hospital after collapsing at home. Diagnosed with end-stage colon cancer, metastatic to his liver and lungs, the patient was a "full code." Placed on a ventilator, his prognosis was poor. A widower with two adult children, he had not designated a health care power of attorney or surrogate decision-maker. When the doctors asked the adult children if their father had made any end-of-life arrangements, such as an advanced directive, they said no. With his capacity to make medical decisions waning, the doctors recommended palliative care. A son agreed, but his daughter wanted "everything done." With the surrogate decision makers divided, the patient remained full code, and all aggressive medical interventions were pursued.

Three days later, with the patient unconscious and imminently dying, the doctors met with the children again. They remained divided on their father's care. The patient was placed on a ventilator and given nutrition through a nasogastric tube. A nurse caring for the man felt increasing moral distress at providing futile treatments and the family division and called for an ethics consult.

The ethicist gathered the clinicians, a chaplain, and family members. She reminded them that they were to make medical decisions based on what the patient, not they themselves, would want done.

The medical team explained that the patient's prognosis had not improved, and they recommended discharge with palliative care. The attending physician asked, "What would your father want done, in this case?" The adult child who wanted palliative care stated, "My father would want to die at home in peace." The adult child who wanted all aggressive measures was quiet.

After a brief pause, she said, "Dad loved being outside. He was an avid fisherman, and before he got sick, used to take us camping. My best memories were of me, my sister, my mom and my dad in the woods. When he got sick with cancer, his doctor told him that he could write down his choices about 'being on machines' and being in a hospital." She continued, "he came home from that appointment and told the family that he wanted to die naturally. He said it would be a waste of God's resources to keep his body alive if his spirit was gone." She turned to the doctors and said, "But I could not accept this answer! His reasons seemed silly to me, and I told him so. Although Dad wanted to write out his wishes for a natural end of life, I prevented him. But now I feel so bad. He was exactly right— I've seen how much garbage the hospital puts out. Every day there are new piles of plastic, tubes, laundry, and wasted food for all the people here. The machines are constantly going to keep Dad's body alive, but his spirit is with God." The daughter concluded, "I want to make things right. Let Dad die in peace, without all these machines and chemicals."

Later that evening, the patient was extubated and transported to his home under the supervision of the palliative care team. A few hours later, he died with his adult children by his side. During rounds the next morning, the medical team passed the room where the patient had been staying. The nurse commented to the attending physician, "If only the patient's wishes had been written down so we could have known what to do! I know talking about end-of-life wishes is hard, but some people don't realize that they have to be vocal about their reasons, even if they seem strange to others. The treatments were futile and, what is worse, they were in direct contradiction to the man's wishes. Why shouldn't a love of nature and care for the planet be a consideration in medical choices at the end of life?"

❖ ❖ ❖ ❖ ❖

Medical treatments, futility, end-of-life care, and health care allocation have hitherto been in the domain of medical ethics. Rarely, however, have such clinical issues come into contact with environmental ethics. Now, carbon dioxide emissions of the medical industry,[1] pressure on health care facilities to provide numerous, resource-intensive treatments, and the need to expand basic health care access worldwide call into question medical models that work in isolation from other global concerns.[2]

In 2018, the United States Conference of Catholic Bishops (USCCB) reiterated that "throughout the centuries . . . a body of moral principles has emerged that expresses the Church's teaching on medical and moral matters . . . proven to be pertinent and applicable to the ever-changing circumstances of health care and its delivery."[3] One component of this body of moral principles is the emerging church teaching on environmental sustainability. This chapter explores connections between environmental ethics and clinical ethics within the Catholic social tradition (CST). After tracing the intellectual foundations of secular biomedical ethics and clinical ethics, I will highlight how Catholic health care ethics—primarily derived from the *Ethical and Religious Directives*—incorporates ecological concerns raised by the Catholic social tradition. I will then outline how these concerns might "green" a central practice of clinical medicine: advanced care and end-of-life planning. My conclusion highlights the potential for green clinical ethics within Catholic health care.

Biomedical Ethics and Clinical Ethics: Erasing Ecological Origins

The most widely accepted articulation of Western biomedical ethics was crafted at the Kennedy Institute for Ethics at Georgetown University. In 1979, Beauchamp and Childress's "Georgetown mantra"— respect for autonomy, beneficence, non-maleficence, and justice—was

---

[1] Jeanette W. Chung and David O. Meltzer, "Estimate of the Carbon Footprint of the U.S. Health Care Sector," *Journal of the American Medical Association* 302, no. 18 (2009): 1970–72.

[2] Erin Lothes Biviano, Daniel DiLeo, Cristina Richie, and Tobias Winright, "Is Fossil Fuel Investment a Sin?," *Health Care Ethics USA* 26, no. 1 (2018): 1–8.

[3] United States Conference of Catholic Bishops, *Ethical and Religious Directives for Catholic Health Care Services*, 6th ed. (Washington, DC: USCCB, 2018), 4.

codified into academic biomedical ethics, and an individualistic approach to health care triumphed.[4] Some bioethicists, however, have taken a broader approach to biomedical ethics, with Gerald McKenny stating that "recognition of the embeddedness of humanity in nature leads [us] to consider issues neglected by standard bioethics and to preserve the initial understanding of bioethics as a field encompassing environmental and population issues as well as biomedicine."[5] This, however, has been the exception rather than the rule. The four principles resonate with modern American society and reflect the mentality that "in the United States, the exaggerated emphasis on individualism has given free rein to the individual to do whatever one wants with regard to nature and ecosystems."[6] This hyper-individualism includes medical care and the environmental impact thereof.

Dissatisfied with the largely philosophical approach to biomedicine and responding to the need for on-the-ground moral guidance in the health care setting, clinical ethics emerged as a praxis-oriented subset of biomedical ethics. Clinical ethics can encompass clinical trials, student learning in teaching hospitals, and organizational ethics of health care systems. However, its fullest development is seen in ethics consultation, like the one in the case above. Clinical ethics consultation (CEC) focuses on the way in which health care decisions are made and incorporate patient care with the patient's values. Instead of beginning with the principles of biomedical ethics, clinical ethicists use a method centered on four discrete topics for organizing ethical reasoning: medical indications, patient preferences, quality

---

[4] The original conception of bioethics was attentive to the environment, following from the work of German minister Fritz Jahr in 1927 and later American oncologist Van Rensselaer Potter in 1971. Both Jahr's and Potter's bioethic extended to the earth and other organisms but fell into disuse for a variety of reasons. Fritz Jahr and Hans-Martin Sass, "Bio-Ethics—Reviewing the Ethical Relations of Humans Towards Animals and Plants," *JAHR-European Journal of Bioethics* 1, no. 2 (2010): 227–31, at 227. Van Rensselaer Potter, *Global Bioethics: Building on the Leopold Legacy* (East Lansing, MI: Michigan State University Press, 1988), 2. See also Van Rensselaer Potter, "Bioethics: The Science of Survival," *Perspectives in Biology and Medicine* 14, no. 1 (1982): 127–53.

[5] Gerald McKenny, *To Relieve the Human Condition: Bioethics, Technology, and the Body* (Albany, NY: State University of New York Press, 1997), 211.

[6] Charles Curran, "Virtue: The Catholic Moral Tradition Today," in *Virtue: Readings in Moral Theology 16*, eds. Charles Curran and Lisa Fullam (New York: Paulist, 2011), 51–78, at 69.

of life, and contextual features.[7] These were developed in 1982 by Albert R. Jonsen, Mark Siegler, and William J. Winslade and remain the standard for clinical ethics today. While the four topics of clinical ethics support and elaborate on the four principles of biomedical ethics, they also leave considerable room for values that are non-Western, non-White, non-male. In short, they embrace people who do not subscribe to the highly inflected principles of biomedical ethics.

Within the four topics of clinical ethics, "medical indications" includes clinical information such as the nature of the disease and possible treatments and correlates with the biomedical principles of beneficence and non-maleficence. In the case above, possible treatments would consider the environmental impact of those treatments. Beneficence could be extended to all living creatures and the ecosystem. Non-maleficence would recognize the often toxic and harmful effects of prolonged hospital stay and nosological infection.

"Patient preferences" seeks to determine what the patient desires in terms of medical interventions or abstention from treatments and are associated with respect for autonomy. In the case above, the patient clearly preferred a life outdoors in harmony with nature. Since his values extended to health care, the patient would have not wanted to be tethered to artificial life support. A respect for autonomy, in this situation, would support those who wish to forgo some, or all, aggressive medical interventions in favor of natural death.

"Quality of life" attempts to predict outcomes of accepting or forgoing available medical treatments and is related to the principles of beneficence, non-maleficence, and respect for autonomy. Quality of life includes not only medical quality of life like pain, cognition, and mobility, but also recreation and simple pleasures like gardening or walking through parks. In the case above, the patient clearly valued opportunities for being in nature. Quality of life is highly subjective, but for many people—particularly outside of the United States—it includes an active lifestyle.

Finally, "contextual features" consider the domains of law, public health, personal and national finances, and institutional policy, and

---

[7] Albert R. Jonsen, Mark Siegler, and William J. Winslade, *Clinical Ethics: A Practical Approach to Ethical Decisions in Clinical Medicine*, 8th ed. (New York: McGraw-Hill, 2015), 3.

are loosely tied to the principle of justice.[8] The environmental impact of medical care fits under this category. In the case above, the patient drew on his dedication to resource conservation as a reason for not wanting many medical treatments. Particularly when tied to eco-justice, and larger concerns about distributive justice, sustainability can be part of clinical ethics.

In both secular and Catholic clinical ethics, value-based conversations could include more emphasis on sustainability. Yet, in many cases, there are missed opportunities because of the default to principles of biomedical ethics. As a corrective, Green Clinical Ethics is an opportunity to synthesize environmental sustainability with already established clinical ethics practices.

Catholic Health Care Ethics, the *Ethical and Religious Directives*, and Environmental Stewardship[9]

For clinicians working in Catholic hospitals and health care facilities in the US, the *Ethical and Religious Directives* (ERDs) provide moral guidance for the physician-patient relationship and for shaping patient care. The ERDs articulate Catholic teachings on biomedical and clinical ethics and were designed for a number of "health care services under Catholic auspices . . . in a variety of institutional settings (e.g., hospitals, clinics, outpatient facilities, urgent care centers, hospices, nursing homes, and parishes)."[10] The latest ERDs, in its sixth edition, was spurred by a need to respond to modern social, medical, and ethical challenges present in larger society that mostly focused on merging health systems. However, the first part of the directives highlights the importance of justice. "A just health care system will be concerned both with promoting equity of care—to assure that the

---

[8] United States Conference of Catholic Bishops, *Health and Health Care: A Pastoral Letter of the American Catholic Bishops* (Washington DC: United States Catholic Conference, 1982), 9.

[9] In this chapter, I highlight the environmental insights found in the ERDs as they apply to clinical care. Subsequent chapters by Ron Hamel, Tobias Winright, and Andrea Vicini detail attention to environmental sustainability found in *Laudato Si'* and the CST more broadly, particularly as applicable to the practices of health care organizations themselves and to the field of bioethics.

[10] United States Conference of Catholic Bishops, *Ethical and Religious Directives*, 28, n. 2.

right of each person to basic health care is respected—and with promoting the good health of all in the community."[11]

While the ERDs do not mention specifically concerns for the environment, environmental justice is central to promoting "the good health of all" and can certainly be read as supporting a clean and sustainable environment. The general introduction to the ERDs states, "the human family shares in the dominion that Christ manifested in his healing ministry. This sharing involves a stewardship over all material creation (Gen 1:26) that should neither abuse nor squander nature's resources . . . through technology it must conserve, protect, and perfect nature in harmony with God's purposes."[12] Catholic health care is aware of the obligations and responsibilities of those in the healing arts to provide medicine in line with the planet's limits.[13]

Climate change causes health problems, which add to human suffering, health care burdens, and economic loss. The World Health Organization records that worldwide climate change poses "potential risks to health [that] include deaths from thermal extremes and weather disasters, vector-borne diseases, a higher incidence of food-related and waterborne infections, photochemical air pollutants and conflict over depleted natural resources."[14] The journal *Health Affairs* recorded that between 2000 and 2009, the US experienced six specific climate change related events which caused more than 760,000 encounters with the health care system and $740 million in health costs.[15]

Outside of the US, climate change affects the health and well-being of vulnerable populations more dramatically. Cheryl C. Macpherson and Muge Akpinar-Elci note that in the Caribbean "geographic and socioeconomic features pose particular vulnerabilities to climate

---

[11] Ibid., 8.

[12] Ibid., 7.

[13] Cristina Richie, "Carbon Reduction as Care for Our Common Home: *Laudato Si'*, Catholic Social Teaching, and the Common Good," *Asian Horizons-Dharmaram Journal of Theology* 9, no. 4 (2015): 695–708.

[14] World Health Organization, *Global Health Risks: Mortality and Burden of Diseases Attributable to Selected Major Risks* (Geneva: WHO Press, 2009), 24.

[15] Kim Knowlton, Miriam Rotkin-Ellman, Linda Geballe, Wendy Max, and Gina M. Solomon, "Six Climate Change-Related Events in the United States Accounted for about $14 Billion in Lost Lives and Health Costs," *Health Affairs* 30, no. 11 (2011): 2167–76.

change."[16] These health hazards disproportionately impact people and communities who are economically and socially insecure. In his landmark encyclical *Laudato Si'*, Pope Francis reminds us that "pollution [is] produced by companies which operate in less developed countries in ways they could never do at home."[17] The compounded pollution and its health effects create an unjust system that exacerbates existing environmental and medical problems.

Environmental exploitation impacts all people, countries, and health care organizations that care for those affected by climate change related medical problems. Given that health is intimately tied to the natural environment—as well as other social factors like race, sex, and income—the dual concerns of personal health and environmental health appear in the ERDs, but little work has been done in Catholic bioethics to strengthen the connection between environmental ethics and clinical ethics. Although there is ample room in clinical ethics to give weight to environmental conservation, certain religious commitments, such as the sanctity of life, have been misinterpreted when applied in health care settings. Particularly at the end of life, the CST and environmental stewardship are consonant with—rather than in opposition to—each other.

Since the natural requirements of all people must be balanced with available resources, creatures, ecosystems, water, and plants should all be considered prior to any human action, including health care development and delivery. In the case above, this recognition would have gone a long way to validating the patient's decisions to avoid aggressive and futile medical interventions at the end of life. Humans are obligated to pursue stewardship, which includes prudent conservation and preservation of the natural world, as well as just allocation of shared resources in medicine. To this end, the ERDs open up the possibility of an internally coherent presentation of ecological conservation within clinical ethics, which are instructive for practi-

---

[16] The six climate-change related events detailed in the article were: United States ozone air pollution from 2000 to 2002, the West Nile virus outbreak in Louisiana in 2002, the Southern California wildfires in 2003, the Florida Hurricane Season in 2004, the California Heat Wave in 2006, and the Red River flooding in North Dakota in 2009. Cheryl C. Macpherson and Muge Akpinar-Elci, "Caribbean Heat Threatens Health, Well-being and the Future of Humanity," *Public Health Ethics* 8, no. 2 (2015): 196–208.

[17] Pope Francis, *Laudato Si'* (On Care for Our Common Home) 51.

tioners, scholars, and patients who are sensitive to responsibilities of environmental stewardship.

Greening End-of-Life Care

As the opening case illustrated, modern medicalized death in the developed world uses numerous natural and medical resources, as patients are connected to multiple machines, housed in intensive care units, given round-the-clock treatments, and subjected to technological supervision. Assessing which life-prolonging measures, such as artificial nutrition and hydration, intubation or tracheostomy, medications to increase blood pressure (vasopressors), experimental therapies, or cardio-pulmonary resuscitation, are medically appropriate belongs to the domain of physician determination. Yet, family members of US patients near the end of life (EOL) often demand extensive use of medical technologies to facilitate a prolonged existence, even when chances for meaningful recovery are slim.

To be sure, health care can and should endorse attentive EOL care. Palliative care and hospice teams often do an excellent job of providing these resources.[18] In particular, these services unearth patient values that are often unrelated to consumerism. Simultaneously, palliative care and hospice reorient families toward a holistic vision for the EOL. A medically laborious death is not the way many people envision their last days, yet they inadvertently find themselves stuck on a treadmill of hospital admissions, futile treatments, and last-chance surgeries until death overtakes them, disconnected from some of the values that mattered most during their life.

Sometimes aggressive medical treatments are chosen based on the erroneous belief that Christians are required to use all available measures to remain alive. However, the ERDs explain, "while every person is obliged to use ordinary means to preserve his or her health, no person should be obliged to submit to a health care procedure that

[18] Committee on Approaching Death: Addressing Key End-of-life Issues, *Dying in America: Improving Quality and Honoring Individual Preferences Near the End of Life* (Washington, DC: National Academies Press, 2015), chap. 2. See also Alfred F. Connors, Neal V. Dawson, Norman A. Desbiens, William J. Fulkerson, Lee Goldman, William A. Knaus, Joanne Lynn, et al., "A Controlled Trial to Improve Care for Seriously Ill Hospitalized Patients: The Study to Understand Prognoses and Preferences for Outcomes and Risks of Treatments (SUPPORT)," *JAMA* 274, no. 20 (1995): 1591–98.

the person has judged, with a free and informed conscience, not to provide a reasonable hope of benefit without imposing excessive risks and burdens on the patient or excessive expense to family or community."[19] The most straightforward interpretation of this directive refers to economic expense.[20] Yet "expense" might take into consideration environmental impacts of prospective medical interventions.

If environmental expense were to be considered in clinical ethics and sustainability were to be part of end-of-life care, a few caveats would be in order. First, it must never be suggested that a patient forgo *ordinary* life-preserving measures, no matter how resource intensive. The USCCB clearly states, "A person has a moral obligation to use ordinary or proportionate means of preserving his or her life." For the bishops, proportionate means are "those that in the judgment of the patient offer a reasonable hope of benefit."[21] Second, the deep tragedy whenever EOL decisions are made must be recognized. Although Christians have faith in the afterlife, surviving family members must still grapple with loss of a loved one. Third, vulnerable populations need extra attention when halting or withdrawing medically futile treatments, and many hospitals have policies to protect these groups. That being said, intensive use of medical technologies in the last stage of life can be enormously resource-intensive and excessively burdensome to patients and the global community. Therefore, environmental "expenses" of medical care are a legitimate factor to be considered in a clinical ethics assessment. This requires collaboration from both practitioners and patients as part of the therapeutic relationship.

[19] United States Conference of Catholic Bishops, *Ethical and Religious Directives*, directive 32.

[20] Prior to subsidized health insurance, the financial cost of a course of treatment would usually be considered by patients. Amish Christians—who reject health insurance—often deliberate within their community whether they can afford to treat a terminally ill patient. They do this with the highest regard for the dignity and value of the person, balanced with the corporate needs of the group. As a communal decision, sometimes aggressive or extraordinary measures are rejected. Jennifer Girod, "A Sustainable Medicine: Lessons from the Old Order Amish," *Journal of Medical Humanities* 23, no. 1 (2002): 31–42, at 34.

[21] United States Conference of Catholic Bishops, *Ethical and Religious Directives*, directive 56.

Practitioners could address environmental impacts of health care as part of the "contextual factors," asserting that environmental burden is a legitimate reason for abstaining from aggressive or futile medical treatments. This process can begin during patient intake and continue throughout the course of medical treatments. Detailed note taking about patient environmental values can bolster stewardship efforts within the hospital. Health care workers often tailor information about medical treatments to the individual's concerns, supporting the values and preferences of the patient and community. Explaining the carbon cost, or projected amount of resource use of any given treatment, would give patients the fullest information about medical procedures available.[22] In fact, one could argue that once carbon expenditure of a given procedure is known, a doctor would be withholding relevant information if she did not provide the patient with environmental data. A 2009 article in *Virtual Mentor*, published by the American Medical Association, indicated that in some cases, educating patients on the environmental effect of various procedures are already integrated into informed consent practices in certain health care facilities.[23] Medical care requires communication between patients and doctors.

From a patient perspective, active participation in health care decision-making surrounding environmental valences is also appropriate. Although from a Catholic perspective, patients should always choose ordinary care, any adult who has mental capacity has the right to refuse any and all medical treatments—even those that prolong life—for any reason. People who feel strongly that resource-intensive medical interventions at the EOL are unacceptable for theological, ethical, or environmental reasons can make their desires and wishes known through advance care planning.

Advance care planning is a broad term that encompasses future arrangements for one's inevitable dying process and includes legal

[22] Compare with the "Choose Wisely" shared-decision making campaign in the UK to minimize use of unnecessary medical procedures. *BBC*, "Doctors Name Treatments that Bring Little or no Benefit," *BBC News*, October 24, 2016, http://www.bbc .com/news/health-37732497. Choosing Wisely, 2016, http://www.choosingwisely .org/.

[23] Louise P. King and Janet Brown, "Clinical Case: Educating Patients as Medicine Goes Green," *Virtual Mentor* 11, no. 6 (2009): 427–33.

and medical documents, conversations with loved ones, and written expressions of desires for medical and social care prior to death. Written advance care planning documents include advance directives and Physician Order for Life-Sustaining Treatment (POLST) forms. Advance directives encompass Durable Power of Attorney for Health Care—a legal document naming a surrogate decision maker—as well as documents outlining general preferences regarding medical care. A POLST is a physician order signed after extensive conversations with the patient that specifies limitations of futile or medically inappropriate treatments. Both advance directives and POLST forms can incorporate patient values with regard to environmental sustainability and help to ensure that the patient's wishes and desires are honored.

In order to be effective, drafting advance care planning documents should not be delayed. In the opening case, the patient could have written down his end-of-life wishes even though his family did not support him. Sometimes friends and family members cannot understand certain environment commitments, even though they themselves may balance competing values in their lives. For instance, one person committed to sustainability might bike to work, another might live off the grid or use natural family planning to limit the number of biological children they have.[24] Some people will choose to avoid medical intervention. All are legitimate and within the CST. Death can happen at any time. Such advance care planning—particularly if it includes environmental values—should thus take place well before the onset of a terminal illness.

Having conversations about death is uncomfortable for many people. It can be more comfortable to avoid the topic of end-of-life care, particularly when opinions differ about quality of life, environmental sustainability, and fear of making our loved ones upset at the prospect of death. Understanding the need for sensitivity, organizations such as Caring Advocates—part of the natural death movement— assist in the first step toward ecological advance care planning. Their

---

[24] Cristina Richie, " 'Green' Reproduction, Resource Conservation, and Ecological Responsibility," *Worldviews: Global Religions, Culture, and Ecology* 18, no. 2 (2014): 144–72. Paul A. Murtaugh and Michael G. Schlax, "Reproduction and the Carbon Legacies of Individuals," *Global Environmental Change* 19, no. 1 (2009): 14–20.

"My Way Cards for Natural Dying" serve as conversation starters for EOL care. These cards act as a step-by-step guide to advanced directive decisions.[25] Carol Taylor and Robert Barnet paraphrase the Caring Advocates natural death movement by remarking:

> Natural dying, like natural child birth, does not depend on high tech medicine, and it requires even less skilled assistance for nature to take its course. When our brains can neither understand how to eat nor appreciate food, natural dying lets three things occur: 1. Cease manual assistance with oral feeding (as ultimately provided by skilled personnel), 2. Withhold/withdraw all life-sustaining treatment, and 3. Provide the best possible comfort care for a peaceful transition.[26]

The natural death movement provides a model of health care that upholds the dignity of the person and the claims of the common good. By focusing on "natural death," which is a phrase that is often invoked in Catholic health care documents,[27] Caring Advocates parallels the ERDs and confirms the legitimacy of an ecologically oriented approach to the EOL.

Conclusion

With growing consensus that environmental sustainability is an urgent priority that deserves attention and action, and with green hospital practices already proliferating in health care facilities—from recycling bins in clinics to local food in cafeterias[28]—greening end-of-life care would be a natural progression for health care institutions

---

[25] Caring Advocates, "A Clear and Specific Living Will can be Effective—If you Cannot Speak for Yourself," 2014, http://caringadvocates.org/card-sorting.php.

[26] Carol Taylor and Robert Barnet, "Hand Feeding: Moral Obligation or Elective Intervention?" *Health Care Ethics USA* 22, no. 2 (2014): 12–23, at 14.

[27] Dignity Health, "Statement of Common Values," (February 12, 2013): 1–3, at 1.

[28] Green Guide for Health Care, "Green Guide for Health Care: Food Service," (2008), 1–40, https://noharm-uscanada.org/issues/us-canada/green-guide-health-care-food-service; Deborah Kotz, "Hospitals Take Steps to Set Healthy Examples for Patients," *Boston Globe*, March 31, 2014, https://www.bostonglobe.com/lifestyle/health-wellness/2014/03/30/hospitals-take-steps-set-healthy-examples-for-patients/k8AdsJDkkdN5qWh8fyKDWL/story.html.

and the individuals they serve. The ERDs provide ample space for integrating sustainability into clinical practice. Indeed, environmental clinical ethics fits within the already established disciplines of environmental bioethics[29] and Green Bioethics[30] in its dedication to sustainable health care, while simultaneously maintaining the immense worth of individual human life, the claims of the common good, and the moral obligations of environmental stewardship.

Today, the environmental crisis presents a unique opportunity for Catholic health care to practice clinical ethics in a way consistent with the ERDs and wider Catholic social thought on justice and the environment. Using environmental clinical ethics to evaluate medical treatments, especially at the EOL, can support the patient and provide a sense of connection to the common good when a dying patient needs it most.

---

[29] Cristina Richie, "A Brief History of Environmental Bioethics," *AMA Journal of Ethics* (formerly *Virtual Mentor*) 16, no. 9 (2014): 749–52; Michael McCally, ed., *Life Support: The Environment and Human Health* (Boston: MIT Press, 2002); Jessica Pierce and Andrew Jameton, *The Ethics of Environmentally Responsible Health Care* (New York: Oxford University Press, 2004); David Resnik, *Environmental Health Ethics* (Cambridge, UK: Cambridge University Press, 2012).

[30] Cristina Richie, *Principles of Green Bioethics: Sustainability in Health Care* (East Lansing, MI: Michigan State University Press, forthcoming).

Chapter 8

Racial Disparities at the End of Life and the Catholic Social Tradition

Sheri Bartlett Browne and Christian Cintron

Angela's tiny, one-pound baby, Faith, arrived unexpectedly at twenty-four weeks gestation after a precipitous labor and delivery.[1] As Faith was alive at birth, Angela requested that every effort be made to save her life. Faith's subsequent prolonged neonatal intensive care unit (NICU) stay was in many ways remarkable. In addition to 175 days of mechanical and noninvasive ventilation, she endured two surgeries, several life-threatening infections, and severe lung disease. Her parents were told to prepare for her death numerous times, but for six months Faith defied the odds.

Faith's Black parents were unmarried, underemployed, and estranged from other family members. Angela's pregnancy had been complicated by poorly managed hypertension, obesity, and infrequent prenatal care. Faith was airlifted a few hours after her birth to a hospital over 100 miles away from the rural town and small apartment Angela shared with Faith's father and her two teenage boys. During this time, Angela had no reliable transportation between home and the hospital, greatly complicating her ability to care for her sons and her new baby.

Angela was fiercely devoted to Faith and distrusted the all-White clinical staff caring for her baby. She demanded that occupational

[1] To protect patient and family confidentiality, identifying information has been removed from this case narrative.

and physical therapists teach her how she could participate in Faith's care, even though she perceived that "They don't like it that I want to do all her care that I can." In addition, she rarely missed morning rounds with the medical team because she wanted to understand what was being done for and to Faith. These meetings, however, caused significant anxiety and frustration on both sides. Often rejecting information the medical team provided as "destroying my hope," Angela developed a reputation for yelling at physicians and nurses. "They think I'm stupid and don't understand, but I do," she reported. From the team's perspective, though, Angela was a problem parent that failed to accept the NICU environment and authority structure.

Committed to her Pentecostal faith tradition, she believed that God would provide complete physical healing if only the medical ·team would not "give up on Faith." The team differed, believing that Faith was likely to survive less than a year and would not leave the hospital without a tracheostomy for long-term mechanical ventilation and a permanent feeding tube. In fact, they presented these two grim realities as a choice for Angela to make. She could accept that Faith would die and explore hospice resources or agree to a tracheostomy and hope that Faith eventually would go home with 24/7 supportive care. These emotionally fraught options only increased the probability that Angela would be, as a social worker put it, "explosive and difficult to manage."

When Faith was six months old, with her condition worsening, Angela made the agonizing decision to approve the tracheostomy. But there really was no other choice to make, as Angela rejected outright ending curative treatment and accepting comfort care. "God and I are not giving up on her," she told the attending physician. The morning before Faith's scheduled surgery, however, she rapidly deteriorated. Early the next day, she went into cardiac arrest. After multiple rounds of CPR inflicted on Faith's ten-pound body, which Angela reported was the "most horrible thing I ever saw," she begged the medical team to stop. Hours later she said, "She didn't want that trach. And now she doesn't have to have it. She's with Jesus."

❖   ❖   ❖   ❖   ❖

Angela's and Faith's heartbreaking story is multilayered and complex, particularly in its psychosocial, medical, and theological dimensions. This family's experience is not unique and illuminates challenges inherent in addressing health care disparities at the end of life (EOL). For example, at several critical junctures in Faith's medical journey, a "comfort care" hospice approach was offered to Angela. That she refused it outright at every point, insisting as well that Faith be treated fully to the end, typifies a Black American approach to EOL care, rooted in a history of racist culture in medicine and reflected in troubling health disparities.

In 1985, the US Department of Health and Human Services (DHHS) issued a report that launched over thirty years of research, clinical interventions, community education, and millions of dollars in health care funding. The Heckler Report acknowledged that "persistent, significant health inequities exist for minority Americans" and further noted that "efforts of monumental proportions were needed" to address disparities in health care. In stark terms, the report presented a health care crisis and national embarrassment that reflected the US racial divide.[2]

As a response, beginning in 1990, Healthy People campaigns brought to the forefront the issue of health disparities.[3] Recognizing that Black Americans, Native Americans, Hispanic Americans, and Asian/Pacific Islanders suffered and died from preventable and treatable illnesses at rates far exceeding those of the White population, policy makers, scholars, and community leaders decided to direct most of their attention to eliminating health disparities among Blacks, then the largest minority group in the country. Yet thirty-three years after the Heckler Report, success in eliminating racial disparities in health care remains elusive. While significant gains have been made in the treatment of and outcomes for Black patients with cardiovascular disease and specific cancers, for instance, many of the problems the DHHS identified in 1985 have been intractable.[4] Black

---

[2] US Department of Health and Human Services, "Report of the Secretary's Task Force on Black and Minority Health" (1985): 2, and opening letter from Secretary Margaret M. Heckler, https://minorityhealth.hhs.gov/assets/pdf/checked/1/ANDERSON.pdf.

[3] See Centers for Disease Control and Prevention (CDC), "Healthy People 2000, 2010, and 2020," https://www.cdc.gov/nchs/products/hp_pubs.htm.

[4] David Williams notes that despite improvements in treatments for heart disease and cancers, the gap between Black and White survivability persists. See Institute of Medicine, *How Far Have We Come in Reducing Health Disparities? Progress Since 2000:*

Americans' lack of access to and utilization of care is therefore a matter of community urgency and social justice.

This essay examines cultural and structural barriers that Black individuals face in utilizing health care, with specific reference to EOL issues such as hospice care and advanced directives. Black Americans bring perspectives to EOL care that reflect their experiences as a historically marginalized and systemically oppressed people; these perspectives help to illuminate more broadly dynamics that underlie health care disparities in the United States. Furthermore, we argue that the Catholic social tradition (CST) provides a liberative paradigm for ethical and equitable treatment that requires relational, intentional, and community-oriented approaches to ending racial disparities in health care.

The Persistence of Racial Disparities at the End of Life

It is well known in the EOL literature that Black patients and families generally eschew hospice care for terminal and life-limiting illnesses. Medicare is the main payer of hospice services for people aged 65 and over, yet in 2015, Blacks represented only 8.2 percent of Medicare-eligible hospice patients when they were 10 percent of the total Medicare-eligible population. State-specific data are even more revealing of the gap between eligibility and utilization; in eight southern states, Blacks are more than twenty percent of eligible beneficiaries. The disparity in accessing adequate EOL care stems from a wide range of factors: socio-cultural, spiritual, and the historical isolation of the Black community within predominantly White medical systems.[5]

Hospice seeks to provide physical and medicinal comfort, counseling and spiritual support, and family bereavement services to individuals whose terminal illness or injury is not viewed as curable.

Workshop Summary (Washington, DC: National Academies Press, 2012), 13, https://www.ncbi.nlm.nih.gov/books/NBK100492/pdf/Bookshelf_NBK100492.pdf.

[5] See National Hospice and Palliative Care Organization, "Facts and Figures," (2016), 3–4, https://www.nhpco.org/sites/default/files/public/2016_Facts_Figures.pdf; The Henry J. Kaiser Family Foundation, "Profile of Medicare Beneficiaries by Race and Ethnicity: A Chartpack," March 9, 2016, https://www.kff.org/report-section/profile-of-medicare-beneficiaries-by-race-and-ethnicity-chartpack/.

Yet entrenched racism and systemic discrimination support Black beliefs in rejecting hospice care.[6] The deaths of Black men, women, and children are portrayed relentlessly as sudden, violent, and/or a product of dysfunctional communities. Black life expectancy is lower than Whites by an average of four years for men and three years for women.[7] Equally alarming, as Aana Vigen's chapter notes, Black women's maternal mortality rate is four times that of White women and Black infants are twice as likely to die before age one.[8]

To live one more day, when Black lives are portrayed as expendable, is viewed as a victory over death itself. Ending potentially curative interventions is perceived often as giving up the battle. "If there is any chance that life is there, I would suggest to go the extra means. Technology is there to keep people alive and give people longer lives."[9] These comments echo the sentiments of Angela with respect to Faith, "We never gave up on her. We did good." However, Angela felt she faced a daily battle to convince the medical team to fight harder for Faith, which created a persistent sense of distrust. Although Angela's feelings and experience were personal, they also reflect a long history of racially based medical abuse.

Black Americans have been targets and victims of medical experimentation from the era of slavery into the late twentieth century, including gynecological and neurological experimentation as well as forced sterilization.[10] Perhaps most egregious was the infamous Tuskegee Syphilis study (1932–72). Four hundred men in Macon

[6] See Annette Dula and September Williams, "When Race Matters," *Clinical Geriatric Medicine* 21 (2005): 240–43.

[7] For Black life expectancy, see Centers for Disease Control and Prevention, "Changes in Life Expectancy by Race and Hispanic Origin in the United States, 2013–2014," https://www.cdc.gov/nchs/products/databriefs/db244.htm.

[8] See Aana Vigen's chapter in this volume for data on disparities in maternal and infant mortality (chap. 5).

[9] Catherine M. Waters, "Understanding and Supporting African Americans' Perspectives of End-of-Life Care Planning and Decision Making," *Qualitative Health Research* 11, no. 3 (May 2001): 390.

[10] Daniel P. Scharff, et al., "More than Tuskegee: Understanding Mistrust about Research Participation," *Journal of Health Care for the Poor and Underserved* 21, no. 3 (Aug. 2010): 880; Irin Carmon, "For Eugenic Sterilization Victims, Belated Justice," *MSNBC*, June 27, 2014, http://www.msnbc.com/all/eugenic-sterilization-victims -belated-justice. Regarding gynecological experiments, see J. Wasserman, et al., "Raising the Ivory Tower: The Production of Knowledge and Distrust of Medicine among African Americans," *Journal of Medical Ethics* 33 (2007): 178.

County, Alabama, suffering from syphilis were studied in a decades-long experiment to investigate the natural course of the disease. Even when antibiotic treatment became widely available, these men did not receive it.[11] As one focus group participant from St. Louis stated, "Just that awareness [about Tuskegee] is enough to stand up generation after generation."[12] Medical mistrust also became a point of contention between Angela and Kevin, Faith's father. He did not want Angela to go home to visit her sons for fear that "these people will do something to [Faith] when we're not here." It is difficult to make critical medical decisions for yourself or a loved one when you lack a fundamental sense of trust in those providing patient care. These tensions can become heightened when discussing patient wishes around DNR (do not resuscitate) orders.

Many studies attest to Black patients' reluctance to sign a DNR form or any type of advanced directive.[13] Rather than viewing a DNR as a means to prevent unwanted, aggressive measures in the dying process, many Blacks view the forms as yet another way that a medical system and its providers can reduce or eliminate care of an expendable Black life. These forms are often referred to colloquially as "death warrants," reflecting Blacks' lived experience of discrimination and historical memories of institutional abuse and betrayal.[14] Angela refused even to discuss a DNR for Faith because she was convinced the doctors "would just let her die." The burden of ad-

---

[11] This research project involved a whole cohort of physicians (both Black and White) and the approval of the US Public Health Service. See Bernice Roberts Kennedy, et al., "African Americans and Their Distrust of the Healthcare System: Healthcare for Diverse Populations," *Journal of Cultural Diversity* 14, no. 2 (Summer 2007): 56.

[12] Daniel P. Scharff, et al., "More than Tuskegee," 884.

[13] Advanced Directives, including Physician Order for Life-Sustaining Treatment (POLST) forms, are common and widely used in hospice and other EOL care situations, because they provide a written record of a dying person's medical wishes, in which a patient often elects to restrict the use of extraordinary medical interventions such as cardiopulmonary resuscitation, mechanical ventilation, artificial hydration, and nutrition that would not provide sufficient benefit. See, for example, Faith P. Hopp and Sophia A. Duffy, "Racial Variations in End-of-Life Care," *Journal of the American Geriatrics Society* 48, no. 6 (June 2000): 658–63; and Kimberly S. Johnson, et al., "What Explains Racial Differences in the Use of Advance Directives and Attitudes Toward Hospice Care?" *Journal of the American Geriatrics Society* 56, no. 10 (October 2008): 1953–58.

[14] Dula and Williams, "When Race Matters," 242.

dressing this mistrust should not rest with the Black population; instead, medical teams and hospital systems must demonstrate through compassionate actions and culturally compassionate communication that they are trustworthy to care for Black patients. Yet these considerations fall often outside of the traditional purview of bioethics.

Inadequate Frameworks for Racial Disparities

EOL care represents a founding set of ethical questions within both a secular and religious bioethical discourse. Within Catholic bioethics, EOL care is equally prominent but negotiated within a distinct moral framework. Issues include an array of technical ethical distinctions regarding forgoing treatment and seemingly uncomplicated topics such as pain management and advanced care planning.[15] While these distinctions and terms can be helpful in discerning what is morally appropriate in light of a patient's situation (health, family, social), the perspectives of Black patients highlight how traditional frameworks such as Tom Beauchamp and James Childress's principles, in which many clinicians and ethicists are trained, obscure critical and operative racial and cultural dynamics.

As the preeminent value in American culture, autonomy's place in biomedical ethics is commensurately privileged as the primary principle toward which patients, physicians, and other health care workers look for guidance. "Respect for the autonomous choices of

---

[15] See part five of United States Conference of Catholic Bishops, "Issues in Care for the Seriously Ill and Dying," *Ethical and Religious Directives for Health Care Services*, 6th ed. (Washington DC: USCCB, 2018), which outlines the traditional list of end-of-life topics in bioethics, both generally and in the Catholic tradition. A primary emphasis in directives 55 and 59 is on the role of informed consent and patient autonomy in the patient's opportunity to choose a morally appropriate treatment. Directives 56 through 58 address ordinary and extraordinary means of care, including the use of artificial nutrition and hydration. Directives 60 and 61 outline the importance of effective pain management in care for the dying, particularly as means of maintaining the patient's dignity. See also "Forgoing Treatment at the End of Life," in *Health Care Ethics: Theological Foundations, Contemporary Issues, and Controversial Cases*, ed. Michael R. Panicola, David M. Belde, John Paul Slosar, and Mark F. Repenshek (Winona, MN: Anselm Academic, 2011).

persons," argue Beauchamp and Childress, "runs as deep in common morality as any principle."[16] While this may resonate with most as a result of an American cultural leaning toward individualism, the priority of autonomy, albeit unintended by Beauchamp and Childress,[17] has caused disagreement among biomedical ethicists about how and why autonomy should be valued over and against other ethical principles and the competing values of health care professionals and/or cultural values of patients. In light of the increased emphasis on autonomy as (unrestricted) individual liberty, patients are more empowered, both intellectually through expanded access to medical and health care information and by exploiting clinicians' fear of legal or administrative censure.

Still, the autonomy of patients of color is stymied by systemic injustices, of which the most basic form is a failure or unwillingness to listen to the patient. Unfortunately, traditional Catholic bioethics implicitly supports this model of care and decision-making insofar as it promotes the autonomy of the person vis-à-vis the synergistic *telos* of the good life that coincides with the grace of free will. Oftentimes, the Catholic tradition turns instead to the language of dignity over autonomy, without considering how the two terms may be used synonymously throughout American society. When dignity is substituted for autonomy and vice versa, the whole of the patient's experience as contextualized subject is lost.

The USCCB's *Ethical and Religious Directives for Catholic Health Care Services* (ERDs) directives 24 and 25 outline a patient's right to an advanced directive (AD) consistent with Catholic teaching, and further stipulate conditions for surrogate decision-making. However, it is no surprise that ADs are underutilized by patients skeptical of the medical system. Similarly, the Catholic tradition encourages hospice care, claiming "patients should be kept as free of pain as possible so

---

[16] Tom L. Beauchamp and James F. Childress, *Principles of Biomedical Ethics* (New York: Oxford University Press), 99.

[17] Ibid. The authors maintain while the first principle appearing in the text is autonomy, it is not an indication of their opinion on the moral priority of autonomy. They argue that while their "critics suggest that the principle for respect for autonomy overrides all other moral considerations," their work is in no way "excessively individualistic."

that they might die comfortably and with dignity, and in the place where they wish to die."[18] Yet, this support from the tradition does not address the systemic reasons underlying reduced availability and use of these services by Black patients. Despite their importance, the traditional teachings of Catholic bioethics prove to be ineffective practically for the patient and the clinician.

In addition to the cultural and historical reasons outlined above, a further issue lies in the theological anthropology that grounds these teachings. Womanist Catholic theologian M. Shawn Copeland argues that the undignified and sinful treatment of the Black community perverts traditional theological anthropology, expressed as *imago Dei*, and rejects the "Black body as a site of divine revelation."[19] Persistent failure to recognize the sacramentality of the Black body has contributed to, and at times legitimized, systems of oppression, and perpetuates bias toward Black persons and has indeed denied their innate human dignity. So, while dignified treatment of persons as an integrated whole is expected, Blacks are denied that type of care, directly or indirectly, through systemic or individually perpetrated violence. Precisely because of persistent and pervasive failures to encompass Black bodies within its theological anthropology, Catholic bioethics has not only turned a blind eye to medical abuse or neglect of Black patients; it also has failed to provide a sufficiently robust framework for championing the specific dignity of embodied Black people. Dignity can continue to offer a critical lens for assessing Black American responses to EOL care as long as dignity is not an abstract principle. Even then, however, dignity alone cannot fully respond to health care systems' unjust practices that contribute to the continued marginalization of Blacks, for dignity is only one component of theological anthropology. Only by incorporating the social nature of the person can we chart a path forward in correcting racial disparities at the EOL and care for Black bodies as sites of divine revelation.

---

[18] United States Conference of Catholic Bishops, *Ethical and Religious Directives*, directive 61.

[19] M. Shawn Copeland, *Enfleshing Freedom: Body, Race, and Being* (Minneapolis, MN: Fortress Press, 2009), 24.

"White Spaces":
Reconsidering the Social Nature of the Human Person

CST illuminates a second essential anthropological feature, namely, people's social being. Persons are relational, only finding fulfillment through "the social ties of family, associations, and political community."[20] Honoring this dimension of an individual's life is as important when one's life is coming to an end as it is at any previous time. Only when persons are considered within their social milieu, and, in the particular case of Black Americans within their historical context, can we begin to appreciate the complex dynamics that Blacks bring to EOL care and how health care as a "White space" often impedes their integral fulfillment.[21]

Elijah Anderson describes White spaces as those which are characterized by the presence of White people and the absence of Black people. When Blacks do enter such spaces, he notes, "others there immediately try to make sense of him or her—figure out 'who that is,' or to gain a sense of the nature of the person's business and whether they need to be concerned."[22] Health care is a White space, and racist treatment has been a dominant feature of US health care. Black bodies have been treated as less than and disposable, resulting in a lack of attention to Black persons as a unified whole; an unwillingness to address them as socially situated perpetuates biases on the part of health care providers and results in inadequate EOL care options. CST challenges these biases by emphasizing "we cannot fight for our lives in isolation . . . we must recognize the biological, social, environmental, and economic conditions that surround us and have profound impacts on our health."[23] The social dimension of the human person counters the White space of health care and its White notions of autonomy that frame EOL conversations.

CST's focus on the social nature of the human person highlights and counters the White Western liberal emphasis on individual au-

---

[20] Charles E. Curran, *Catholic Social Teaching: A Historical, Theological, and Ethical Analysis* (Washington, DC: Georgetown University Press, 2002), 133, summarizing *Gaudium et Spes* 24–25.

[21] Jamelle Bouie, "White Spaces," *Slate* (April 17, 2018); Elijah Anderson, "The White Space," *Sociology of Race and Ethnicity* 1, no. 1 (2015): 13–15.

[22] Anderson, "The White Space," 13.

[23] Emilie Townes, *Breaking the Fine Rain of Death: African American Health Issues and a Womanist Ethics of Care* (Eugene, OR: Wipf and Stock, 2006), 119.

tonomy that pervades traditional bioethical discourse and its inherent bias that tends ironically to "disregard innovative and good ideas that might come from non-privileged groups."[24] In the individual model, the clinician remains susceptible to viewing patients as a condition-to-be-treated, rather than cared for as a person in the context of a community. A focus on the relational dimension of autonomy incorporates the patient's context, perceived and real, addresses power dynamics existing between autonomous patient and clinician, and confronts the assumption that patients' understandings of autonomy coincide with those of traditional bioethics. The relational dimension of autonomy at the EOL does not magically resolve the myriad issues facing Black patients; it represents, rather, an important turn in caring for patients as socially situated or relational beings, an important first methodological insight of CST.

Second, the CST's response to marginalized persons and communities aims to correct both acute and systemic causes of injustice in pursuit of the common good. The pursuit of the common good, validated in the preferential option for the marginalized, is further elucidated in the CST's principle of solidarity. In *Sollicitudo Rei Socialis* (1987), Pope John Paul II called solidarity the remedy for social sin. "Solidarity is a firm and persevering determination to commit oneself to the common good, that is to say, to the good of all."[25] Black patients experience inequitable treatment at the EOL for numerous reasons: power dynamics that exist between providers and patients, social determinants of health contributing to patients' conditions at the EOL, and discriminatory practices that limit access to hospice and other EOL services to name a few. Solidarity, coupled with the preferential option for the marginalized, mandates an obligation to care for those who have been subjected to systemic oppression or denied basic rights.

The preferential option obliges health care providers and relevant political organizations to improve care available to these patients, ensures that care is equal to the care of others, and also corrects the very social structures that have created an environment in which Blacks at the EOL do not choose or are not offered adequate and equitable care. Responses to structural sins of racism, socioeconomic

---

[24] Copeland, *Enfleshing Freedom*, 14.
[25] Pope John Paul II, *Sollicitudo Rei Socialis* 38, para. 5.

oppression, and racial disparities in health care must comprise fortitude to seek lasting societal change and commitments to love and serve one another, to see our common humanity as fundamentally interconnected. These liberative dimensions of the CST are bound to the very mission of health care, and such an approach may also well lead to changes in EOL paradigms, as Black perspectives and experiences bring correctives to standard White practices.

Moving Forward Together

The historical, cultural, theological, and ethical complexities surrounding racial disparities in EOL care are obviously daunting. Indeed, there is no "band-aid" that can heal the wounds of racism, slavery, segregation, disfranchisement, medical experimentation, and forced sterilization. Yet, there are approaches to EOL care, informed by CST, that promote physical, spiritual, and psychosocial healing and foster relationships of trust. These include the reevaluation and expansion of cultural humility curricula; the adoption of aggressive measures to racially and ethnically diversify the clinical workforce; and advocacy and promotion of palliative care as a holistic and compassionate approach to chronic and life-limiting illness.

First, medical schools and health care systems must be committed assertively to cultural diversity. They must offer robust training and curricula in cultural humility rooted in pedagogies of solidarity and the obligation to care for and improve the condition of the marginalized. These curricula ought to replace current approaches to "cultural sensitivity" training that by design undermine its significance by reinforcing racist stereotypes about "the other" and present minority cultures and beliefs as a problem to overcome. Contrary to what many employees and administrators may think, the purpose of training in cultural humility is not to help us be nice to each other but is meant to help us truly care for one another.[26] In caring for one another, the entirety of the health care ministry engages in the praxis of solidarity.

---

[26] Aana Vigen, "'Keeping it Real' while Staying out of the 'Loony Bin': Social Ethics for Health Care Systems," in *On Moral Medicine: Theological Perspectives in Medical Ethics*, 3rd ed., ed. M. Therese Lysaught and Joseph Kotva (Grand Rapids, MI: Eerdmans, 2012), 172–74; and Carolyn Waters, "Understanding and Supporting African Americans' Perspectives," 396.

Indeed, as Copeland argues, the praxis of solidarity begins with "anamnesis—the intentional remembering of the dead, exploited, despised victims of history," which imposes an obligation upon Christians to shoulder "responsibility for that history."[27] Approaching culture in the spirit of solidarity places the emphasis on an encounter with the other, while at the same time recognizing and addressing the structural injustices that affect the Black community.

These curricula for Catholic health care systems should be designed to challenge learners' assumptions and understandings of systemic racism and structural oppression. CST emphatically states that racism and poverty are social and structural sins that must be acknowledged and eradicated. Doing so provides an opportunity for health care systems to learn from Black Americans' sociocultural history within medicine and their current social location, as clinicians and health care systems strive toward models of health care delivery that truly embody solidarity. Preferably, this curriculum would be taught by specifically trained practitioners who are not majority White and could be developed or expanded based on cultural sensitivity resources already present within Catholic health care systems.

Another possible approach to this curricula, which honors people's relational and social ties to family and community, is through shared partnership opportunities in neighborhood clinics, organizations, or churches, enabling clinicians to listen to and learn from people whose sociocultural and medical experiences are different from their own.[28] One such model that immerses participants in the praxis of solidarity is the "Neighborhood-Engaged Care" curriculum developed for medical students participating in the Urban Bioethics Program at Temple University in Philadelphia. Students enrolled in a semester-long Community Engagement course are integrated as learner-practitioners into neighborhood health clinics and nonprofit organizations serving specific diverse urban populations.[29] In so

[27] Copeland, *Enfleshing Freedom*, 100.
[28] Aana Vigen, "'Keeping it Real,'" 172–74.
[29] Norma Alicea-Alvarez, et al., "Impacting Health Disparities in Urban Communities: Preparing Future Healthcare Providers for 'Neighborhood-Engaged Care' Through a Community Engagement Course Intervention," *Journal of Urban Health: Bulletin of the New York Academy of Medicine* 93, no. 4 (2016): 732–43; see also Copeland, *Enfleshing Freedom*, 94.

doing, participants are confronted by and challenged to address oppressive causes of suffering and bear that burden for the other.

In developing partnerships, insights and tools of clinical pastoral education (CPE) prove helpful for reimagining competency curricula. CPE long has been recognized as a necessary educational component of health care chaplaincy and is also highly recommended for community pastors who wish to serve capably their ailing and dying congregants. It is a model for the type of solidarity advocated by the CST, caring for one another with dignity, respect, and informed awareness of a patient's relational, social, and theological milieu. CPE's hallmark learning style is praxis oriented, focusing on action-reflection-action in clinical settings. It requires that the learner/practitioner embrace self-critique, particularly in challenging of one's sociocultural assumptions and how those assumptions affect care provided to others.[30] Perhaps most important, CPE requires that practitioners build skills in attentiveness and deep listening. To truly listen signals respect and empathy for the speaker's circumstances; it indicates a desire to be fully present and attuned to another's tone and body language. Especially in reference to death and dying, Black patients feel keenly that they are not worth the time, that their stories are a waste of time, that their family members will take too much time.[31] Recall that one of Angela's primary frustrations with the physicians caring for Faith was that she believed they did not listen; therefore, she felt their attitude toward her was patronizing and dismissive. Listening is one of the most significant ways in which to honor the life story and dignity of a fellow human being.

Our second recommendation addresses the structural change that needs to happen among educators, medical schools, health systems, and Black communities to mentor, recruit, and retain qualified clinicians who are not majority White.[32] The mistrust and unease that Angela and Kevin expressed about leaving Faith alone in the hospital was partly related to the racially stratified staffing they saw around

[30] See Logan C. Jones, "You Learn it in Your Heart: Transformative Learning Theory and Clinical Pastoral Education," *Journal of Pastoral Care and Counseling* 64 (December 2010): 1–10.

[31] See Carolyn Jenkins, et al., "End-of-Life Care and African Americans: Voices from the Community," *Journal of Palliative Medicine* 8, no. 3 (2005): 585–92.

[32] For more on the importance of diverse staffing for patient care and satisfaction, see Robert Gordon's chapter in this volume (chap. 10).

them. "The only Black people I see here are the ones cleaning the floor," Angela said. National trends in Black medical student graduates have held steady at roughly ten percent of the total graduate population, but these figures will result in a shortfall of tens of thousands of Black physicians by 2025, especially in southern states where the majority of Blacks reside.[33] One prototype for increasing racial diversity among practitioners comes from a partnership between Ohio Hearts and Minds and Mercy Health in Cincinnati. They have implemented a mentoring program for Black youth from fifth through tenth grade to introduce them to Black medical professionals and careers in health care.[34]

Third, health care systems must embrace fully a model of comprehensive EOL care that is underutilized and poorly understood within society: palliative care. The philosophy of palliative care is multilayered and interdisciplinary, with teams including various subspecialties as well as chaplains and social workers. Palliative approaches focus on holistic and dignified health consistent with the Catholic tradition for those in chronic pain, with multiple co-morbidities, and those who are or will soon be experiencing the dying process.[35] Unlike hospice, it offers opportunities to continue curative therapies while addressing such factors as pain management and emotional support. It also can be effectively delivered in multiple medical venues as well as at home.

For Black patients, barriers to palliative care mirror those of hospice described above and require careful analysis to overcome.[36] However, a main objection that these patients voice regarding hospice

[33] See the Association of American Medical Colleges, "Enrollment, Graduates, and MD-PhD Data," https://www.aamc.org/data/facts/enrollmentgraduate/; and Robin Warshaw, "Priming the Medical School Pipeline: Schools Reach Out to Teens in Minority and Underserved Communities," *AAMC News* (Association of American Medical Colleges), September 29, 2016, https://news.aamc.org/diversity/article/schools-minority-underserved-communities/.

[34] Kathleen Nelson, "Doctors Capture 'Hearts and Minds' of African-American Boys," *Catholic Health World* (Catholic Health Association of the United States, February 15, 2017).

[35] For a definition of palliative care, see National Hospice and Palliative Care Organization, "An Explanation of Palliative Care," https://www.nhpco.org/explanation-palliative-care; and USCCB, *Ethical and Religious Directives*, 55–59, 61.

[36] See, for example, LaVera Crawley and Richard Payne, et al., "Palliative and End-of-Life Care in the African American Community," *Journal of the American Medical Association* 284, no. 19 (November 2000): 2518–21.

are perceptions that one is "giving up" on treatment and therefore giving up on life. Opportunities to continue curative measures and participate in palliative therapies must be clearly and compassionately discussed with patients and their families. The meaning of hospice and palliative care often are conflated, which increases the chance that palliative care also will be rejected. For these reasons, it is imperative to work in and through existing community structures to provide information regarding EOL care.

These three recommendations require collaboration with local communities, draw from the CST's emphasis on solidarity and subsidiarity, and could be administered effectively through partnerships between Catholic health care ministries, local parishes, and community centers, possibly as part of community benefit programs. The programs not only would address the EOL concerns raised above, but would also facilitate improved relationships between community members and local health care ministries in an effort to address thoughtfully and compassionately lingering effects of medical mistrust. One example of this type of health care community collaboration is Samaritan Center, a facility that formerly housed Detroit Mercy Hospital. The center hosts primary care and dental clinics as well as seventy other tenants providing "a platform for addressing social determinants—including homelessness, hunger, joblessness, illiteracy and poverty—that have a significant impact on people's health." While its focus is not specifically on EOL care, the center is a model for social service and health care outreach. According to its Executive Director Mark Owens, "This is a place that gives people hope."[37]

Initiatives such as Samaritan Center additionally would provide an opportunity to address the general health of the neglected Black population toward improving the aging process itself. With this outreach and focus, the EOL process would not be a shock to patients and their families. These programs also would provide a familiar and comfortable environment for communicating more effectively the

---

[37] Julie Minda, "Repurposed Trinity Hospital is Health, Social Service Hub for Detroit's East Side," *Catholic Health World*, Catholic Health Association of the United States, March 15, 2018, https://www.chausa.org/publications/catholic-health -world/article/march-15-2018/repurposed-trinity-hospital-is-health-social-service -hub-for-detroit's-east-side.

purpose and benefits of palliative care. Ecumenical collaboration with Black pastors in the community, including the requisite medical ethical training of the pastors themselves, would allow for Catholic health ministries to serve better their Black patients who have established relationships with leaders of their respective congregations. A community-based approach such as this can truly illuminate and respond to concerns of Black patients approaching or already dealing with the EOL in a manner consistent with the CST.

Finally, from a health care systems and leadership perspective, addressing and eliminating racial disparities in EOL care requires that resources for palliative care must be a priority, not only in terms of expansion and funding but in terms of commitment to executing high quality care. It is especially unfortunate that palliative care is not always available in communities with large populations of vulnerable and marginalized people. Recent data demonstrate an acute shortage of palliative care resources in areas where the vast majority of Black patients live.[38] Pediatric palliative care has been available for only a few years in many large teaching hospitals, though its availability is even more limited in the South. At the southern hospital caring for Faith, the only pediatric palliative care physician had been hired just a few days before her death. One wonders what difference a culturally sensitive palliative approach might have made in medical decision making for Faith and in the bereavement support provided to her parents.

Conclusion

Racial disparities in health care have been a blight on the American health care system for decades. Resolving inequities in access to and utilization of treatment, particularly at the EOL, requires a holistic approach, one that takes into account Black Americans' lived and historical experiences as well as their cultural and theological perspectives. This brief essay is an attempt not only to understand the general problem and persistence of disparities and their possible

---

[38] Center to Advance Palliative Care, "America's Care of Serious Illness: 2015 State-by-State Report Card on Access to Palliative Care in Our Nation's Hospitals," https://reportcard.capc.org/wp-content/uploads/2015/08/reportcard-2015-table-a.pdf.

solutions but also to bring specific underserved voices into the discussion. Indeed, the voices of Black individuals often have been disregarded in the search for an end to disparities, and their specific health care needs frequently go unmet. For these reasons, we assert that CST's liberative dimension, as evidenced in the principles of solidarity, the option for the marginalized, and the pursuit of the common good, united with a theological anthropology that embraces human beings as social, relational, and interdependent, provides an ethical path forward on the journey toward ending disparities.

PART THREE

Incarnating a Just Workplace

Turning the lens of Catholic social thought on the practice of Catholic health care brings into view not only new community-based issues or subtle dynamics of patient-physician encounters; it also illuminates the often ethically fraught work context of health care associates. How an organization treats its employees—be they providing direct patient care or serving in less direct capacities—has a direct impact on the identity of the organization as well as its ability to embody that identity in practice. Questions of workers' rights, racial equality, and how to fairly organize a work environment to meet the needs of health care professionals remains a constant struggle. These questions are properly the purview of Catholic bio-ethics not only due to the long history of attention to the rights of labor and the integral meaning of work for human fulfillment in the Catholic social tradition. They are highlighted, again, in the *Ethical and Religious Directives*:

> A Catholic health care institution must treat its employees respectfully and justly. This responsibility includes: equal employment opportunities for anyone qualified for the task, irrespective of a person's race, sex, age, national origin, or disability; a workplace that promotes employee participation; a work environment that ensures employee safety and well-being; just compensation and benefits; and recognition of the rights of employees to organize and bargain collectively without prejudice to the common good.[1]

[1] United States Conference of Catholic Bishops (USCCB), *Ethical and Religious Directives for Catholic Health Care Services*, 6th ed. (Washington DC: USCCB, 2018).

But, as Daniel P. Dwyer notes in his chapter, how often does the bishop query Catholic health systems on how well they are adhering to or fulfilling directive seven?

As each chapter in part III makes clear, these concerns are not just human resource dilemmas. These concerns bear significantly upon the way that Catholic health care lives up to the demands of CST and the necessity of standing up for the rights of those maligned and marginalized with structures of sin. Each author expands and challenges Catholic bioethics to take up questions that CST raises with respect to workers' rights, sexism, racism, and Catholic health care's responsibility to support associates in maintaining the global mission work of the broader church. This section calls mission and ethics leaders to consider how they might ensure that their hospitals and systems do not simply replicate these societal problems but rather witness to alternative possibilities.

In chapter 9, "Unions in Catholic Health Care: A Paradox," Daniel P. Dwyer recounts the process that led to the establishment of a nurses' union at Queen Valley Medical Center in California. His narrative juxtaposes the clear support of unions in CST with the opposition that can arise when unions attempt to organize within Catholic institutions. This resistance is ironic given that the historical locus that gave birth to CST was workers' rights, specifically the rights to organize for justice in the work place. However, Catholic health care, like Catholic universities, has not been immune to often creating an at best unhealthy and at worst an unjust work environment for employees. Dwyer asks whether it has been the neglect of CST within Catholic institutions that has resulted not only in a felt need for unions but also sparked vociferous opposition from health care leadership when they are formed. He urges mission leaders and ethicists to serve as a bridge between senior management, associates, and unions.

Creating an organization that lives the Catholic social tradition requires not only attending to how work is structured; it requires attending to who is included in the workplace. Chapter 10, "Inviting the Neighborhood into the Hospital: Diversifying our Health Care Organizations," offers the narrative of how a small community hospital located on the Southside of Chicago embodies the tenants of CST in the work that they do and in who does the work. Robert

Gordon tells the story of St. Bernard Hospital and Health Center, a "Safety-Net Hospital," in which over 50 percent of their patients depend on Medicaid and almost all their patients are Black. In most hospitals, however, the physician and nurses these patients would meet would not be. Committed to their local community and to CST, the leadership of St. Bernard's made an unusual commitment—to hire from the community and to diversify their staff. As a result, St. Bernard's now boasts a staff that is 69 percent diverse, drawn largely from the surrounding Englewood neighborhood. Gordon's chapter offers a narrative-based critique of the racial inequality among providers in health care. He challenges Catholic health care organizations to focus on the importance of diversity, not only for better patient care, but to fulfill a vital community role that builds up the common good by developing hiring practices that strengthen employee engagement and draw on the local communities.

CST both illuminates how our health care institutions replicate the racial sins of our culture and raises questions regarding the treatment and role of women in Catholic health care. Attention to women's health in Catholic bioethics and health care has long been reduced to a few reproductive questions. In chapter 11, "The Rocky Road of Women and Health Care: A Gender Roadmap," Jana Bennett seeks to nuance how we consider the role of women within Catholic health care institutions as both patients and professionals. While other chapters describe health care as a "White space," Bennett could qualify that further by arguing that it is a "White male/heteronormative space." Women, she notes, are underrepresented in health care leadership positions; as patients they are often misdiagnosed or more easily caricatured than their fellow male patients. While admitting that the CST has its own rocky tradition when it comes to women, she encourages organizations to consider Pope Francis's emphasis on "how everything is interconnected." The interconnectedness of health care, absent women's voices, not only skews what decisions are made, but how they are made. She encourages ethicists to nuance not only the range of issues discussed with respect to women's health, but to explore the social implications of those questions related to both patient care and hospital staffing.

The integral human development of associates concerns not only working conditions within a system; it also concerns the ways in which our systems enable associates to fully pursue the mission of Catholic health care, even beyond the parameters of our local hospitals. In chapter 12, "Continuing the Ministry of Mission Doctors," physicians Brian Medernach and Antoinette Lullo expand how we conceptualize Catholic health care's global responsibility in providing care beyond US borders. Their narrative account reviews the historical emergence of "mission doctors" who served both a spiritual and physical role in remote parts of the global south. Mission doctors have traditionally been women and men religious and priests who trained as physicians and took their skills and ministries to locations in need. Across the globe, they established local Catholic health care clinics that embedded themselves in the realities of the people whom they served. Medernach and Lullo offer an account of one such clinic, Centro de Salud Santa Clotilde, founded in Peru in the 1940s. After tracing the development of this center, they propose that Catholic health care has an organizational responsibility to continue the legacy of mission doctors by creating a new paradigm of teaching, research, and service with partner institutions in the global south. They challenge Catholic health care systems and physicians to discern what it might look like to live out the preferential for the poor without institutional, organizational, or national borders.

Chapter 9

Unions in Catholic Health Care: A Paradox

Daniel P. Dwyer

For more than fifty years Queen of the Valley Medical Center in Napa, California (or "The Queen," as it is known locally), has played an essential role as the county's only Level III trauma center, with specialized programs in oncology, cardiology, and neurosurgery that provide a breadth and quality of care far more sophisticated than its size and location might suggest. The hospital is nationally recognized as a leader in community benefit, with strong programs in public health and social services outreach. Generations of Napa locals have strong ties to the hospital: many residents (and their children and grandchildren) were born at The Queen, and many beloved family members drew their last breaths there. The importance of this hospital to the city of Napa and to the region is reflected by extremely generous local financial support generated by The Queen's fundraising initiatives. Queen of the Valley Medical Center (QVMC) is also the largest employer in Napa County.

Despite decades of successful community service and support, QVMC—like most health care institutions—has not been immune to external financial pressures and changes in organizational structure. In 2011, the loss of a lucrative contract with the California prison system to provide inmate care resulted in a staggering loss of $23 million in annual revenue. The resulting budget gap led to layoffs, the discontinuation of popular community and employee initiatives, and an increased emphasis on productivity and cost reduction. Internally, the perception grew that quality of care was being compromised to save money and that employees—especially nurses—were doing much better elsewhere. Attrition rose.

At the same time, corporate restructuring shifted the locus of decision-making from the local ministry to regional and system leaders. Cost-containment pressures originating at the system level were perceived as insensitive to local realities and challenges and, in some cases, an unfair reallocation of local resources to support system initiatives of uncertain local value. Rebranding efforts (e.g., changing the name of the hospital on signage from Queen of the Valley to St. Joseph Health and, eventually, Providence-St. Joseph Health) were perceived by local board members, donors, and employees as diminishing the unique character of a beloved local institution. The Queen's community identity, and the sense of community within the hospital itself, began to fracture.

Amidst this financial and cultural upheaval, the California Nurses Association (CNA), a powerful nursing union with a string of successful union campaigns throughout the state, turned its attention to QVMC. The Queen's nurses, unsettled by financial setbacks and cultural changes, were receptive to union promises to raise pay, improve benefits, and address ongoing concerns about patient and worker safety brought about by revenue loss, corporate mandated productivity requirements, and attrition of their nursing colleagues. In 2013, after a contentious two-year campaign that met resistance from management and divided hospital employees, CNA proponents succeeded in winning an election to represent over 450 nurses at Queen of the Valley.[1] Their excitement was short-lived.

The vote to organize was followed by a protracted and adversarial contract negotiation. Acrimony grew on both sides as talks stalled repeatedly around the issues of wages and nonmedical benefits. Frustrated nurses responded with picketing and, finally, the unthinkable: a day-long walkout in the summer of 2014. The union accused hospital and system negotiators of bad faith, unfair labor practices, and dragging their feet. The hospital accused union organizers of intimidation tactics, smear campaigns, and strategic maneuvering

---

[1] Of the 450 nurses on staff at the Queen, 388 were eligible to vote, and 248, or 64 percent, voted to unionize.

designed to leave Catholic health systems unacceptably vulnerable to potentially crippling statewide nursing strikes. The rancor played out in the press, and a confused and divided Napa was relieved when both sides returned to the table and, finally, signed a contract in the summer of 2016. From all perspectives—management, labor, and community—the fallout was significant: between the vote for unionization and the signing of a contract, nearly 200 frustrated nurses left Queen of the Valley, as did many of the hospital's top administrators.

❖ ❖ ❖ ❖ ❖

Historically, the social justice tradition within the Catholic church has been a strong proponent of unionization in the United States, citing the rights of workers to organize for fair wages, decent working conditions, and meaningful participation in the decision-making processes that affect their lives and livelihoods. Since the publication of Pope Leo XIII's *Rerum Novarum* in 1891, numerous papal decrees, as well as statements by US Catholic bishops, have grounded strong support for unionization in principles of Catholic social teaching (CST). Given the church's pro-labor history, it may be surprising to encounter the conflicted response of Catholic health care organizations to the rise of unions in their own industry. Why have unionization efforts at many Catholic hospitals been, paradoxically, so contentious? Even more pressing, why have unionization efforts been necessary in the first place, if these organizations are "healing ministries of Jesus" dedicated to the principles of human dignity, subsidiarity, and solidarity, and historically cognizant of and supportive of workers' rights?[2]

This chapter attempts to answer several questions related to this seeming paradox. What is the ideal relationship between Catholic health care organizations and their own employees, from the perspective of Catholic social teaching? How can we understand the complicated social and business context of contemporary Catholic health care that may give rise to labor unrest? What can we learn from

[2] Katherine Gray, "Jesus, Formation, and Transition in Leadership," *Health Progress* (July-August 2014): 9–13.

studying the QVMC narrative that can be generalized to other Catholic health care organizations? What is—and perhaps more important, what should be—the role of Catholic mission leaders and ethicists in bridging the gap between employers, workers, and unions? And, finally, we address the heart of the paradox itself: Is a failure to live up to foundational principles at the root of unionization in Catholic health care?

Catholic Health Care and Directive 7

The Catholic Health Association (CHA) describes Catholic health care as a ministry "rooted in our belief that every person is a treasure, every life is a sacred gift, every human being a unity of body, mind, and spirit." From this foundational perspective of the sacredness of human life, Catholic health care ministries in their myriad roles "as provider, employer, and citizen . . . work to bring alive the Gospel vision of justice and peace."[3] That Gospel vision is articulated in numerous key principles and core values, collected and reaffirmed over time, that together constitute the body of work referred to as Catholic social teaching.

Catholic ethicists working in a clinical setting frequently access principles of CST to guide behaviors of Catholic health care ministries in their role as *provider*, including those principles that guide decisions related directly to patient care such as reproductive issues, end-of-life care, and (more recently) care of transgendered persons.[4] Much less frequently accessed, or even referenced, are CST principles that focus on Catholic ministries in their role as *employer*, despite a clear acknowledgement of this responsibility in directive 7 of the *Ethical and Religious Directives for Catholic Health Care Services* (ERDs). Directive 7 states:

> A Catholic health care institution must treat its employees respectfully and justly. This responsibility includes equal employment

---

[3] Catholic Health Association, "A Shared Statement of Identity for the Catholic Health Ministry," https://www.chausa.org/mission/a-shared-statement-of-identity.

[4] For more on care of transgendered persons, see Michael McCarthy's chapter in this volume (chap. 6).

opportunities for anyone qualified for the task, irrespective of a person's race, sex, age, national origin, or disability; a workplace that promotes employee participation; a work environment that ensures employee safety and well-being, just compensation and benefits; and recognition of the rights of employees to organize and bargain collectively without prejudice to the common good.[5]

Ethicists who do recognize a responsibility to employees of Catholic health care ministries have cited the principles of subsidiarity and solidarity, the dignity of work, and furtherance of the common good to support positions on labor issues, including the role of unionization.

Social Context of Unionization in Catholic Health Care

Each health care ministry has a unique story, often rooted in the early founding of hospitals and clinics by small groups of sisters in remote locations with very limited resources. These foundational stories, shared by local formation leaders, become part of the ministry's identity, providing inspirational touchstones that resonate with employees at all levels and instill a sense of pride and ownership in the communities they serve. These stories of shared sacrifice for the common good also provide moral justification for the expectation that an employee of a Catholic health care institution would see their work as more than just a job and a paycheck. They would see it as service. Many local ministries are not far removed from the days when a Sister of Mercy or a Sister of St. Joseph played a very visible role within the institution, either as CEO or as an influential vice president of mission, helping to ensure—at least in principle—that CST remained front and center in hospital governance and decision-making, including employee relations.

Today's health care landscape has changed drastically. Mirroring developments in for-profit health care, Catholic institutions are becoming fewer in number but larger in size, as corporate executives negotiate mergers of large-scale systems and acquisitions of smaller,

[5] United States Conference of Catholic Bishops, *Ethical and Religious Directives for Catholic Health Care Services*, 6th ed. (Washington, DC: USCCB, 2018), directive 7.

independent hospitals, many of them non-Catholic. Several reasons are given for these mergers, most of them economic and many of them compelling, but the subsequent diminution of local historical identity and often imperfect attempts to marry different organizational cultures and modes of governance can result in confusion and even alienation for local employees trying to ascertain where they belong—or even *if* they belong—in these new, impersonal, increasingly margin-driven ministries.

At the same time, the inspirational stories of the founding sisters' personal sacrifices for the common good are coopted by new corporate leadership eager to appropriate (but not necessarily emulate) their examples of communitarian behavior. Principles of CST are presented as part of ministry formation programs for leaders, but with limited attention directed at applying these principles. The role of mission leaders and ethicists in Catholic health care governance, especially at the corporate level, is growing increasingly thin as lay leadership, often recruited from for-profit industries far removed from nonprofit health care, is brought on board to steer these increasingly complex businesses. Many of these leaders, if not outright resistant to the role of mission and ethics on leadership teams, are unfamiliar with the histories of the ministries they lead or the foundational principles, anchored in CST, designed to inform business decision-making, including employee relations.

It is within this context of growing corporatization, decreasing identification with local ministries and their foundational stories, and decreasing reliance on moral discernments grounded in CST, provided traditionally by mission leaders and ethicists, that the union movement has gained a foothold in Catholic health care. This observation is not a judgment for or against unions: as the Catholic Health Association has pointed out, "The presence of a union does not make an organization just, nor does the absence of a union make it unjust."[6] Instead, many of the usual reasons for joining a union cited by employees intent on organizing—better pay and benefits, job security, and the ability to contribute meaningfully to the governance of the organizations they serve—take on new urgency and resonance.

---

[6] Catholic Health Association Just Workplace Task Force, "The Church, Social Justice, and the Health Care Ministry," *Health Progress* (January–February 2012): 22.

Catholic health care employees are no longer convinced that local leadership has the power to advocate effectively on their behalf and doubtful that distant corporate leadership is "walking the talk" when it comes to mission and values, which is what played out at QVMC.

Just as each ministry has its own story, so does each instance of a successful union campaign. How does a mission-driven community hospital become susceptible to labor unrest and subsequent unionization? From the opening narrative, one could argue persuasively that a powerful element in the success of the union was the perception that conditions that supported Catholic social teaching, particularly the principles of subsidiarity and solidarity, were missing. Where were the voices of mission and ethics leaders during unionization? More important, where were they *before* a union became likely, asking discerning questions about the culture of the organization and the ethics of corporatization?

The Role of Ethics in Catholic Health Care

Despite the church's unambiguous affirmation of the dignity of workers in ERD 7, in practice too little attention is sometimes paid to the impact on frontline employees of decisions made by health care leadership, particularly at the system level. Solidarity—a foundational commitment to the common good—is often sacrificed as Catholic health care organizations grow in size and complexity. Rather than perceiving workers at all levels of an organization as partners in the shared mission of providing quality health care, leadership too often separates itself by rank, appearing to apply standards and award benefits to those at the top at the expense of other employees. The workplace becomes divided into "us" and "them," and subsidiarity—a foundational recognition that individuals have a right to participate in decisions that directly affect them—is compromised when important decisions are made by "us" for "them" without seeking employees' input or buy-in.

In principle, Catholic health care ethicists are well-placed to address this discrepancy between words and practice. Traditionally, however, ethicists have focused primarily on applying the *Ethical and Religious Directives* to a select group of theological and ethical issues confronting medicine in its care of the individual human person in a clinical setting. Much less attention has been paid to the social contexts within which ethical conflicts arise, such as family and cultural systems (including the culture of work), and organizational ethics. This is problematic, because a too-narrow focus on clinical ethics may overlook or ignore workplace dynamics and institutional inequities that contradict CST principles and leave Catholic health care vulnerable to union organization.

If clinical ethicists are not attuned to social and organizational ethical challenges, it may be in part because they have not been invited by leadership to participate. Ethicists, too, are employees of Catholic health care, often straddling the line between "us" and "them." Their job descriptions and role statements naturally focus on clinical issues important to the organizations that pay them and encourage acceptance of the cultural assumptions and espoused values of their ministries. Focused almost exclusively on bedside ethics, many ethicists fail to question or even see organizational inequities, including those that may contribute to unionization. Ethicists who do recognize these challenges and accept the responsibilities conferred by ERD 7 may nonetheless find their roles circumscribed and limits placed on their ability to speak out on behalf of other employees.

Finally, the field of health care ethics itself has narrowed the frameworks for identifying core competencies of ministry ethicists, perhaps unintentionally. Priority is given to academic credentials in philosophy and theology while overlooking valuable real-world expertise in organizational management, clinical experience with family and cultural systems, training in resiliency and conflict management, and a pastoral commitment to upholding principles of social justice and the common good in an organizational setting, informed by core principles of CST.

A critical challenge facing Catholic health care is the discrepancy between an espoused self-identity as a values-based healing ministry and actual behaviors that appear to contradict those values. To acknowledge and address this discrepancy requires understanding the distinction between ethics *in* Catholic health care and an ethics *of* Catholic health care. The narrower role of clinical ethicist reflects the bias of ethics *in* Catholic health care, with attention directed primarily to applying ERD guidelines to clinical challenges affecting individual patients and their physicians. This is of course a crucial undertaking, intrinsic to the mission and values of Catholic health care ministries.

An ethics *of* Catholic health care, by comparison, would continue to address clinical challenges while expanding the scope of ethical inquiry to include governance itself, training a wider lens on an organization's values-based decision making to assess compliance with Catholic Social Teaching, including ERD 7, and the organization's own mission and values. A more socially oriented ethics would consider, among other things, how nurses and other frontline employees are treated, listened to, supported, and walked with well before union organizing takes place—and if necessary, during and after unionization.

Practical Suggestions for Ethicists and Leaders

The principles of CST, regularly and consistently applied in Catholic health care ministries, have the potential to produce a deeper sense of community and, with community, a stronger commitment to the workplace, with or without a union presence. Independent of the contractual demands of union contracts, these principles treat all employees as "us"—invested colleagues with inherent dignity and an equal desire for work with meaning and purpose. Unions still may have a role to play, but it need not be an adversarial role. As co-champions of employee rights, Catholic health care ethicists and mission leaders can provide a compassionate and prophetic voice in union negotiations, helping to ensure that the guidelines set forth in *Respecting the Just Rights of Workers* are adhered to by all parties and lessening the acrimony and divisiveness that too often greets union outreach.[7]

In the end, a commitment to live out the principles of CST, with or without a union presence, calls for virtuous leaders who have operationalized these principles. A culture of the workplace inspired by these principles depends on leaders who display virtues of

---

[7] United States Conference of Catholic Bishops Committee on Domestic Justice and Human Development, *Respecting the Just Rights of Workers* (Washington, DC: USCCB, 2009).

wisdom, humility, and love. These are leaders who feel called to serve a ministry of committed persons; leaders who can self-reflect, question their assumptions and biases, and embrace their hypocritical selves. Leading with the principles of dignity, the common good, subsidiarity, and solidarity requires a capacity to live in the tensions and weigh the competing goods of organizational life. The health care ethicist can be a partner in that endeavor, helping leaders navigate the challenges of operationalizing the principles of CST while addressing the ethical tensions inherent in organizational management.

Two important processes are required to effectively embed CST's commitments to subsidiarity, solidarity, and dignity of the worker into the structures and cultures of complex health care ministries: (1) formation programs that include every employee, from administrative leadership to frontline workers, and (2) ethics and mission discernments of every key decision that affects employee well-being. In principle, these processes are already operative in most ministries, but in practice their reach is often limited. For example, virtually all Catholic sponsored systems provide formation programs for senior leadership and middle management, but fewer provide substantive formation opportunities for frontline workers too. In Catholic health care ministries, formation programs introduce employees to the heritage, mission statement, and core values of their organizations and include presentations on CST, including the ERDs. Instituting a more inclusive formation process helps to create a shared vision and a commitment to the common good of the organization that transcends rank and job title.

Extending the reach and improving the effectiveness of formation programs can have a profound impact on the workplace cultures and lived values of these ministries, with or without a union presence. However, merely teaching leaders and employees how to *talk* about CST without assessing the effectiveness with which those teachings are operationalized is ineffective. Formation programs supported by ethicists must include opportunities for all employees to demonstrate skills and perspectives that reflect CST in practice as well as principle.

The crucial process of discernment is another important opportunity for ethicists to contribute to an organizational culture that reflects its commitment to CST. Discernment in Catholic health care is a process for examining decisions that impact patients, employees, and the community in significant ways. Lay-offs, consolidations or closure of programs, affiliations and mergers should be subjected to a discernment process. Ethicists can identify "triggers" for decisions that should be subjected to a discernment. Along with mission leaders, they can help gather the appropriate participants and facilitate the discernment process. Discernments should be frequent demonstrations of an organization's commitment to reflecting its values and mission in action.

Other opportunities for ethicists to contribute to a just workplace culture include collaborating with talent management and organizational development to ensure that key employees are "hired for mission," especially senior leaders tasked with operationalizing the mission and values of the organizations they serve. Ethicists can also help craft policies and procedures that include workers in decisions that significantly impact their jobs and workplaces and participate in organizational assessments that evaluate the degree to which the ministry's labor relations reflect its Catholic identity. Ethicists can also co-partner with community benefit and advocacy to ensure a balanced perspective on issues of social ethics, including those that involve the poor and vulnerable, the mentally ill, and marginalized individuals such as undocumented immigrants and transgendered persons, some of whom may be employees.

Conclusion: Confronting the Inconvenient Truth

Ron Hamel, former senior director of ethics at the Catholic Health Association, has noted that the moral requirement to live up to the principles of CST in our ministries is neither easy nor inexpensive, a truth that for many is "inconvenient."[8] The most inconvenient of all truths may be that Catholic health care, divorced from the mission that legitimizes it and justifies its nonprofit status, becomes just another corporate institution focused on cutting costs and maximizing

---

[8] Ron Hamel, "Human Dignity in the Workplace: An Inconvenient Truth," *Health Progress* (September-October, 2007): 4–5.

profits. Already, executive leaders in Catholic health care are compensated as if they were running for-profit ventures. The buying up of local hospitals by distant corporate entities and the concerted effort to consolidate profits by moving money out of the communities that generate those earnings and into corporate coffers echoes corporate America's for-profit ethos and practices. In theory, redistribution enables less prosperous health care organizations within a larger system to continue to serve their populations, and this does happen—to an extent. But the subtraction of money upward into regional and system level enterprises, which funds increasingly large corporate leadership structures, appears at times to benefit top-level leaders at the expense of the ministries they lead.

The trends in Catholic health care merely echo an ethos all too common in today's pro-corporate business environment which places profits first and people a distant second. System leaders' resistance to expanding community benefit programs, for instance, may echo the claims of some political leaders that our nation cannot afford crucial social welfare programs, despite unnecessarily large tax breaks for corporations and the wealthiest Americans. Legal strategies that pit Catholic health care management against labor and treat its own employees as adversaries reflect current government policies that undercut unions and workers in favor of Big Business. By increasingly favoring margin over mission, Catholic health care is in danger of following corporate America over a moral precipice, undermining employee well-being and contributing to the economic inequality that threatens to destabilize our democracy. But it does not have to be that way.

Currently, Catholic health care finds itself in the "tragic gap" between what is and what could and should be.[9] The answer is not to ignore the tension of inconvenience or deny the difficulty of fundamental change, but to openly acknowledge that we cannot achieve the healing goals of our ministry without opening our hearts to each other. Learning how to live and lead creatively means renewing our commitment to consensual decision making, rules that enforce collaborative and not adversarial processes, and "listening with new

---

[9] Parker Palmer, "The Broken-Open Heart: Living with Faith and Hope in the Tragic Gap," *Weavings* 24, vol. 2 (2009).

ears to hold the tension of opposites," which permits the synthesis that allows us to move forward.[10] As provider, employer, and—most important—as *citizen*, Catholic health care can reclaim its prophetic role as a ministry of Jesus Christ, dedicated to serving the common good. With foundational principles grounded in Catholic social teaching that recognize the dignity of human life and the dignity of work, Catholic health care leadership can lead a margin-sensitive but mission-driven counter-revolution in US health care—if the will to "walk the talk" is truly there.

[10] Ibid., 10.

Chapter 10

Inviting the Neighborhood into the Hospital: Diversifying Our Health Care Organizations

Robert J. Gordon

St. Bernard Hospital and Health Care Center is a 202-bed hospital whose emergency department serves approximately 37,000 patients annually. It provides high quality health care without discrimination and regardless of inability to pay. It offers a wide range of services—a dental clinic for children, adults, and special needs persons; a prenatal women's wellness clinic; a pediatric asthma and allergy center; a diabetes clinic; and orthopedics, an immediate care clinic, imaging and diagnostic services, MRI, and outpatient behavioral health to name a few.[1] On paper, it looks like any community hospital.

St. Bernard's, however, is unique among Catholic hospitals in the United States. It is located in the Englewood neighborhood of Chicago, a three square-mile community on the South Side of Chicago, inhabited by roughly 30,000 residents, 97 percent of whom are Black. In 2013, 42 percent of the Englewood population lived below the poverty level and the unemployment rate was 21 percent; it is often characterized as one of the most dangerous neighborhoods in the

---

[1] A full list of services can be found at St. Bernard Hospital and Health Care Center, https://www.stbh.org.

city.[2] It is in this community that St. Bernard's serves as "Safety-Net Hospital," meaning that 50 percent or greater of its patients depend on Medicaid.[3] In 2017, Medicaid comprised 76.3 percent of payer reimbursement and Medicare 19.6 percent (for a total of 95.9 percent), 3.9 percent was self-pay (often no-pay), and only .02 percent of the patients had private insurance.[4] Without St. Bernard there would be no local health care option, leaving residents to travel miles by public transportation or use emergency services to receive quality life-saving care.

Clearly, St. Bernard's finds itself immersed in the social and structural inequalities that wrack the US. But it is what is happening *within* St. Bernard's—in its workforce and its relationship to its local community—that makes it particularly unique. In contrast to national trends, St. Bernard's has made a conscious effort to employ a diverse workforce to serve its local patient population. Nationally, only 4.8 percent of physicians and 10 percent of nurses are African American.[5] Conversely, for decades St. Bernard's has made a commitment to diversified staffing, maintaining an average 55 percent or more total Black workforce, with records from 2017 showing the percentage at 69.6 percent (see table 1). African American physicians and nurses are also represented at higher than the national average: 18 percent of its physicians and 43.6 percent of its nurses are Black.[6] What is

---

[2] Mark Suppelsa, "'It's Englewood': 12 Hours in one of Chicago's Most Dangerous Neighborhoods," *WGN 9*, August 25, 2013, http://wgntv.com/2013/08/25/its -englewood-12-hours-in-one-of-chicagos-most-dangerous-neighborhoods/; and Chau Tu, "An Economic Breakdown of Chicago's Englewood Neighborhood," *Marketplace*, February 11, 2013, https://www.marketplace.org/2013/02/11/wealth-poverty/guns -and-dollars/economic-breakdown-chicagos-englewood-neighborhood. As a counterpoint to this story, see Joseph Erbentraut, "Don't Believe Everything You've Heard About Chicago's Most 'Dangerous' Neighborhood," *Huffington Post*, May 23, 2014, https://www.huffingtonpost.com/2014/05/23/whats-good-in-englewood_n _5360688.html.

[3] Medicaid assistance program provides health insurance for low-income families and individuals. Illinois Medicaid covers more than 3 million people annually.

[4] The statistics were provided by Charles Holland, current president and CEO of St. Bernard Hospital and Health Care Center.

[5] US Department of Health and Human Services, "Sex, Race, and Ethnic Diversity of U.S. Health Occupations (2011–2015)," August 2017, https://bhw.hrsa.gov/sites /default/files/bhw/nchwa/diversityushealthoccupations.pdf.

[6] This data was provided by St. Bernard Hospital Department of Human Resources on June 19, 2018.

more, St. Bernard's workforce is comprised largely of local residents. Of the total 592 African American employees, 305 live within the local community.[7]

The hospital's commitment both to diversity and the local community serves as a paradigmatic example for challenging the status quo hiring practices within Catholic health care that result in a predominately White leadership and medical staff caring for communities of color. This achievement reflects a conscious choice on the part of St. Bernard's. In the early 1960s, Englewood rapidly changed from a mid-income majority White community to a low-income majority Black community. The religious congregation of women who founded the hospital— the Religious Hospitallers of St. Joseph—made a pledge of Christian service and a bond of solidarity with the poor and vulnerable.

❖ ❖ ❖ ❖ ❖

St. Bernard's provides three lessons for Catholic health care institutions. The first is an acknowledgment that safety-net hospitals are truly mission hospitals running on the barest of budgets striving to provide the highest quality of care while sharing in the same ministry of healing as every Catholic health care institution. No doubt, this ongoing dedication to manifest Catholic social teaching (CST) through the healing mission of Jesus Christ makes St. Bernard vulnerable to the funding decisions of civil government. Second, the mission of these institutions cannot run on goodwill alone—they need participation from the local community. If the highest quality of patient care is delivered by those who can relate to and understand the needs of the community, St. Bernard's serves as a model for the ways in which effective patient care can be delivered in the midst of limited economic means. Thirdly, it highlights why diversity in staffing is important for patient care, employee satisfaction, community benefit, and hospital fiscal health.

The story of St. Bernard's is one of the best-kept secrets in US Catholic health care. This chapter offers the narrative of St. Bernard's as a paradigm for how its intentional commitment to Englewood

[7] Ibid.

provides a model for other Catholic hospitals. This chapter demonstrates that it is *possible* to staff our institutions with a workforce that reflects our patient populations, and that diversity results in better care and a better living and working community grounded in the healing ministry of Christ. It challenges Catholic health systems to recognize that solidarity begins at home, through accompaniment of the poor near at hand, and that a primary beneficiary of such solidarity will be not only the poor but our institutions themselves, which will find themselves gifted, changed, and transformed.

St. Bernard *Hotel Dieu* and a Necessary Discernment

In 1903, Englewood was an expanding community just seven miles south of downtown Chicago, settled by mostly German and Irish immigrants who laid rail line.[8] Reverend Bernard Murray, pastor of St. Bernard Catholic parish in Englewood, invited the Religious Hospitallers of St. Joseph (RHSJ), a community of women religious, to build a hospital in the parish.[9] Later that year seven sisters arrived from Kingston, Ontario. They immediately sought funds and resources. Ground breaking for the new structure began in 1904. On November 21, 1905 (Feast of the Presentation of the Blessed Virgin Mary), the hospital was dedicated as St. Bernard *Hotel Dieu*, "house of God," in honor of Father Murray's patron saint. "The Sisters admitted their first patient on 27 December 1905."[10]

St. Bernard's sat at the intersection of Harvard and 64th Street, near the second busiest shopping district in the city located at Halsted and 63rd Street, second only to downtown Chicago's Loop. Englewood was an all-White economically thriving community. However, the Great Migration of 1915 to 1950 brought millions of southern Blacks

---

[8] Clinton E. Stockwell, "Englewood," in *Encyclopedia of Chicago* (Chicago, IL: Chicago Historical Society, 2005), http://www.encyclopedia.chicagohistory.org /pages/426.html.

[9] For a history of the Religious Hospitallers of St. Joseph, see www.rhsj.org. Their founder, Jerome Le Royer, is also the founder of the City of Montreal in 1642 in what was then known as New France. In that same year, a lay woman and nurse, Jeanne Mance under the guidance of Le Royer established Ville-Marie Hotel-Dieu in Montreal, for the recently formed Religious Hospitallers of St. Joseph.

[10] For a brief history, see "St. Bernard Hospital (Chicago, Ill.) Records, 1881–1991," http://explore.chicagocollections.org/marcxml/luc/42/3b5xf9s/.

north to Chicago and other northern and west coast cities, changing neighborhood demographics decade by decade.[11] By 1930, Blacks comprised 1.3 percent of the population.[12] By 1950, the Great Migration increased the number of Blacks to 11 percent. Whispers of "White flight" had begun and a decade later were in full effect.[13] By 1960, the racial demographics of this community of 97,000 had shifted dramatically from nearly 90 percent White in the 50s to 70 percent Black in a decade. Although the neighborhood demographics had shifted, Whites were still the largest portion of the patients at St. Bernard's.

Nevertheless, in the early 1960s, the sisters of St. Bernard were committed to expanding and staying in Englewood. Even before the opening of the Second Vatican Council, they were "reading the signs of the times . . . in the light of the Gospel."[14] What was always the constant was the sisters' concern for the poor and their belief that "everyone should look upon his neighbor (without any exception) as another self, bearing in mind above all his (sic) life and the means necessary for living it in a dignified way."[15] The sisters wholeheartedly believed in this mission.

[11] For a detailed history of the migration, see Isabel Wilkerson, *The Warmth of Other Suns: The Epic Story of America's Great Migration* (New York: Vintage Books, 2010).

[12] Stockwell, "Englewood."

[13] The Great Migration resulted in population shifts in which immigrant populations that were west and southwest of Bronzeville moved further out. "Slumlords made the most of it by subdividing what housing there was into smaller and smaller units" (Wilkerson, *The Warmth of Other Suns*, 289). The Black population filled these vacancies and kept moving south searching for more housing. See also Mick Dumke and Chanel Polk, *A Brief History of Englewood* (Chicago Reporter, December 1999). More displacement followed the building of the Dan Ryan Expressway during the 1950s. The expressway ran along Wentworth Avenue. Properties were claimed for its construction. See "Properties Claimed for Construction of Dan Ryan Expressway, 1953–1954," in *Encyclopedia of Chicago* (Chicago, IL: Chicago Historical Society, 2005), http://www.encyclopedia.chicagohistory.org/pages/11536.html. The creation of the federally subsidized Interstate Highway program instituted in 1956 under Dwight D. Eisenhower was one of a series of post-war interventions that disrupted vibrant Black neighborhoods, displacing their residents and contributing to the development of contemporary urban ghettos. For more on this history see David Hilfiker, *Urban Injustice: How Ghettos Happen* (New York: Seven Stories Press, 2002), chap. 1.

[14] Vatican II, *Gaudium et Spes* 4. Quotations of Vatican II documents from Austin Flannery, ed., *Vatican Council II: Constitutions, Decrees, Declarations; The Basic Sixteen Documents* (Collegeville, MN: Liturgical Press, 2014).

[15] *Gaudium et Spes* 27, para. 1.

Extracts from the chronicles of the community kept in the provincial archives in Kingston, Ontario, Canada give a real-time window into the sisters' discernment. In an entry dated September 12, 1958, an analyst comments on the local community's mission in Englewood:

> Just another thought on our changing neighborhood here at St. Bernard's in Englewood, for over the last decade since 1949 the [Negro] Race [have been coming] in and the White Race moving out at this present writing we have about 98 percent Negro and 2 percent White left. No doubt our Foreign [mission] is right here in Englewood, the people are very poor and illiterate and overcrowded housing conditions and other unfortunate circumstances.[16]

These letters demonstrate the recognition by the religious sisters on what today would be described as the social determinants of health. Thus, their commitment to the health of the community extended beyond those patients that walked through the door and into concerns about the health of the community. Therefore, when the opportunity to move the hospital out of Englewood presented itself, the sisters argued against it vociferously.

A request had been made to the Provincial Council in Ontario to close the hospital's School of Nursing. "The debt being incurred had an impact on their ability to secure loans."[17] The Provincial Council sent a letter, dated September 12, 1960, to the local superiors and local councils of St. Bernard and St. George hospitals.[18] In the letter, it proposed two options. First, consider combining the resources of St. Bernard and St. George hospitals and build a new hospital in Palos Park.[19] The council did realize that making a financially based deci-

---

[16] St. Bernard Community, *Annals and Minutes April 1954–December 1968,* RHSJ St. Joseph Region Archives (Hotel Dieu Hospital, Kingston, ON). The sisters requested that the author of this chapter replace the word "coloured" with [Negro], which they used interchangeably in 1958. While neither would be acceptable today, it is important to read the language used within that particular historical locus.

[17] Rodney Carter, comments on extracts from *Minutes of the Provincial Council (1954–June 1969)* in an email dated April 9, 2018.

[18] Auburn Park Community Hospital was purchased by St. Bernard in 1939 and renamed St. George through a need to expand.

[19] The RHSJ's owned property in Palos Park. A farm provided produce, poultry, and dairy to the hospital.

sion to relocate could be mistaken as a move from a racially changing neighborhood. This was not their intention.[20] The second consideration was to ask the Archdiocese of Chicago to take over the financial management of the hospitals and employ the sisters to operate them.[21] Both hospitals rejected these options, and in response the local superior and council of St. Bernard Hospital stated in a letter dated September 21, 1960:

> Several years ago, when the building program at St. Bernard's had just begun to develop, the doctors and the sisters were asked if they wished to remain at our present location or if they would rather build a new hospital in Palos. The sisters expressed their desire to remain on Chicago's southside. The doctors also requested that the sisters continue to serve in the area that they have served for so many years, and in their turn, they promised to support the hospital and to continue to send their patients to St. Bernard's. So it was decided to add to and renovate the old hospital. . . . Several drives for the building fund have been undertaken, and all donations have been given for an addition to the existing St. Bernard's Hospital. If we went to Palos now, we would be going back on our promise to our sisters, to our doctors, and to all the benefactors who have donated to our building fund. We would also be obliged in justice to return the money so received.[22]

St. Bernard Hospital responded that the two proposals would go against a commitment already made. They reaffirmed their mission by acknowledging that few hospitals have the privilege of sharing at such a level of charity. They realized this level of work, however, could be improved upon by relying even more on the support of the local community and sought to integrate the hospital staff in the early parts of the 1960s.

In a letter dated January 16, 1961, the Provincial Council, while referring to Cardinal Meyer's views[23] on integration, suggested the

---

[20] *Minutes of the Provincial Council (1954–June 1969)*, RHSJ St. Joseph Region Archives (Kingston, ON: Hotel Dieu Hospital).

[21] Ibid.

[22] Ibid.

[23] Cardinal Albert Meyer was archbishop of Chicago from 1958 to 1965. He favored integration of Catholic schools.

hiring of a Black physician in view of increasing Black patient admissions.[24] Discussions continued around the status of St. Bernard and St. George hospitals.[25] Then in February 5, 1963, a letter was sent from the Provincial Council to the local superior and local council of St. Bernard.

> The Provincial Council is very much aware of, and in sympathy with your current problems, especially the large debt on the new wing, the low patient census, and the question of racial integration. In reality, all three seem to stem from the one root cause, namely, integration. We must face the inevitable fact that St. Bernard's is, and will continue to be, in a predominantly [Negro] area of Chicago, and until patients, doctors, and other personnel of the hospital are completely integrated, the problem of debt and low census is about to remain . . . the Provincial Council strongly urges that you take immediate steps to procure at least three more fully qualified Negro doctors on your staff. The Sisters of St. Bernard's will have to take a prominent lead in breaking down the existing prejudices, even at the risk of personal feelings.[26]

While the context of the letter is concerned with stimulating the patient census, the lived reality for the religious sisters was their commitment to justice and equity of care for their patients and their providers. Does Catholic health care today address racism on an individual and structural level as directly as the Sisters of St. Bernard's?

Their decision to forge ahead with diversifying their staff was particularly prophetic in the midst of the civil rights era. The decade of the Sixties was a turbulent time for America, and the changes which the sisters were initiating met resistance in both overt and in subliminal ways. The sisters devised an integration policy that they thought was sensible and sensitive to the whole community. A May 6, 1963, letter of response to the Provincial Council reads:

[24] *Minutes of the Provincial Council (1954–June 1969).*
[25] St. George Hospital eventually built Palos Community Hospital on the Palos property and closed its Chicago location in 1972.
[26] *Minutes of the Provincial Council (1954–June 1969).*

We at St. Bernard's are proud of what we have been able to accomplish, with the help of God's Grace, in the past few years. Slowly we have introduced Negro doctors, patients, and personnel into our hospital in such a way that they are accepted and loved as an integral part of an integrated hospital. All hospital facilities are open to our Negro patients, including wards and semi-private rooms. Successfully integrating a hospital is not an easy task and our sisters have willingly and lovingly, without complaint, borne the brunt of the burden of recognizing in it the Cross of Christ.[27]

As an integrated hospital, it promoted itself within the community. In a newsletter published in 1971, "St. Bernard Hospital . . . 66 Years of Health Care in Englewood" recognized these important changes, including the first Black physician elected to serve as president of the medical staff. "For the first time a Black doctor was elected to the position of president of the medical staff. Other firsts for the hospital were the appointments of a Black doctor to the Administrative Board and of a Black doctor to the chairmanship of a major hospital department."[28] The election of the first Black physician to a chair indicated not only a different way of governing then—it still represents the exception rather than the rule. Black leaders in health care are unfortunately still rare.

Dr. Ephraim Grier was elected president of the medical staff. Dr. Jasper Williams was appointed the new administrative board member, and his brother Dr. James Williams was appointed the head of the department of surgery.[29] Dr. James T. Johnson was appointed vice chairman of the department of medicine. All of these were African American physicians. The article also notes that at the time, "20 of the 60 most active physicians on the St. Bernard medical staff are Black. The facility is actively recruiting additional Black doctors."[30] The intentional promotion of qualified and capable physicians

[27] Ibid.

[28] Constance A. Howard, "St. Bernard Hospital . . . 66 Years of Health Care in Englewood: Medical Staff Changes Reflect a Changing Community" (Chicago: Charles A. Davis, 1971).

[29] The Williams brothers were both graduates of Creighton University, Omaha, NE, a Jesuit institution, per Sr. Elizabeth van Straten, RHSJ.

[30] Howard, "St. Bernard Hospital."

of color to lead the staff was revolutionary. But it did not come from a utilitarian perspective of better patient care, rather it came out of sense of justice and fairness to the community. The sisters saw racial inequality as an injustice and envisaged reforming their system as a way to address this glaring inequality so as to better meet the needs of their community as foundational to their mission. In 1973 an active African American business leader in Englewood who had also served on St. Bernard's board of directors, Joseph H. Thomas, was appointed administrator of the hospital.

Out of the sisters' dialogue arose the word *integration*. Here integration was understood through the lens of solidarity with the community, a community that had been pushed to the margins of society. Since the hospital was in the neighborhood, the sisters would fully invite the neighborhood into the hospital. They practiced solidarity at all levels, building a hospital community that represented the local community they served while providing the best medical care available which the community deserves. The motivation behind all of their efforts was a hope that their tender mercies would be a compelling sign of God's love. "I give you a new commandment, that you love one another. Just as I have loved you, you also should love one another" (John 13:34).

Inviting the Neighborhood into the Hospital: The Benefits of a Diverse Hospital Staff

St. Bernard Hospital stands as a beacon of the possible in a country where racial polarization silently infects so many cultural spaces, including health care institutions. As data make clear, the racial and ethnic diversity of the US continues to increase at an exponential pace, with projections suggesting that by 2044, the US will be a "majority-minority" nation.[31] Yet segregation persists, both geographically and within the health care professions.[32] A 2017 study con-

---

[31] Jordan J. Cohen, Barbara A. Gabriel, and Charles Terrell, "The Case for Diversity in the Health Care Workforce," *Health Affairs* 21, no. 5 (September/October 2002): 91.

[32] Aaron Williams and Armand Emadjomeh, "America is More Diverse than Ever—but Still Segregated," *The Washington Post*, May 10, 2018, https://www.washington post.com/graphics/2018/national/segregation-us-cities/?noredirect=on&utm _term=.1d4c563f7c1a.

ducted by the US Department of Health and Human Services charts diversity within the health care professions from 2011 to 2015.[33] They find that across thirty health care professions studied,

> Whites make up the majority of the U.S. workforce (64.4 percent) compared to Hispanics (16.1 percent), Blacks or African Americans (11.6 percent), Asians (5.3 percent), and individuals reporting Multiple and Other races (1.8 percent). American Indians and Alaska Natives, and Native Hawaiians and Other Pacific Islanders represent less than 1 percent of the U.S. workforce (0.6 percent and 0.2 percent, respectively). Compared to their representation in the U.S. workforce, Whites are overrepresented in 23 of the 30 occupations.[34]

Such occupational segregation renders hospitals what sociologist Elijah Anderson refers to as "White spaces." Such spaces, characterized by the overwhelming presence of White people, creates a dual dissonance.

> When present in the white space, blacks reflexively note the proportion of whites to blacks, or may look around for other blacks with whom to commune if not bond, and then may adjust their comfort level accordingly; when judging a setting as too white, they can feel uneasy and consider it to be informally "off limits" . . . .When the anonymous black person enters the white space, others there immediately try to make sense of him or her—to figure out "who that is," or to gain a sense of the nature of the person's business and whether they need to be concerned.[35]

St. Bernard's has taken steps, long before it was a priority, to recognize this racial dynamic takes a toll on patients and associates alike.

[33] US Department of Health and Human Services, *Sex, Race, and Ethnic Diversity of U.S. Health Occupations (2011–2015)*, (Rockville, MD: US Department of Health and Human Services, 2017), https://bhw.hrsa.gov/sites/default/files/bhw/nchwa/diversityushealthoccupations.pdf.

[34] Ibid., 5.

[35] Elijah Anderson, "The White Space," *Sociology of Race and Ethnicity* 1, no. 1 (2015), 10, 13. Anderson uses lowercase letters for the terms black and white, and we follow his usage when citing his work.

It certainly impacts patient care. Biases imported into the clinical context by health care providers contribute significantly to unequal treatment and negative health outcomes. As Cohen notes, "even when insurance status, income, age, and severity of condition have been adjusted for, minorities tend to receive lower quality of care than whites do."[36] In addition to those detailed elsewhere in this volume, disparities exist with regard to medically indicated bypass surgery, pain management, and medications for HIV infection. Members of minority groups generally have lower life expectancy and are more likely to suffer from HIV, uncontrolled hypertension, cardiovascular disease; and die from stroke, cancer, diabetes, infant mortality, homicide, cervical cancer, and complications from asthma.[37] "Minorities are also more likely to undergo procedures such as bilateral orchiectomy (removal of the testicles) and amputation, which are generally avoidable with optimal medical care."[38]

Such experiences encountered in the clinical setting discourage minority patients from seeking treatment. Not surprisingly, when given a choice, minority patients are more likely to select health care professionals of their own racial or ethnic background and are more likely to report receiving higher-quality care.[39] At the same time, minority and female caregivers are more likely to care for patients from underserved communities, increasing access to health care.[40] "According to the Sullivan Commission's report, Black patients are significantly more likely to receive their care from Black dentists (who treat almost 62 percent of Black patients) than from White dentists (who treat 10.5 percent of these patients)."[41]

---

[36] Cohen, et al., "The Case for Diversity in the Health Care Workforce," 90. See also Health Professionals for Diversity Coalition, "Fact Sheet: The Need for Diversity in the Health Care Workforce," www.aapcho.org/wp/wp-content/uploads/2012/11/NeedForDiversityHealthCareWorkforce.pdf.

[37] Cohen, et al., "The Case for Diversity in the Health Care Workforce," 93.

[38] Ibid.

[39] Health Professionals, "Fact Sheet."

[40] Ibid.

[41] Dennis A. Mitchell and Shana L. Lassiter, "Addressing Health Care Disparities and Increasing Workforce Diversity: The Next Step for the Dental, Medical, and Public Health Professions," *American Journal of Public Health* 96, no. 12 (December 1, 2006): 2093–97.

Working within a White space takes a toll on clinicians and other health care associates as well. As Anderson details, constantly having to negotiate White spaces creates a source of stress—either subliminal or conscious—for persons from diverse backgrounds, particularly African Americans. Within professional spaces like hospitals, African Americans must first prove that they have transcended the "deficit of credibility" associated with the ghetto stereotype. Even today, "the most easily tolerated black person in the white space is often one who is 'in his place'—that is, one who is working as a janitor or a service person or one who has been vouched for by white people in good standing. Such a person may be believed to be less likely to disturb the implicit racial order—whites as dominant and blacks as subordinate."[42] From housekeeping to the board room, this credibility must be established through constant performance or negotiation, "what some blacks derisively refer to as a 'dance.' "[43] "This performance can be as deliberate as dressing well and speaking in an educated way or as simple as producing an ID or a driver's license in situations in which this would never be demanded of whites."[44] Successful performance provides provisional acceptance, but only person-by-person; no matter how established the person is, new encounters with unknown White people require them to "dance" anew. As a result, women and members of racial and ethnic minorities are more likely to feel excluded, and that exclusion is linked to job dissatisfaction and lower sense of well-being.[45] Diversity has a balancing effect on clinician well-being and performance because different sociodemographic groups respond to stress and errors differently. If there is a sense of belonging and cohesion among diverse peers, there is less burnout and better clinical performance.

What is more, diversifying hospital staff by hiring locally may bring financial benefits to both the community and the hospital itself. Urban planning scholars Mara Nelson and Laura Wolf-Powers found

[42] Anderson, "The White Space," 13.

[43] Ibid.

[44] Ibid.

[45] Michàl E. Mor Barak and Amy Levin, "Outside of the Corporate Mainstream and Excluded from the Work Community: A Study of Diversity, Job Satisfaction and Well-being," *Community, Work and Family* 5, no. 2 (2002): 133.

that health care is the single best industry for moving people from poverty to middle class.[46] Growth in hospital employment in urban areas—especially among low- and semi-skilled workers—outstrips the potential for poverty reduction and economic growth impact of other hiring sectors, including that growth in accommodations, legal services, and securities and commodities.[47] Local hiring enhances the common good by infusing capital into the community, quietly strengthening the web of economic security. In other words, one of the best forms of community benefit—or better, community building—that a not-for-profit Catholic hospital can engage in is hiring from the local community. Thus, the solidarity that the RHSJs worked for with their local community, yielded benefits beyond their "diversifying the workforce." They created an intentional community of care.

Such good may well redound to the hospital itself. Rightly or wrongly, health care insurance in America is primarily a function of employment.[48] Compared to private insurance, government reimbursement is low and slow, and health care providers with too many publicly insured patients are said to have an adverse payer mix.[49, 50] Helping unemployed people in a hospital's local community find full-time employment promises to improve its bottom line by improving its payer mix. This approach also has the potential to strengthen a health system's brand among patients who are increasingly adopting a consumer mindset. And, as detailed in the *Harvard Business*

---

[46] Laura Wolf-Powers and Marla Nelson, "Chains and Ladders: Exploring the Opportunities for Workforce Development and Poverty Reduction in the Hospital Sector," *Economic Development Quarterly* 24, no. 1: 33.

[47] Ibid.

[48] Centers for Medicaid and Medicare Services, "The Nation's Health Dollar ($3.2 Trillion), Calendar Year 2015: Where It Came From," https://www.cms.gov/Research -Statistics-Data-and-Systems/Statistics-Trends-and- Reports/NationalHealthExpend Data/Downloads/PieChartSourcesExpenditures2015.pdf.

[49] Avery B. Nathens, Ronald V. Mayer, Michael K. Copass, and Gregory J. Jurkovich, "Payer Status: The Unspoken Triage Criterion," *The Journal of Trauma* 50, no. 5 (2001): 776–83.

[50] Intermedix Staff, "The Importance of Understanding Your Payer Mix," October 20, 2016, https://www.intermedix.com/blog/the-importance-of-understanding -your-practices-payer-mix.

Review, studies have shown that managerial diversity significantly drives both innovation and financial performance.[51] Workforce diversity is not just a good thing to do (to eliminate disparities and disparate treatment); it is beneficial for everyone, and hence enhances the common good. Patients, providers, and local communities will be better off.

St. Bernard's Today: Living the Mission

The sisters' love for the community has shown itself not only in their commitment to keeping St. Bernard's in Englewood but has expanded to an array of community-building projects. In 2018, this once prosperous and highly populated neighborhood is experiencing a gradual rebuilding and recovery. To cite a few of the hospital's initiatives: Bernard Place, a housing development in collaboration with St. Bernard Hospital, the City of Chicago and Chicago Neighborhood Initiatives built seventy-seven new affordable single-family homes beginning at 64th Street and the Dan Ryan Expressway. St. Bernard Hospital is also a founding member of Teamwork Englewood, a community organization whose mission is to facilitate comprehensive community development to raise the quality of life for each resident.[52] In 2016, the hospital opened its ambulatory care center, which provides easy access to an immediate care clinic, physicians' offices, diagnostic testing (MRI), rehabilitative care, school physicals, and more. The hospital also participates in local job and health fairs and a mobile pediatric unit serves neighborhood schools.

Curious as to the effects of their commitments, St. Bernard's conducted a survey in 2018 to assess employee perspectives on St. Bernard's commitment to reflect the demographics of its surrounding area in the diversity of its staff. The survey invited responses from associates who had been employed at St. Bernard's twenty or more

---

[51] Rocio Lorenzo and Martin Reeves, "How and Where Diversity Drives Financial Performance," *The Harvard Business Review*, January 30, 2018, https://hbr.org/2018/01/how-and-where-diversity-drives-financial-performance.

[52] Team Work Englewood, "Team Work Englewood," http://www.teamworkenglewood.org/index.html.

years (10.8 percent of its workforce). A partial table representation of the survey can be found in table 2.[53]

The findings indicate several important trends that positively affect the work environment that lead to better patient care and more engaged employees. A quick summary of key findings indicates that those working at St. Bernard's find it to be an environment in which CST is embodied. Further, 94.1 percent of respondents consider it an important part of the Catholic mission of the hospital to hire local employees and train those employees for leadership opportunities (question 10), while 88.2 percent of respondents affirm that the Catholic mission of the hospital has manifested itself in the local community (question 11).[54] What is striking about these numbers is that the health care staff identify the diversity of the hospital community and its commitment to the local community as a foundational piece of the hospital's mission. This identity is foundational to the culture and mission that the RHSJs saw as vital to the development of the St. Bernard's ministry. In Catholic health care, it has become increasingly rare for the health care institutions to maintain such a strong connection to the mission of its religious founders. In developing the founders' instincts as leadership shifted, St. Bernard's serves as paradigm for creating an alternative to the "White space" of healthcare and a model for both employee and community engagement.

As Catholic institutions, we are mission oriented. It would be wise for our members to also be oriented to the founder's mission. May we not only read but also pray and act with our mission and values

---

[53] There was a 36.8 percent return of the surveys (34 out of 94 invitations). Of these, 50 percent were Asian, 32.4 percent were Black or African American, 11.8 percent Caucasian and 2.9 percent Hispanics. The average years of service for Asians who responded was 29.8 years. For Blacks or African Americans, it was 32.8 years. For Caucasians, it was 24 years. One Hispanic who responded has been at St. Bernard for 42 years; one African American who responded has served for 48 years.

[54] A comment from respondent no. 22: "St. Bernard Hospital has met its mission in numerous ways: By caring for the health of its patients that are present to us, from caring for the poor and less fortunate regardless of ability to pay, providing and promoting health education to the patients, providing social services support by connecting patients to community partners, aiding patients who are seeking housing and food programs, improving the community by building homes and meeting its Mission, Vision and Values."

statements so that the words of these statements come alive and in turn read us and transform us. Like our founders who were informed and transformed by the spirituality or charism of their religious communities, rooted in the Word of God, our Lord Jesus Christ, so the contemporary community and its lay leadership today may be similarly informed and transformed by the spirit of its founders. Such a transformation reaches out to the local community it serves, inviting it to enter within its walls, transforming it from a White space to one where diverse cultures may meet, embrace, and learn to serve each other in mutual hospitality and shared objectives, creating a new space that is vibrant, inclusive, and resonant of the Gospel.

Table 1

Percentage of Black or African American Workforce
of Total Workforce at St. Bernard Hospital

Year of Report	Black/African American Workforce	Total Workforce	Percentage of Workforce
2007	458	795	57.6 %
2008	466	796	58.5 %
2009	495	833	59.4 %
2010	498	853	58.3 %
2011	514	858	59.9 %
2012	524	825	63.5 %
2013	560	849	65.9 %
2014	541	831	65.1 %
2015	574	876	65.5 %
2016	581	857	67.8 %
2017	592	850	69.6 %

The data in this table was provided by St. Bernard Hospital Department of Human Resources on April 6, 2018. The April 2018 Management Roster shows a 55.4 percent ratio of Black or African Americans in leadership positions in comparison to the total number in leadership. The roster includes supervisors through officers.

Table 2

ST. BERNARD HOSPITAL AND
HEALTH CARE CENTER QUESTIONAIRE

(Employed 20 years or more.)

Name _____ I would rather remain anonymous: ___

Race: ☐ Asian   ☐ Black   ☐ Caucasian   ☐ Hispanic

1. What year did you start working at St. Bernard Hospital? ____

2. What position did you hold when you started at St. Bernard Hospital? _____

3. What position do you hold now? _____

4. Briefly describe the Englewood community at the time you started at St. Bernard Hospital. Include racial mix and economic levels in your description. _____

5. Did the workforce at St. Bernard including its leadership and officers reflect the local community when you started here? Yes _____ No _____   If "No" what is different?

   _____

   _____

6. Briefly describe the Englewood community of today:

   _____

   _____

7. Does the workforce at St. Bernard including its leadership and officers reflect the local community of today? Yes _____ No _____   If "No" what is different?

   _____

   _____

8. Do you believe that St. Bernard Hospital has demonstrated a practice of hiring employees including its leadership and officers from the community (neighborhood) and/or a practice of hiring individuals that reflect the community (Englewood) that the hospital resides in?   Yes _____ No _____

   Please explain your answer: _____

   _____

9. Acknowledging that all employees including leadership cannot come from the local neighborhood due to unavailability or the need of certain skills, do you think the hospital can better serve its community and understand its needs if it reflects the community through local hiring, when possible?
Yes _____ No_____   Give example: _____

10. Do you consider it an important part of the Catholic mission of the hospital to hire local employees and train those employees for leadership opportunities? Yes _____ No _____

11. Please comment: Given the Catholic mission of St. Bernard Hospital and Health Care Center, how has this mission revealed its self; that is, manifested itself in the local community? In other words, how has the hospital served the community? Please give examples. _____
_____

Thank you for taking this survey.

Chapter 11

The Rocky Road of Women and Health Care: A Gender Roadmap

Jana Marguerite Bennett

While studying for my Master of Divinity degree some decades ago, I worked full time for several months for a chaplaincy department at 400-bed Presbyterian/St. Luke's Medical Center with several level one units. I rotated through high-risk labor and delivery, women's surgery and oncology, and medical telemetry. Most of my time was spent visiting patients, attending patient rounds, and doing case notes. But I did visit another floor: adult oncology. Effectively a hospice overflow floor for when there were no hospice beds, these patients were moving through the final stages of their dying processes. Only open when there were patients who needed it, this unit was tucked away in a very out-of-the-way space—up and down several stair cases and through a tunnel. It was a forgotten unit for largely forgotten patients.

I vividly remember two dying patients. One was a sixty-year-old woman who had fallen from her bed and broken her wrist. She was in a great deal of pain from the break and the end-stage ravages of ovarian cancer. She kept begging for surgery to fix her arm, even as cancer took over her body. Her life prognosis was two weeks, however, and surgery on the break was contraindicated. As I accompanied her in her final weeks, I was disturbed by the way the health care staff treated her. They dismissed her complaints and labelled her as a whiny woman who needed to just get with the program, face the fact that she was dying, deal with it, and move on. They treated her grudgingly; a nurse or intern might heave a large sigh while rising from their chairs at the nurse's station, and say, "Well, I guess I'll go deal with 4B." I never saw any visitors; she was an older widowed woman. Even in the unit of the forgotten, this woman was doubly forgotten.

A male patient provided a stark contrast. About seventy years old, he appeared robust and healthy at first, but then showed a precipitous decline from his lung cancer. He, also, had only weeks to live, but he had visitors who would exclaim, "Gosh, amazing, he doesn't even complain about his pain!" He was in a room that would often contain not only family members, but also at least one smiling medical professional, joking and laughing.

❖ ❖ ❖ ❖ ❖

These two patients might not be the first to come to mind when one thinks of gender and Catholic bioethics. Yet this anecdote—and a growing body of evidence from research—highlights the myriad of ways that our implicit and explicit biases about gender impact the care of patients.[1] Gender seems a relatively simply term for something that is actually quite complex. Gender includes consideration of sex, which is specifically tied to a person's biological sex chromosomes and physical characteristics. It also broadly includes social and cultural understandings of what it means to be considered male or female, what kinds of gendered roles exist, and how our cultural assumptions about gender impact political and economic participation, family structure, health care access, and more.

This chapter provides a "roadmap" for plotting this multilayered landscape of gender, providing signposts along the long, sometimes rocky, road that describes relationships between gender, Catholic social teaching, health care, and bioethics, particularly concerning women.[2] Gender concerns touch on a number of volatile subjects—

---

[1] For some of the many articles dealing with this topic, see fn. 6–11 in the following.
[2] Gender also relates to LGBTQ+ concerns, and there are additional questions related to gender and sexuality that I do not discuss in this chapter due to restrictions

including the more traditional issues of abortion, contraception, and same-sex attraction. Yet each individual patient—and each individual health care professional—brings gender into the mix of the clinical encounter and health care delivery. Thus, questions of gender pervade health care in powerful ways that are often less visible or less often considered topics but are important because of how gender biases influence even the most mundane everyday activities.

I begin the chapter with a brief snapshot of the status and role of women in health care, both as professionals and as patients. Next, I consider how CST can both help and hurt consideration of women. I argue that attention to CST can improve how we think about gender and medical care. Finally, I consider CST in relation to traditional topics in bioethics, as well as less-often discussed questions including treatment of health care workers, women's access to leadership in health care, and the omnipresence of hetero-male norms throughout health care.

Hiding in Plain Sight:
The Rocky Road of Women and Health Care

Considering the status and role of women in health care requires attention to both health care workers and patients. In some respects, the field of medicine looks enterprising for women. In modern medicine, the first female doctor, Elizabeth Blackwell, began practicing in the 1850s. She eventually opened a women's and children's clinic, as well as a school for training other women doctors.[3] Today, more than 75 percent of workers in health care are women. Yet women typically occupy fields that are often considered to be of lesser prestige (or at least, lower pay),[4] such as nursing, speech therapy, audiology, and

---

on length and subject matter. Questions about heteronormativity and reproductive technologies are discussed further in this volume in the chapters by McCarthy (chap. 6) and Vigen (chap. 5), respectively.

[3] See Ephraim Fischoff, *Elizabeth Blackwell: First Woman MD* (Springfield, IL: Department of Medical Humanities/Southern Illinois University, 1981).

[4] Sociologists and a number of research organizations offer survey data discussing occupational prestige. Physicians nearly always top the list of most prestigious jobs; nurses often do not make the top 20, or they display a large gap in prestige. Consider the 2014 Harris Poll, which shows doctors as having top prestige (88 percent of poll

midwifery.[5] Among the more often-considered prestigious job of physician, only 34 percent are women.[6] Women also occupy far fewer top level administrative posts in medical schools (16 percent of dean-ships) and health care systems (26 percent of CEO-level positions).[7] Lack of women's participation is detrimental to health care and is also a likely reason why gender issues in health care have been overlooked.

In addition, patient care has been highly focused on men to the detriment of women. Medical diagnoses have frequently been biased in favor of cultural assumptions. For example, in the nineteenth century, "hysteria" gained special prominence as a diagnosis, especially among White middle class women.[8] Part of the working presumption in this diagnosis was that women were the "weaker" sex. Feminist scholars have identified how specific norms for men and women have contributed to gender-specific illnesses—such as corsets, which likely contributed to a number of physical ailments for women. Physician researchers such as M. Irené Ferrer and Marianne Legato have been at the forefront of researching how gender impacts the way people respond to medical treatments.[9]

While particular women's diseases like hysteria are no longer routine diagnoses, enormous gender inequality still surrounds the conceptualization, diagnosis, and treatment of diseases. For example, women are most likely to be diagnosed with autoimmune conditions,

---

responders seeing the occupation as prestigious), while nurses show an 18 percent gap, with 70 percent of responders seeing that occupation as prestigious. See also Tracey L. Adams, "Gender and Feminization in Health Care Professions," *Sociology Compass* 4, no. 7 (2010): 454–65.

[5] Linda H. Pololi, et al., "Experiencing the Culture of Academic Medicine: Gender Matters, A National Study," *Journal of General Internal Medicine* 28, no. 2 (2013): 201–7.

[6] Henry J. Kaiser Family Foundation, "Professionally Active Physicians by Gender," October 2017, https://www.kff.org/other/state-indicator/physicians-by-gender/.

[7] Elizabeth Travis, "Academic Medicine Needs More Women," *AAMC News*, January 18, 2018, https://news.aamc.org/diversity/article/academic-medicine-needs-more-women-leaders/; and Annette Walker, "More Female Leadership: A Different Kind of Health Care Reform," *Stat News*, July 10, 2017, https://www.statnews.com/2017/07/10/female-leadership-health-care-reform/.

[8] Andrew Scull, *Hysteria: The Biography* (New York: Oxford University Press, 2009).

[9] For further information, see The Foundation for Gender-Specific Medicine, https://gendermed.org/.

but the very symptoms that indicate many autoimmune diseases (like fatigue) are often dismissed as being in women's imaginations.[10] Studies note gendered disparity in knee replacement patients, with women being three times less likely than men to receive knee arthroplasty when clinically appropriate.[11] Studies of heart disease in relation to gender (and race) have famously demonstrated disparities in treatment, as has the diagnosis of COPD.[12, 13] This marginalization has resulted in a distortion of medical practices and priorities in patient care.[14]

Gender and Catholic Social Teaching

Women are not only marginalized with regard to research, diagnosis, treatment, and profession; these same distortions are present in the male dominated world of Catholic social teaching (CST). Through much of its history, the documents of the social tradition have rarely mentioned women specifically. Older documents use the general term "man" or "men," terms presumed to cover all of humanity.[15] While this may seem in keeping with the time period, many documents speak specifically of women as weak people in need of protection in their homes.

[10] See Maya Dusenbery, *Doing Harm: The Truth About How Bad Medicine and Lazy Science Leave Women Dismissed, Misdiagnosed, and Sick* (New York: Harper Collins, 2018).

[11] G. A. Hawker, et al., "Differences Between Men and Women in the Rate of Use of Hip and Knee Arthroplasty," *New England Journal of Medicine* 342, no. 4 (2000): 1016–22.

[12] See K. R. Chapman, et al., "Gender Bias in the Diagnosis of COPD," *Chest* 119, no. 6 (2001): 1691–95.

[13] S. Weitzman, et al., "Gender, Racial, and Geographic Differences in the Performance of Cardiac Diagnostic and Therapeutic Procedures for Hospitalized Acute Myocardial Infarction in Four States," *American Journal of Cardiology* 79, no. 6 (1997): 722–26.

[14] See Elizabeth N. Chapman, et al., "Physicians and Implicit Bias: How Doctors May Unwittingly Perpetuate Health Care Disparities," *Journal of General Internal Medicine* 28, no. 11 (2013): 1504–10.

[15] See Maria Riley's discussion of women's appearances in social encyclicals in her article "Theological Trends: Catholic Social Thought Encounters Feminism," *The Way* 31 (1991): 150–62.

Rerum Novarum, considered the first major document of CST, focuses on the plight and rights of workers. It presumes that men are the primary referent for labor concerns and political involvement. Women are presumed *not* to be working outside the home, yet millions of women—especially poor women—fueled the nineteenth-century industrial revolution as factory workers and domestic servants and often suffered its worst abuses. Within much of the CST, women and their work are invisible, or they are understood as too weak for the public sphere. It is not until the 1960s that CST starts mentioning women and their specific needs in their own right.[16]

However, even though women's concerns have slowly entered the social tradition, the CST often avoids questions of sexuality. Many Catholics, including the magisterium, tend to divide church teaching into two parts: sexual/personal ethics and social teaching/economics/politics. This structure presumes a division of spheres—a private domain of women in the home concerned with sex and children and separated from the public social sphere populated by men.[17] This fuels a problematic division in health care in which gender concerns frequently seem limited to volatile private sphere issues (such as abortion, contraception, artificial reproductive technologies) at the expense of social determinants of health.[18] While sex and sexuality remain important, related social questions about economic and political conditions that adversely affect women's health—such as the fact that women often take double or triple shifts or work in countries far from home—need a more prominent stage in Catholic ethical reflection on health care.

Yet the CST contains resources for challenging gender myopia. One of the most important is the conviction that each human person is made in the image of the Triune God. This image calls us to recog-

---

[16] Ibid.

[17] See, for example, Christine Firer Hinze's essay, "US Catholic Social Thought, Gender, and Economic Livelihood," *Theological Studies* 66 (2005): 568–91.

[18] See, for example, Charles Curran's descriptions of moral theology in *The Moral Theology of Pope John Paul II* (Washington DC: Georgetown University Press, 2005), in which he divides the late pope's teachings into a social teachings category, and a "marriage, sexuality, gender, and the family" category. In Curran's view, these two categories demonstrate severe inconsistencies in John Paul II's thought. I am not convinced such a divide is present, especially such a sharp inconsistent divide.

nize the dignity of each human person, including women. Americans often conflate the dignity of the human person with particularly American conceptions of individual rights and freedoms, especially as guaranteed in the US constitution. Thus, we value the individuality and autonomy of each particular person—individually. Autonomy is also a bedrock of health care ethics; consequently, the CST's commitment to the dignity of the human person seems to map neatly onto respecting individual autonomy.

In CST however, the dignity of the human person centers on human interrelatedness. Each individual person matters because we already exist in relationships to other human beings, through family, friendships, and social institutions. Our interrelatedness also extends to the whole of creation, as we see in Pope Francis's recent environmental encyclical *Laudato Si'*: "It cannot be emphasized enough how everything is interconnected. Time and space are not independent of one another, and not even atoms or subatomic particles can be considered in isolation."[19] The dignity of being human beings in relationship therefore connects to the CST concept of "the common good." While CST never denies the importance and beauty of each individual person, it highlights the common life that humans have together.

As seen in the opening narrative, via CST, dignity and the common good might have differently shaped how health care providers interacted with the woman dying of cancer. For example, we could consider how various people involved in the woman's care might have developed different relationships, relationships that emphasized the woman's dignity. Focusing on dignity in relationships does not mean sugarcoating or overlooking medical issues; it might instead mean having a frank conversation (or several) with a patient about her pain, about why surgery was not a good solution, and so forth.

In addition, the notion of the universal destination of goods, and the principles of solidarity and subsidiarity impact the view of health care and gender. Women are often overrepresented among impoverished populations (especially single mothers and widows). They have a far more difficult time receiving the goods (property, jobs, and wages) that are due to them, that would enable them to have full

---

[19] Pope Francis, *Laudato Si'* 138.

dignity.[20] As noted in the introductory narrative, women also may receive differential treatment for similar health care concerns, and less empathy for their plight, which reflects a lack of solidarity. Solidarity in the woman's case might have meant more directly acknowledging her pain and not associating her feelings with "whininess." It might also mean creating, or tapping into, community resources to respond to the woman's loneliness; in this particular case, a more direct connection with hospice volunteers earlier in the woman's treatment, would have been beneficial.

Women may also (depending on geographical location) have fewer options to make choices regarding the health care needs of themselves and people related to them—including poor access to information and lack of legal rights to make health care decisions.[21] For example, women living in areas where early marriage among young girls is normative are also less likely to have access to information about their reproductive systems. Poverty is a major driver (both in the US and internationally) in gender disparities for women, since women are much more at risk for being impoverished, which impacts their access to health care. Subsidiarity enables the development of social relationships and of each person's dignity. When women and men are unable to make valued contributions and good decisions regarding the social groups of which they are part, the principle of subsidiarity has been denied.

CST and Health Care:
Reframing Traditional Gender Issues

Traditionally, Catholic bioethics has limited attention to gender and health care to a narrow range of issues, almost entirely related to reproduction. At front and center have been, of course, abortion and contraception. Yet despite 125 years of development of the CST, Catholic health care ethics does not frequently consider how human dignity, the common good, the universal destination of goods, and

---

[20] See, for example, the United Nations report, "The World's Women: Poverty," https://unstats.un.org/unsd/gender/chapter8/chapter8.html. Depending on area of the world, women have lower access to cash, inheritance, and a say in household expenditures.

[21] United Nations Report, *The World's Women*, chap. 2.

the principles of solidarity and subsidiarity might help us to see previously invisible facets of these volatile issues, which might assist us in envisaging new ethical responses. In addition, it is important to consider specific questions related to obstetrical care, the one field that is solely devoted to care of women.

Abortion

The oversimplified framework of pro-life and pro-choice is typically posed as the two, and only two, options regarding abortion. This frame pits the individual human dignity and rights of the human fetus against the individual human dignity and rights of the mother. This standard framing also locates abortion under the heading of sexual ethics, seeing it as a personal, private, ethical dilemma for women, separating it from essential social and economic questions.

Such a framing neglects a host of issues. It fails to articulate the *common* good of mother and child, instead seeing them as adversaries. It also neglects their connections to the father, other children, extended relations, and society as a whole. By contrast, the CST calls us to consider the ways that abortion is a social issue that impacts not only our view of the dignity of all people, including mother and baby, but also asks us to interrogate the ways in which society fails women and children. CST calls us to look at how lapses in the common good—particularly lack of jobs, education, and resources for women or their families—make many women feel they have "no choice" but abortion. CST asks us to stand in solidarity with women and children, especially in cases of spousal abuse and rape. Rather than accepting the oversimplified framework of personal choice of a mother-versus-her child, CST suggests that the primary way to address abortion is by promoting policies and practices that enhance interconnectedness, the common good, and families—such as paid family leave and universal child care and kindergarten, while emphasizing laws against coercion of abortion, strengthening laws against domestic abuse, and promoting development of education and resources for women.[22]

---

[22] For a discussion of legal avenues in the United States that might aid women and their unborn children, see the last chapter of Charles Camosy, *Beyond the Abortion Wars: A Way Forward for a New Generation* (Grand Rapids, MI: Eerdmans, 2015).

Contraception

Catholic teaching on contraception is often viewed as nonsensical, evidenced by the fact that most Catholic women dissent against the teaching by using artificial contraception, according to a Guttmacher Institute report.[23] Catholic women have written incisive essays about this teaching.[24] Still, the Guttmacher Report suggests that perhaps 13 percent of Catholic women are currently either using natural family planning or not using contraception at all. While a minority, this figure represents approximately 5 million Catholic women.[25] It is thus worth considering this issue as a small signpost on this gender roadmap.

First, it is important to note some common misconceptions regarding the church's teaching. The church does *not* teach that people should have as many children as they can.[26] There are many reasons to postpone or not have children at all, and the church encourages couples to make those decisions, partly as an embodiment of subsidiarity. The church permits physicians to prescribe oral contraceptives to treat and heal bodies. A classic example is for the treatment of endometriosis. In addition, some Catholic researchers aim at finding non-contraceptive ways of treating endometriosis and polycystic ovarian syndrome.[27]

---

[23] According to a Guttmacher Institute Study, 98 percent of Catholic women have used artificial methods of contraception at least once in their sexual activity, 2 percent currently use natural family planning methods, and 11 percent use no form of contraception. See Rachel K. Jones and Joerge Dreweke, "Countering Conventional Wisdom: New Evidence on Religion and Contraceptive Use," The Guttmacher Institute, April 2011, https://www.guttmacher.org/report/countering-conventional-wisdom-new-evidence-religion-and-contraceptive-use.

[24] See Christina Traina, "Papal Ideals, Marital Realities: One View from the Ground," in *Sexual Diversity and Catholicism: Toward the Development of Moral Theology*, ed. Patricia Beattie Jung and Joseph A. Coray (Collegeville, MN: Liturgical Press, 2001), 269–88.

[25] This number derives from Pew Forum Survey suggesting that about 72 million Americans identify as Catholic, and 54 percent of Catholics are women. See Pew Forum Research Center, "Religious Landscape Survey: Catholics," http://www.pewforum.org/religious-landscape-study/religious-tradition/catholic/.

[26] See Pontifical Council for Justice and Peace, *The Compendium of the Social Doctrine of the Church* (Washington, DC: USCCB, 2005), 234.

[27] According to NaPro, the technology is designed to work in concert with women's fertility cycles; women track their fertility and are treated for a range of gynecological problems, including infertility, PCOS, repeat miscarriages, ovarian cysts, and more.

In addition, an increasing number of people—Catholic and otherwise—share the church's concern that artificial contraception objectifies women's bodies, impacting views of the dignity of women.[28] Others have noted gender disparities in researching and marketing contraceptives. This disparity relates not only to questions of human dignity, but also the common good, and to subsidiarity. At least one study of an injectable male hormonal contraceptive was discontinued because male participants reported pain at the injection site and increased depression, perhaps due to hormonal effects.[29] Women have acerbically noted these are the same kinds of effects *they* encounter with hormonal contraceptives, yet their concerns have often been dismissed.[30, 31] The principle of the common good suggests examining connections between contraception, social issues, and the environment. For example, some feminists have articulated concerns that focusing on contraception for women conveniently means that businesses do not have to think about instituting family-friendly policies, including paid family leave. Others have raised questions about potential effects of excess hormones being released into the water cycle and the impact on wildlife.[32]

Obstetrical Care

Labor and delivery is most clearly women's purview. Over the past few decades, feminists have highlighted the ambivalence of

[28] See, for example, Pope Paul VI's discussion of the objectification of women's bodies in *Humanae Vitae* 17; and Parsemus Foundation, "Male Contraception Attitudes: Summary of Surveys and Research," March, 2016, https://www.parsemus.org/wp-content/uploads/2016/03/Male-Contraception-Attitudes-Surveys-and-Research-7-8-16.pdf.

[29] Parsemus Foundation, "Male Contraception Attitudes."

[30] See Hermann Behre, et al., "Efficacy and Safety of an Injectable Combination Hormonal Contraceptive for Men," *The Journal of Clinical Endocrinology and Metabolism* 101:12.

[31] See, for example, Rachel Krantz, "Why It's Time for Women to Question the Pill," *Bustle*, February 2, 2015, https://www.bustle.com/articles/58288-why-its-time-for-women-to-question-the-pill; see also Holly Grigg-Spall, *Sweetening the Pill or How We Got Hooked on Hormonal Birth Control* (Alresford, UK: Zero Books, 2013).

[32] See Elizabeth Bahnson, "The Pill is Like . . . DDT? An Agrarian Perspective on Artificial Birth Control," in *Wendell Berry and Religion: Heaven's Earthly Life*, ed. Joel James Shuman and Roger Owens (Lexington, KY: The University Press of Kentucky, 2009), 85–97.

many pregnant women toward health care technologies.[33] While women tend to appreciate technologies that make them feel more assured about the health of their fetuses, they often also feel like medical care is done *to* them rather than *with* them, especially during labor. The labor and delivery ward is frequently a place where interconnectedness and dignity can get sidestepped. Nurses and doctors are busy; labor takes time; women often report feeling pressured to make decisions about fetal-maternal care without quite having a good sense of possible outcomes.[34] Patients do not always understand the hard choices that medical care professionals find themselves having to make, especially in and around the principle of patient autonomy, which can make adversaries of health care workers and their patients. In the postpartum phase, women describe alternately being "pushed" into breastfeeding when they do not want to do so or not being supported enough.[35]

CST might alleviate such tensions in obstetrical medical care in a number of ways. For example, focusing on the common good and interrelatedness might encourage practitioners to find ways to establish longer term relationships between patients and caregivers. The current system of 48- to 72-hour stays in hospital, followed by visits to the pediatrician, meet certain health care criteria, yet this kind of postpartum care does not necessarily foster good mother-baby relationships, especially since much of what affects a mother-baby relationship is the day-to-day tasks present once a mother has returned home. In-home visits (perhaps by postpartum doulas) provide a better sense of how women are sleeping, doing daily tasks, and otherwise coping with the arrival of a new baby.[36] Such care might reduce the incidence of postpartum depression and create structures that

[33] For one early voice, see Frances Evans, "Managers and Labourers: Women's Attitudes to Reproductive Technologies," in *Smothered by Invention: Technology in Women's Lives*, ed. Wendy Faulkner and Erik Arnold (London: Pluto Press, 1985), 109–27.

[34] One narrative of laywomen's ambivalent views of labor and delivery, medical interventions, and women's work is found in Jennifer Block, *Pushed: The Painful Truth about Childbirth and Modern Maternity Care* (Philadelphia, PA: Da Capo Press, 2007).

[35] J. Graffy and J. Taylor, "What Information, Advice, and Support Do Women Want With Breastfeeding?" *Birth*, no. 32 (2005): 179–86.

[36] See Canadian Pediatric Society, "Maternal Depression and Child Development," *Paediatrics and Child Health* 9, no. 8 (2004): 575–83.

connect, rather than isolate, women with their communities. Yet time is money, and these kinds of solutions are often seen as impractical. This is one way health care systems (among others) foster a view of childbirth as a private sphere concern. Yet CST's focus on economic and political issues should ask all of us to address how our health care systems and practices are implicated in the broader economic and political structures of society.

Differentiated Health Care for the Right Reasons

Beyond abortion, contraception, and obstetrical care, many additional areas of health care involve gendered concerns, but this aspect is obscured. As Catholic feminist bioethicist Lisa Cahill writes, "Catholic advocates for health care justice seem to keep getting sidelined by public debates that reduce Catholic moral commitments to the protection of embryos and fetuses. . . . Individual bioethics decisions cannot be and never have been separated from social ethics."[37] Additional signposts on the gender landscape include: treatment of health care workers; women's access to leadership in health care; and the omnipresence of hetero-male norms throughout health care.

One broader issue is treatment of health care workers. Some of health care jobs that are staffed predominantly by women are low paying, which disenables their full participation in society. More family-friendly leave policies would enable women—and men—to take a genuine family leave for births and adoptions, rather than having to short circuit medical residencies, or be expected to be back on the job within two weeks. Over the past few decades, demands on health care workers have increased, especially in relation to the volume of documentation and other paperwork required.[38] Patient loads have often risen as well. Both of these factors increase the risk of stress and burnout, and do not promote an atmosphere where either patients or health care workers treat each other with appropriate respect for

---

[37] Lisa Sowle Cahill, *Theological Bioethics: Participation, Justice, and Change* (Washington, DC: Georgetown University Press, 2005), 1–3.

[38] A. George, "Nurses, Community Health Workers, and Home Carers: Gendered Human Resources Compensating for Skewed Health Care Systems," April 17, 2008, http://www.who.int/hrh/documents/gender/en/.

the common good and economic concerns. Furthermore, women health care workers are filling in gaps in existing health care systems. Home health aides and nurses (the vast majority of whom are women) disproportionately bear the weight of double-checking physician orders or taking care of ill patients who have been sent home from the hospital with numerous medical concerns that are difficult to treat at home. As the World Health Organization reports, female health care workers often undertake this care to the detriment of their own health, their wages, and the care of their own families and social communities. Yet again, CST's discussions of the common good and economic and political considerations enable criticizing this unbalanced gendered system.

Catholic social teaching sees connections between the ways women health care workers are treated and the ways patients are treated. It is imperative to create working environments that support and celebrate women, including the women who are part of the house-keeping and dining staffs. Fostering dignity and solidarity might include some of the suggestions I have made above, including more flexible work schedules; clearer and longer family leave policies; and support groups or other structures that enable women to discuss and share the challenges of raising families, care for ailing parents, and also work full-time jobs. Yet fostering dignity and solidarity also means telling the stories of women who are often forgotten, including and especially home health aides, janitors, and other such female-dominated jobs. Telling stories about women may also mean high-lighting a hospital's or health care system's origins more directly: many hospitals and health care systems in the US have their origins in Catholic women's religious groups. Thus, one way of celebrating women is to celebrate those strong, but often overlooked founders. Another possibility is to feature women role models wherever possible. In remembering those workers who are often overlooked, we foster an environment where female patients can also be remembered.

Related to this concern is the point alluded to above about the lack of women leaders and role models across health care. When 26 percent of hospital CEOs are women,[39] and no women are leaders of

---

[39] Annette Walker, "More Female Leadership."

Fortune 500 health care companies,[40] it is more difficult to enable and envision better policies and treatment for female health care workers. While women are well represented in health care overall (74 percent), there are structural challenges that prevent them from moving toward top-level positions. That means that women's voices are often left out of top-level economic and political discussions about health care laws, reforms, and funding. One telling example was the 2017 *New York Times* report that noted there were no women on the committee charged with developing an alternative to the Affordable Care Act.[41]

In order to practice solidarity with women and in relation to women's issues, women need to be better represented in high levels of administration, academia, and governments from the local, state, and national levels. Gender diversity is also a matter for the common good, for we all reap the benefits of a more diverse society. Contemporary workplaces have noticed that gender diversity "can translate to increased productivity, greater innovation, better products, better decision-making, and higher employee retention and satisfaction."[42] Moreover, gender diversity makes the gender disparities, like the ones I have named here, much more visible. Creating avenues for women in administrative and other leadership roles requires the same kinds of tools as for health care workers generally: flexible schedules, better family leave policies, and more visibility of women role models. In addition, creating mentorship and leadership programs that target women might enable women to imagine themselves in leadership positions.

Finally, but not exhaustively, we need to consider more fully the impact of hetero-male norms in health care. Journalist and feminist Maya Dusenberg recently investigated US health care systems and their impact on women, noting a number of issues. For instance, "it felt like every disease that experts described as an overlooked, and

[40] Halle Tecco, "Women in Healthcare 2017: How Does Our Industry Stack Up?" *Rock Health*, https://rockhealth.com/reports/women-in-healthcare-2017-how-does-our-industry-stack-up/.

[41] Robert Pear, "13 Men, and No Women, Are Writing New GOP Health Bill in the Senate," *New York Times*, May 8, 2017, https://www.nytimes.com/2017/05/08/us/politics/women-health-care-senate.html.

[42] Morgan Stanley, "Investor's Guide to Gender Diversity," https://www.morgan stanley.com/ideas/gender-diversity-investor-guide.

often growing, 'epidemic' disproportionately affects women."[43] Leading causes of death like heart disease, cancer, and Alzheimer's disease affect far more women than men, but their differing impact on women is not often studied. Women may well be receiving overdoses of pharmaceuticals, since dosage is determined and often tested via White men's bodies.

Dignity of women and solidarity with people are best served when health care research involves more differentiation, and thus specifically addresses individuals' needs. Moreover, the common good is better enabled because more research across populations enables a much broader and holistic picture of health care concerns. Medical schools and research hospitals should financially and structurally support research programs that examine gender differentiation.[44] People should be further encouraged to do scientific research that examines gender concerns; discussion of how research addresses and investigates gender concerns needs, additionally, to become more fully part of research prospectuses and Institutional Review Board (IRB) requests.[45]

Conclusion

My female patient with ovarian cancer represented the wide-ranging issues related to CST. She was a woman, a widow who was statistically more likely to be poor. Her health care concerns were dismissed, in comparison to the male patient just down the hall. She had fewer social resources and fewer connections to society. Witnessing her marginalization by the hospital staff and neglect of her dignity and worth as a human continues to disturb me many years later. Yet what I hope I have shown in this essay is that this woman's health care was not only about her and the clear gender disparities of her

---

[43] George, "Nurses, Community Health Workers, and Home Carers."

[44] For example, supporting groups like the Foundation for Gender-Specific Medicine might be one approach, https://gendermed.org.

[45] On my view, this would go far beyond the current ways IRB proposals describe gender, which is primarily to note vulnerable populations. I think that we could develop more positive criteria for thinking about gender too, by discussing specifically how research intends to overcome gender bias and examine potential gender differentiation.

case. It is also about the nurses on that forgotten floor, who may have been experiencing high rates of depression and burnout. It is about the housekeeping staff and the nutrition staff, who are often women, more likely to be impoverished, and who are often also disparaged. It is about making sure that women role models are more visible, and that women are encouraged to seek higher level positions in health care. Thinking about CST in health care means thinking holistically about the status and role of all women, so that we can encourage dignity, solidarity, and the common good of all.

Chapter 12

Continuing the Ministry of Mission Doctors

Brian Medernach, MD, and Antoinette Lullo, DO

One afternoon during Holy Week, on the Napo River in the Amazon jungle of Peru, we received news from a health outpost of a woman who was having complications during her delivery. She was six hours away by boat. The patient, a young mother, planned to have her baby in her home with the assistance of her husband and family members. However, after several hours, the baby still was not born. The family sent for the local midwife who arrived at the house to find that the child was lying horizontally in the womb; the arm and shoulder impeding the baby from being delivered. The mother's vital signs were stable, she noted, and the child still had a heartbeat; understanding the gravity of the situation and the risk to both baby and mother, the midwife and nurse technician loaded the patient and her husband into a small boat and began the long journey to the Centro de Salud Santa Clotilde. That day, our physician most skilled in obstetric surgery was away on a ten-day vaccine campaign and attending to patients in the rural outlying communities. That left one of us and Father/Doctor Jack MacCarthy awaiting the patient.

Upon entering the triage room, the patient was alert and in pain, receiving fluids through an IV in her arm. More striking was the child's purple arm protruding out from her mother. We placed the Doppler machine on mother's abdomen, desperately seeking a heartbeat and wondering if the child had survived the long journey. Before we were able to hear any heartbeat, the baby's hand miraculously squeezed the midwife's finger. We rushed to the operating room and performed an emergency cesarean section under local anesthesia. The newborn baby, born limp, came to life after resuscitation. After several days in the hospital, mother and baby boarded a canoe with the new father, and they returned home, a healthy family of three.

❖ ❖ ❖ ❖ ❖ ❖

Global health physicians face a variety of challenges around the world, not unlike those on the Napo River. Although each country presents a unique set of issues, many can be generalized to lack of resources and infrastructure. Resources include medical supplies like sutures, gloves, surgical instruments, imaging equipment such as x-ray and computed tomography (CT) scanners, and medicines. Lack of human resources, namely health care professionals and administrators, are an ongoing challenge. Hospitals and clinics depend on well-trained technicians, nurses, and physicians to function. However, there are often limited educational opportunities or institutions to educate and train sufficient workforce to meet the country's demand. The effect of brain drain can dramatically affect low- and middle-income countries. Physicians and nurses leave to seek further education and training available in other countries, and many do not return home for a variety of reasons: monetary benefits, safety, and improved living conditions. Losing talented members of the community contributes to the infrastructure challenges many low- and middle-income countries face.

Part of the reason trained health care professionals leave is the lack of infrastructure to support their work. Many countries have insufficient funds to support a robust health care system. Oftentimes ministries of health use the limited resources they have to appropriately focus on preventative care, such as vaccines and public health measures, in order to make the largest health impact with the resources available. This in turn affects the ability to appropriately attend to acute medical issues and emergencies. In addition to the inability to sustain an emergency response system, more pressing needs such as inadequate roads and public transport present a major barrier to patients' abilities to access care that is available. These present just some of the challenges in an urban setting. All of these factors are magnified in rural settings, where brain drain of physicians from rural areas to the country's major cities is increased and cost for access to education and health care is often too expensive to even consider.

In response to these challenges, women and men religious have historically entered into these rural communities, attempting to fill both a religious and social service need. However, the number of these capable practitioners is dwindling. Given that communities like Santa Clotilde have relied on the work of Catholic religious missionaries, our question is: do Catholic health systems and their physicians have an opportunity and responsibility to continue the work in these communities grounded in the preferential option for the poor?

This chapter explores how Catholic health systems can extend their mission of ministry by supporting and continuing the ministry of physician missionaries in areas of the world, like the Napo River. US Catholic health systems are well-positioned to be leaders in global health work due to the surfeit of resources they possess relative to our global counterparts and the foundational role that Catholic social thought (CST) ought to play in witnessing to their mission. First, we describe a crucial component of this work—the call to global health work specific to Catholic physicians. Second, we discuss ways in which physicians with commitments to social justice can find strategies and support to allow them to pursue a vocation in global health within the structure of current health care systems. Third, we offer specific recommendations to address how physicians and health systems can work toward sustainable access to quality patient care in remote, global areas, using Santa Clotilde, Peru, as an example. Finally, we detail how the global void in health care allocation provides Catholic health care systems with an opportunity to advance their mission of healing in the spirit of the Gospel with service directed by the preferential option for the poor at home and abroad.

The Church's Call to Lay Missioners

Our small rural hospital and health network, Centro de Salud Santa Clotilde, was developed and expanded by two priest-physicians, Jack MacCarthy, OPraem, and Maurice Schroeder, OMI. The story of how two missionary priest-physicians arrived in the

Peruvian Amazon traces its roots back to the many changes that occurred on the world stage in the late twentieth century. In the Amazon region of Peru, the discovery of rubber at the turn of the century created a boom, and the world's demand led rubber barons to the enslavement and genocide of many indigenous peoples along the Napo and Putamayo Rivers. These atrocities were addressed by Pope Pius X's 1912 encyclical *Lacrimabili Statu*. In that encyclical, Pope Pius X denounced the rubber barons and called on the bishops of Latin America to encourage missions to the indigenous people, showing charity not only in word but in deeds.[1]

The Amazon jungle region was within the Vicariate Apostolicó of Iquitos which was under the direction of the Augustinians. In 1945, the Holy See created the prefecture Apostolicó de San José del Amazonas, and this mission was received by Canadian Franciscans who expanded to several more mission sites including Santa Clotilde in 1946. With health care as the foundation of their charism, the Franciscans began Catholic health care services on the Napo River.

Centro de Salud Santa Clotilde felt the effects of mid-twentieth century changes in Catholic missions. One of the most significant changes in overseas work was the papal call for missionaries and the acceptance of lay missioners. In 1951, Pope Pius XII advocated for the support of the laity in his encyclical *Evangelii Praecones*. This opened the door for the foundation of lay mission organizations in the United States, including Lay Mission Helpers and Mission Doctors Association. The changes brought about by Vatican II further opened the doors for lay persons to participate more fully in the work and mission of the Catholic Church both within the local church, but also in mission communities globally.[2]

The church's engagement in Latin America was also deeply influenced by a group of Catholic bishops from the Americas, among them Archbishop Antonio Samoré who posed a challenge to the United States at the National Catholic Welfare Conference. At that conference, Samoré asked the US church what it was prepared to do for the church's brothers and sisters to the south. This question made to a

---

[1] Pope Pius X, *Lacrimabili Statu* (Vatican City: Libreria Editrice Vaticana, 1912).

[2] Dana L Robert, *American Women in Mission: A Social History of Their Thought and Practice* (Macon, GA: Mercer University Press, 2005).

group of bishops at Georgetown in November of 1959 started discussions that led to a proposal in 1961 calling for 10 percent of all religious congregations to serve for a time in Latin America.[3] The 1961 proposal was endorsed by Pope John XXIII and became known as "the pope's proposal." Many dioceses, congregations, and lay missionary programs responded to the call of John XXIII, including St. Norbert Abbey in DePere, Wisconsin.

In 1963, a Norbertine mission was founded in Lima, Peru, and the Canadian Oblates followed suit in 1966. In 1986, the Norbertine prior in Lima, Father Dave Strenski, had been contacted by the Franciscan bishop working in the Peruvian Amazon who was looking for a physician. This conversation ultimately resulted in Father Jack MacCarthy's arrival at Santa Clotilde in the spring of 1986 and the extension of this invitation to the arrival of Oblate priest-physician Father Maurice Schroeder later that year.

In 1986, Father Jack, Father Maurice, two nursing nuns, and two government workers began the transformation of the small dispensary into what today is an expansive health network along four hundred kilometers of the Napo river. Thanks to these founders and the tireless energy and collaboration of a number of local employees, the health system currently is comprised of thirteen outposts, a rural hospital, and over one hundred health care workers. Over the course of three decades, the priest-physicians, along with nurse-nuns, built this network with the help of countless agents including their congregations and individual donors. Many in this workforce now have stable contracts from the ministry of health. To help meet the needs of remote and growing populations, health promoter trainings were established within the communities. Over the past several years since the retirement of the priests-physicians, there has been continued collaboration between San José del Amazonas, the local Catholic vicariate, and the local ministry of health. However, given the reality of brain drain, the shortage of religious missionaries able to carry out this work, and the immense needs, community missions like Santa Clotilde are an endangered species.

---

[3] Tom Quigley, "The Great North-South Embrace: How Collaboration Among the Churches of the Americas Began," *America: The Jesuit Review* (December 7, 2009).

Today, with declining numbers in vocations, many religious congregations are no longer in a position to send their religious community members overseas. In Santa Clotilde, the last of the nursing nuns was reassigned to another mission in 1993. Father Maurice went to Lima in 2008 as a superior of the Peruvian Oblates and then to retirement in 2015. At the same time, Father Jack returned at the abbot's request to the Norbertine Abbey in Wisconsin. Thus, within the span of a decade the core of the constant health provider presence in this community was forced to move on. While lay missionary groups continue their work, the majority continue doing so in small organizations, such as the Mission Doctors Association, or on an ad-hoc basis. What is really lacking is the presence of Catholic physicians and nurses capable of carrying out the healing ministry of Jesus, where it is needed most.

Short-Term Interest, Long-Term Challenges

Long-term religious missionaries spent their entire lives providing Catholic health care and building up local systems. Their role was to be fully integrated into the community, serving mind, body, and spirit. The roles of priest and physician were not separate roles, but rather complementary. Much like Saint Luke, the patron saint of physicians, the medical service of the priests allowed them to attend to the physical, spiritual, social, and psychological needs and was a core part of their ministry. They were able to perform the sacraments of baptism, Eucharist, and anointing of the sick in the setting of being a physician and healer. They played a role in educating those interested to fill staffing roles at the health system. As physicians, they both treated and taught the local community members how to physically take care of themselves, issuing cautions about river water, waste contamination, and ensuring a safe work environment. Finally, they were a source of spiritual support, not only in their role as women and men religious, but in accompanying families amidst grief and loss. In short, they embodied what Catholic health care aspires to be at its best. They addressed many needs, and their absence creates a void that is not filled adequately by the small organizations mentioned.

One way to address the growing global need has been through short-term medical missions. Approaches to short-term medical mission trips vary widely.[4] Generally, a team of ten to twenty persons, from a parish, health system, or a university spend a week to ten days in a particular location, dispensing what medical assistance they can. Some of these teams are comprised entirely of health professionals; other teams may include primarily persons with no professional health training. Some organizations may visit the same site each year; others will visit different sites each time.

An estimated 6,000 short-term medical missions are launched from the US each year at a cost of over $250 million USD.[5] Short-term mission numbers continue to grow for a variety of reasons: exposure to other cultures and communities via news and social media; easier and cheaper travel; and more available mission opportunities in earlier education such as high school or university. While we would like to say these trips have stemmed from individuals discerning a move or developing long-term partnerships with international communities, these short-term medical missions are largely a result of a surge in global health interest that has skyrocketed among students and physicians-in-training.

In 2017, the Association of American Medical Colleges (AAMC) surveyed graduating US medical students. Of the 15,609 that completed the survey, 27.1 percent had participated in a global health experience, a significant increase from the 6 percent found in the initial AAMC survey in 1978.[6] This amounts to over 4,000 medical students exposed to the global realities of health care and will hopefully translate to more interest in making global health a part of their vocation. This increased exposure in medical school has led to increased interest in global health experiences for resident physicians-in-training. While medical student interest is commendable, they are virtually unable to contribute to the complex health needs in these communities. Resident interest has led residency training programs and graduate medical education to explore ways to provide these

---

[4] For more on short-term medical mission trips, see Bruce Compton's chapter in this volume (chap. 18).

[5] Jesse Maki, et al., "Health Impact Assessment and Short-Term Medical Missions: A Methods Study to Evaluate Quality of Care," *BMC Health Services Research* 8, no. 1 (2008): 121.

[6] American Association of Medical Colleges, "Medical School Graduation Questionnaire 2017 All Schools Summary," https://www.aamc.org/download/481784 /data/2017gqallschoolssummaryreport.pdf.

experiences to their resident physicians who can assist, but only for a short term. While this may lead a resident doctor to consider this type of work, there are many barriers that make a move like Father Jack's or Father Maurice's logistically challenging.

For trained physicians interested in serving in global contexts, the current US health care system poses numerous barriers that are both personal and professional. Perhaps the most obvious obstacle to pursuing global service is the monetary cost. Data from the AAMC shows that 75 percent of the medical school class of 2017 graduated with a median debt of $192,000.[7] Debt is the major logistical obstacle preventing physicians from participating in global health. Recent graduates cannot afford a period of time where they do not earn sufficient salary to meet loan reimbursement costs. In addition, volunteering entails costs for travel, food, lodging, evacuation insurance, health insurance, liability insurance, workmen's compensation, and more. Living and working internationally also removes one from the traditional physician workforce and may make it difficult to re-enter afterwards. The credentialing process at hospitals often relies on the numbers of procedures done and competencies that may not be accepted if performed outside of a US-approved site. Also, time away may lead to inability to keep up with continuing medical education, new medicines, or treatment recommendations due to lack of opportunities and the logistics of living and working in another country.

In order to avoid some of these challenges, physicians may initially carve out time to devote to global health. Employer expectations also hinder this work. Although highly encouraged and verbally supported by their employers to pursue global health interests, physicians are rarely given any time or financial support. As a result, physicians must look for ways to shoulder the personal, monetary, time, and career costs. These costs have been referred to as "the global health tax" that "many global health doctors willingly assume . . . demonstrating the extent to which they are driven by a sense of purpose."[8] An example of this "tax" would be physicians who use vaca-

---

[7] Ibid.

[8] Daniel Palazuelos and Ranu Dhillon, "Addressing the 'Global Health Tax' and 'Wild Cards': Practical Challenges to Building Academic Careers in Global Health," *Academic Medicine* 91, no. 1 (2016): 30–35.

tion or personal time to do work abroad. Physicians may use as much as half or more of their yearly vacation time to do mission work, which may have consequences for their personal life as they now have less time during the year to recharge and reconnect.

Additionally, there are clinical costs. Physicians are obligated to ensure their patients at home have coverage and continued access to care during their absence. Asking others to provide coverage places an increased burden on colleagues at home. While colleagues who are unable to go abroad will happily cover for a mission doctor, some resent the flexibility given to these doctors to perform "non-clinical" responsibilities. In discussions with colleagues looking for jobs that would allow for global health, we found that many hospitals require the traveling physician to work double shifts or make up for time missed on their return, in order not to increase the workload on others in the system. Alternatively, a colleague shared that she could also accept decreased salary for her decreased productivity at her US clinic.

However, given the increased attention and global awareness that many Catholic health care systems have, medical schools and residency programs are pressed to find attending physicians who are both interested in and actively participating in global health initiatives. Finding interested doctors is predicated on creating a structure in which their domestic and international work is compatible with academic or system-based medicine. Few institutions alter their requirements to accommodate the responsibilities of global health physicians. Often, physicians can spend significant time abroad, but this does not immunize them from their own "global health tax." Greysen et al. found many working in global health have output consisting of web-based materials or NGO or government reports but lack traditional peer reviewed publications. "It's pretty significant to have given two or three years of service" notes a faculty member, "but . . . academically that counts for nothing. We have to put in place [systems] to make this a reasonable choice. . . . I don't want people getting stuck because they did something really good for humanity, but it really didn't help them career-wise in the end."[9]

---

[9] Greysen, et al., "Global Health Experiences of U.S. Physicians: A Mixed Methods Survey of Clinician-Researchers and Health Policy Leaders," *Globalization and Health* 9:19 (2013), http://www.globalizationandhealth.com/content/9/1/19.

Catholic institutions, both academic medical centers and health systems, are in a unique place to emerge as leaders in creating a work environment that allows global health physicians to thrive in their mission. While it will require a shift of resources, Catholic health care's mission provides the institutional justification for realigning priorities to live up to the legacy of the first and second generations of Catholic religious missionaries in order to better meet the needs of the global health community.

Centro de Salud Santa Clotilde as a Paradigm

Despite its success, the Centro de Salud Santa Clotilde has weathered many struggles over the years. The most limited resource is well-qualified health professionals willing to commit to the long term. Santa Clotilde is a long distance from the city of Iquitos, and it takes six hours of travel by river to get there. The Napo district is a world of impoverished farmers and fishermen, and Santa Clotilde, its capital, counts on only five hours of electricity a day, has no drinkable water, limited internet access, no access to continuing medical education, or even a bank to cash a check. Inconsistent government funding leads to insufficient funds to cover the exorbitant cost of gasoline needed to transport patients and supplies up and down the river. There are difficulties in maintaining accurate accounting, due in part to the simple reality that local shops are unable to provide receipts. Government reimbursement often is paid late or not at all, and the regional referral hospitals often go on strike limiting access to care.

Despite these many day-to-day challenges, the work has continued. The priests, with a passion for equity and justice, worked tirelessly to obtain contracts and funds from the Peruvian Ministry of Health to support their locally trained workers who wanted to stay, live, and work on the river. The fathers endeavored to recruit young Peruvian professionals from all parts of the country to complete their year of government service within the health network on the Napo river. They also partnered with two North American medical schools to allow their students a month-long supervised rotation. After more than thirty years of presence in the town of Santa Clotilde, the priest-physicians remain involved from afar. Their continued work now relies on the extended commitments of young Peruvian doctors, missionary physicians from Mission Doctors Association, a group that sponsors Catholic doctors and their families to serve abroad, and other volunteer physicians to work alongside local health workers. This work in Peru has continued through many efforts and affiliations and is an example of one of the many places worldwide where health systems could establish lasting and sustainable collaborations to effect change and sustainability.

Our own work in Peru has been sustained by the long-term support of Mission Doctors Association. After completing four years of mission service, we now are able to return on an annual basis to Peru supervising residents and students. As faculty in academic medicine and residency training programs, we have been given support and acknowledgement of the benefits of the experience in Peru. In turn, the patients are able to see caring trained specialists who otherwise they never have access to locally.

One of the explicit ways Catholic health care institutions can continue the support of these missions is through establishing collaboration between an organization like Mission Doctors Association or another institution committed to developing ties to the local community. Both of our institutions' graduate medical education departments have identified a global health focus as key for prospective resident trainees. Part of our role has been to help create and develop a curriculum-based program with a global health experience for residents. This has enabled us to make a sustainable impact in Peru, but it has also allowed us to help our institutions think organizationally about our social responsibilities in supporting global health sites.

Physician groups, for example, could create a work structure for global health with job-sharing programs, allowing for continued patient coverage at home and sustainable presence at a partner overseas site. In this model, a group would take a slightly lower salary and carry a patient load that would always allow for one member to be away for a set amount of time each year. In other words, a primary care group of six physicians could agree to split the total amount of five salaries and share a patient panel. Each of the six physicians could rotate two to three months per year at a partner site. Each doctor would make one-sixth less of their normal salary but could maintain their benefits and provide sustainable care locally and abroad with the intention of capacity building and system building at the partner site, while also establishing institutional history and continuity.

Conclusion:
Continuing the Legacy of Mission Doctors

The checkered past of the first Catholic missionaries to Latin America is well documented. They were tied to colonialism, conversion, and imposing a particular way of life on indigenous communities. The post-Vatican II missionaries called for by John XXIII exhibited a different kind of spirit and a focus on coming to learn from and with the communities in which they were missioned. The spirit that led to the founding of missions like Centro de Salud Santa Clotilde is needed again.

Global health care ministry finds no foothold in the for-profit health care environment; global health mission work does not bring a dollar-to-dollar return. However, for Catholic health care, developing a system that supports these missions grounds the ministry globally in the option for the poor. It is the faithfulness to the mission that provides the clearest benefits to the health care system. In our experience, mission work helps reignite the underlying motivations of health care professionals who chose to enter medicine to care for others, improve the health of their community, affect health policies, and solve difficult medical and scientific questions. The ability to practice a purer form of medicine with intimate patient care without the electronic medical records and insurance bureaucracy brings a refreshing change to patient care. Physicians and trainees who go on missions acknowledge that global health activities can enhance the quality of their domestic work, improve physical exam skills, and increase their level of involvement with vulnerable populations, health policy advocacy, or research on the social determinants of health.[10, 11]

[10] Nelson, et al., "Developing a Career in Global Health: Considerations for Physicians-in-Training and Academic Mentors," *Journal of Graduate Medical Education* 4, no. 3 (September 2012): 301–6.

[11] Drain, et al., "Global Health in Medical Education: A Call for More Training and Opportunities," *Academic Medicine* 82, no. 3 (March 2007): 226–30.

With the significant increase in short-term mission in the past thirty years, the evidence and research continues to grow about the efficacy of such programs. However, what these programs provide is an entrée into the world of global health and the lives that missionary physicians have led. Catholic social teaching and broader commitments to social justice should catalyze Catholic health systems to not only value those most in need around the world but to create structures that foster these relationships for all who are called to these ministries.

PART FOUR

Leading for Social Responsibility

Each of the foregoing chapters calls for a shift in leadership priorities within Catholic health care. While most of the topics raised in this book can be taken up by individuals within a health system, the chapters in part IV note the importance of executive leadership in creating a socially responsible culture. Each chapter challenges leadership to think beyond the status quo of accepted business practices and to evaluate each aspect of the organization from the perspective of the Catholic social tradition. Here, the virtue of fortitude should not be underestimated as a value in health care leadership. Questions of environmental responsibility, practical support for and advocacy around immigration, and the function of health care as both a business and a social agent are not politically neutral topics. Mark Kuczewski's chapter, perhaps most succinctly, points to the risks of taking a stance on a controversial issue. However, Catholic health care—as it is fond of saying—continues the healing ministry of Jesus. Not only has this ministry always stood on the side of those who were marginalized and maligned by society. Following in the footsteps of Jesus presents risks. Jesus' healings were one of the things that led to his crucifixion.[1] Catholic health care—following in the footsteps of Jesus—is required to take stances that may pose challenges to the

---

[1] As early as Mark's third chapter, Jesus heals the man with the withered hand on the Sabbath and because of this, "The Pharisees went out and immediately conspired with the Herodians against him, how to destroy him" (Mark 3:6; see also Matt 12:9-14).

institution's margin, may unsettle certain political constituents, and may require a bold public relations backbone—all of which are necessary costs of living out the mission of Catholic health care.

One question, of course, is: what are the costs of *not* embodying the CST? In chapter 13, "A Call to Conversion: Toward a Catholic Environmental Bioethics and Environmentally Responsible Health Care," Ron Hamel argues that there is global and environmental cost to the awareness gap that exists among leadership in Catholic health care who do not take seriously CST's emphasis on caring for the environment. Health care in and of itself can be a wasteful practice. Immense resources are consumed in daily and routine patient care as well as the overall operation of a hospital. Hamel notes that the environmental impact of caring for patients has indirect consequences on the health of the environment that equally affects the health of the community. While both Catholic and secular bioethics are late to the game on environmental ethics, the continued lifting of environmental questions within the CST—particularly in light of Pope Francis's major encyclical *Laudato Si'*—should call Catholic health care leadership to a higher standard. Hamel's chapter offers a framework to better understand the role that Catholic health care can play at the intersection of environmental ethics and health. He concludes by offering multiple examples of institutions that prioritize Pope Francis's efforts to care for our common home through solidarity, the common good, and integral human development.

While the current political climate surrounding environmental consciousness is fraught, the climate surrounding immigration is fevered. Mark Kuczewki's chapter, "DACA and Institutional Solidarity," may be read as both a call to action and a warning of what that action may entail. Chapter 14 details the plight of immigrants due to federal neglect of this issue for the better part of three decades. The cost of neglecting immigrants has resulted in a sizeable population of undocumented children, adolescents, and young adults who were brought to the US by their parents, and who until 2012 and Deferred Action for Childhood Arrivals, lived in fear of deportation. Despite the current administration's claim to the contrary, Kuczewski notes that DACA has opened possibilities unforeseen by these high achieving students that create opportunities both for the individual and the community. He encourages those in leadership positions to take a stand, just as the American Medical Association and American

Association of Medical Colleges have, for DACA recipients and on behalf of migrant rights. He notes that CST does not permit us to be indifferent to the plight of the poor and marginalized. When false witness, false imprisonment, and injustice plague our patients, staff, and students, will Catholic health care stand on the right side of (salvation) history?

Chapter 15 likewise might be read as a warning about following the status quo with respect to business practices. Here, in their chapter "Reframing Outsourcing," M. Therese Lysaught and Robert DeVita take up "outsourcing," a standard business practice that offloads certain institutional activities to external suppliers. Most frequently food, environmental services, business processes, and IT might be sourced outside of the institution. However, with ever-thinning margins facing Catholic health care, other operational costs are also considered for outsourcing, including physician services. While noting that outsourcing is an accepted business practice, Lysaught and DeVita argue that CST raises the ethical threshold for Catholic institutions. Drawing extensively on Benedict XVI's final encyclical, *Caritas in Veritate*, they establish a process for discerning under what circumstances outsourcing can function as a socially responsible business practice that prioritizes persons (both associates and communities) over profits and integrates mission with margin.

Too often, profits and margin win. In chapter 16, "Population Health: Insights from Catholic Social Thought," Michael Panicola and Rachelle Barina take executive boards to task for focusing more on ROI than restoring or protecting the health of persons and communities. They challenge Catholic health care to more boldly make the shift from a fee-based model that privileges high-tech, high-profit, acute interventions for the wealthy and insured to one that focuses on population health. Thus, rather than treating a patient only when she presents in the hospital, they argue that greater attention should be given to promoting healthy communities so that patients do not need to come to the hospital in the first place. For the US, this represents a significant shift in business practice. In fact, if Catholic health care is guided by the principles of human flourishing, the common good, and justice, then prioritizing population health should become an even greater priority for Catholic health care insofar as it promotes health equity, advocates for universal health care, and critiques the current system centered on high cost specialty care.

Chapter 13

A Call to Conversion: Toward a Catholic Environmental Bioethics and Environmentally Responsible Health Care

Ron Hamel

"Go to something more useful!" I overheard a large urban hospital CEO saying to one of his senior leaders at a Catholic health care conference a few years ago. The senior leader was planning to attend a breakout on environmentally responsible health care. The CEO continued, "We're in the business of providing health care, in a very challenging environment. That's where our complete attention needs to be. This environment stuff is just another flavor of the month! A distraction! Health care is what we do, not tree hugging!"

The senior leader was, in fact, the organization's mission leader. I talked to him after the breakout, and he mentioned that he had just completed a course in bioethics as part of his degree program at a Catholic institution. When I asked why he was interested in environmentally responsible health care, he responded that his interest was piqued by what he had been reading and hearing about various other health care organizations' efforts in this area. "Did the bioethics course play a role?" I asked. "Not at all."

❖ ❖ ❖ ❖ ❖

Links between health care, the environment, and bioethics need to be made more explicit. The narrative above vividly illustrates two challenges with regard to health care and the environment. One is an "awareness gap." The CEO was unaware of the significant ways health care contributes to environmental degradation and the intimate connections between the environmental impact of health care and the very diseases that health care seeks to treat. He additionally failed to consider the integral bond between care for the environment and the mission and values of Catholic health care and, likely, of his own facility. The second omission stems from the frequent oversight of environmental issues in bioethics and health care ethics. While this essay will note some strides have been made, much work remains to be done.

This chapter will briefly address the neglect of the environment in bioethics along with more recent developments, as well as three dimensions of the CEO's awareness gap. Second, the chapter identifies major themes from Catholic social teaching that call Catholic health care to environmental responsibility and can shape a Catholic environmental bioethics. Finally, the chapter concludes with a brief review of initiatives in health care that have been and are beginning to exercise ecological responsibility.

Neglect of Environmental Issues in Bioethics

In *The Future of Bioethics*, Howard Brody devotes an entire chapter to "Environmental and Global Issues."[1] He locates the neglect of environmental issues in the very origins of bioethics by drawing on the work of Van Rensselaer Potter.[2] Potter seems to have been the first person to employ the term "bioethics" in the US.[3] According to Brody, Potter intended "bioethics" to refer to "the questions about

---

[1] Howard Brody, *The Future of Bioethics* (New York: Oxford University Press, 2009), 178.

[2] See also Daniel Callahan, "Bioethics," *Encyclopedia of Bioethics, Vol. I*, ed. Warren Reich (New York: Simon and Shuster Macmillan, 1995), 248, 250; Albert R. Jonsen, *The Birth of Bioethics* (New York: Oxford University Press, 1998), 27.

[3] Potter was a cancer biochemist in Madison, Wisconsin, who published a volume in 1971 titled *Bioethics: Bridge to the Future* (Englewood Cliffs, NJ: Prentice-Hall) in which he describes his project. The term "bioethics" was actually first employed by a German Protestant pastor, Fritz Jahr, in 1927. For a discussion, see H. M. Sass, "Fritz Jahr's 1927 Concept of Bioethics," *Kennedy Institute of Ethics Journal* 17 (2007): 279–95.

humankind's relationship with its environment, and the survival of the human species in the face of environmental threats, such as pollution, overpopulation, and nuclear war."[4] However, around the same time, the Kennedy Institute of Ethics was founded at Georgetown University. They, too, employed the term "bioethics" to describe the focus of the institute, but, as Brody points out, they meant something very different from Potter. For the Kennedy Institute of Ethics, bioethics concerned ethical issues arising out of the practice of medicine and research in the biological sciences. The Georgetown model prevailed and defined the scope of the field moving forward, narrowing it considerably.[5] Brody laments this missed opportunity and calls for the development of an "ecological bioethics" that engages environmental issues as they relate to health care.[6]

Interestingly, in 2001, a few years after the second edition of the *Encyclopedia of Bioethics* that contained an entry by Daniel Callahan on bioethics and an entry on "environmental ethics," philosopher Jessica Pierce (together with Andrew Jameton) published what appears to be the first volume that connects the environment with health care—*The Ethics of Environmentally Responsible Health Care*.[7] She published subsequently (with George Randels) a text in bioethics, *Contemporary Bioethics: A Reader with Cases*, that she describes as "the first to cover the emerging area of environmental bioethics."[8] Pierce explains elsewhere that "environmental bioethics is a sub-field of bioethics that focuses on the complex interactions between humans, health, health care, and the natural environment."[9] Her efforts are an attempt to get back to Potter's vision. Pierce describes that the "environmental turn" in bioethics involves exploring

---

[4] Brody, *The Future of Bioethics*, 178.

[5] Ibid.

[6] Ibid., 181.

[7] Jessica Pierce and Andrew Jameton, *The Ethics of Environmentally Responsible Health Care* (Oxford University Press, 2001).

[8] Jessica Pierce and George Randels, *Contemporary Bioethics: A Reader with Cases* (Oxford University Press, 2009).

[9] Jessica Pierce, "Environmental Bioethics—A Manifesto," https://healthafteroil .wordpress.com/2009/11/13/environmental-bioethics—a-manifesto/.

what an environmentally sustainable health care system might look like, how doctors might take environmental values seriously within their practice, how climate change might shape the conversation about health care priorities, what concepts from ecosystem science are applicable to the conversation about human health, and whether the moral vocabulary developed within the field of environmental ethics might have something to offer bioethics.[10]

Pierce's attention to this neglected field in bioethics does not seem to have caught on widely either in secular or religious bioethics. Likewise, bioethics texts by Catholic authors have largely focused on traditional topics.[11] Even texts in organizational ethics do not address environmental issues and health care delivery.[12] The environment has been a neglected area in the literature and is a gap in the training of Catholic health care leaders.

The CEO's "Awareness Gap"

Perhaps the CEO in the above narrative does not reflect the attitudes of a majority of his colleagues in leadership positions in Catholic health care today. Nonetheless, to the extent such attitudes do exist, they undermine attention to environmental responsibility in the

---

[10] Ibid.

[11] See, for example, Raymond R. Devettere, *Practical Decision-Making in Health Care Ethics: Cases, Concepts and the Virtue of Prudence,* 4th ed. (Washington, DC: Georgetown University Press, 2016); David Kelly, Gerard Magill, Henk ten Have, *Contemporary Catholic Health Care Ethics* (Washington, DC: Georgetown University Press, 2013); Michael Panicola, David Belde, John Paul Slosar, and Mark Repenshek, *Health Care Ethics: Theological Foundations, Contemporary Issues, and Controversial Cases* (Winona, MN: Anselm Academic, 2011); Nicanor Austriaco, *Biomedicine and Beatitude: An Introduction to Catholic Bioethics* (Washington, DC: Catholic University of America Press, 2011); Benedict Ashley, Jean DeBlois, Kevin O'Rourke, *Health Care Ethics: A Catholic Theological Analysis,* 5th ed. (Washington, DC: Georgetown University Press, 2006). There is at least one exception—*An Introduction to Bioethics* by Thomas Shannon and Nicholas Kockler (Mahweh, NJ: Paulist Press, 2009) who include a final chapter titled "A Whole Earth Ethic."

[12] See, for example, Philip Boyle, et al., *Organizational Ethics in Health Care: Principles, Cases and Practical Solutions* (San Francisco, CA: Jossey-Bass, 2011); Leonard Weber, *Business Ethics in Healthcare: Beyond Compliance* (Bloomington, IN: Indiana University Press, 2001); Robert T. Hall, *An Introduction to Healthcare Organizational Ethics* (New York: Oxford University Press, 2000).

delivery of health care. They also reflect a lack of awareness of several critical considerations that lead to an "awareness gap" comprised of three elements.

Drawing from my overheard conversation with the CEO, his first "gap" results from a lack of knowledge. It is now a well-established fact that health care contributes in significant ways, both directly and indirectly, to environmental harm. This harm occurs in a myriad of ways: health care's use of energy (heating cooling, ventilation, illumination, running equipment) and water (estimated to be about 315 gallons per day per hospital bed), waste production (approximately 3.4 billion pounds annually), food production, packaging, transport, use and disposal, the use of certain toxic chemicals (e.g., mercury, PVC, DEHP), and through the production, transport, use, and disposal of equipment.[13] This environmental harm also has direct and indirect impacts on human health, contributing to respiratory conditions, cancer, birth defects, developmental disabilities, reproductive issues, and many other diseases and conditions.

The second gap, while flowing from a lack of knowledge, is ironic: by contributing to environmental degradation, health care directly and indirectly exacerbates those very illnesses and diseases it is committed to preventing, alleviating, and curing. Environmental harm factors into respiratory conditions, cancer, birth defects, developmental disabilities, reproductive issues, and many other diseases and conditions.[14] By failing to see linkages between its operations and human health, health care daily does harm to patients, employees, and the communities it serves. It undermines its good work.

Third, the CEO fails to see that environmental responsibility is integral to Catholic health care's mission. At its core, Catholic health care carries on the healing mission of Jesus, God's healing work in the world. Neglecting environmental impacts of health care delivery undermines this fundamental mission, as well as core commitments of Catholic health care: respecting life and human dignity, promoting the common good, caring for the poor and the vulnerable, and stewarding resources responsibly.

---

[13] See Matthew J. Eckelman and Jodi Sherman, "Environmental Impacts of the U.S. Health Care System and Effects on Public Health," *PLoS One* 11, no. 6, June 9, 2016, http://journals.plos.org/plosone/article?id=10.1371/journal.pone.0157014.

[14] Ibid.

In sum, Catholic bioethics, like secular bioethics, has largely over-looked ethical dimensions of environmental and health impacts of health care delivery. Interestingly, theologians writing on environmental ethics have also overlooked bioethics.[15] While Catholic bioethics has made significant contributions to the clinical side of health care delivery, it has failed to attend to ethical dimensions of the broader context of clinical care, including its environmental situatedness. These oversights are aggravated when leaders in Catholic health care see environmental impact only as a negative externality or a "flavor of the month."

How can this void in Catholic bioethics be addressed? What might a Catholic bioethics attentive to the environment draw upon for guidance? Traditional bioethics principles are not adequate to this issue; however, environmental ethics and Catholic social thought (CST) yield important insights.[16]

Toward a Catholic Environmental Bioethics: Contributions of Catholic Social Teaching

The field of environmental ethics, which emerged in the 1960s and 1970s, has become a robust and mature area of study. Scholars offer a variety of values, principles, and virtues—sustainability, solidarity, interconnectedness, common good, temperance, stewardship, prudence, and more—that could be imported into an environmentally conscious bioethic and assist environmentally responsible health care.

Papal and episcopal teaching on environmental responsibility can significantly shape a worldview that can serve both to motivate toward environmental responsibility and provide value-laden guidance for addressing various aspects of the problem. John Paul II calls for a "morally coherent world view."[17] Pope Francis's *Laudato Si'*

---

[15] See, for example, Richard W. Miller, ed., *God, Creation, and Climate Change: A Catholic Response to the Environmental Crisis* (Maryknoll, NY: Orbis Books, 2010); Tobias Winright, ed., *Green Discipleship: Catholic Theological Ethics and the Environment* (Winona, MN: Anselm Academic, 2011); David Cloutier, *Walking God's Earth: The Environment and Catholic Faith* (Collegeville, MN: Liturgical Press, 2014).

[16] Pierce, "Environmental Bioethics—A Manifesto."

[17] John Paul II, "Peace with God the Creator, Peace with All of Creation: Message for the 1990 World Day of Peace" (Message of His Holiness Pope John Paul II for the Celebration of the World Day of Peace, January 1, 1990), 2, http://w2.vatican.va

chorus that everything is connected resonates with previous papal insights and hints at what an environmentally responsible worldview would consider.

Creation

Grounding this worldview is the affirmation of creation, the story that opens Genesis and all of the Judeo-Christian tradition. First and foremost, all of creation is *gift* of the Creator. As Benedict XVI points out, "[Nature] is prior to us, and it has been given to us by God as the setting for our life."[18] "The environment must be seen," he says elsewhere, "as God's gift to all people."[19] And this gift is *good*. "And God saw everything that he had made, and indeed, it was very good" (Gen 1:31).

Understanding creation as gift of God and as fundamentally good leads to a sense of *responsibility* for this good gift. Recent teaching sees creation as our common heritage,[20] our common home,[21] and a shared inheritance and a collective good.[22] As a common home and a common heritage, its care is the *responsibility of all*.[23] The US bishops sum up well what this responsibility entails.

/content/john-paul-ii/en/messages/peace/documents/hf_jp-ii_mes_19891208_xxiii -world-day-for-peace.html. Tobias Winright and Andrea Vicini expand on this notion of an ecological worldview in their chapter in this volume. Winright also speaks of "a basic orientation or fundamental direction for how one should think about who one ought to be and how one ought to live," in his " 'Go Forth in Peace to Love and Serve the Lord,' " in Tobias Winright, ed., *Green Discipleship*, 427.

[18] Benedict XVI, *Caritas in Veritate* 48 (Charity in Truth).

[19] Benedict XVI, "If You Want to Cultivate Peace, Protect Creation: Message for the 2010 World Day of Peace" (Message of His Holiness Pope Benedict XVI for the Celebration of the World Day of Peace, January 1, 2010), 2, http://w2.vatican.va/content /benedict-xvi/en/messages/peace/documents/hf_ben-xvi_mes_20091208_xliii -world-day-peace.html.

[20] John Paul II, "Peace with God the Creator," 8.

[21] Francis, *Laudato Si'* 3 (Praise Be to You).

[22] Ibid. 93, 95.

[23] John Paul II, "Peace with God the Creator," 15; United States Conference of Catholic Bishops, "Renewing the Earth: An Invitation to Reflection and Action on Environment in Light of Catholic Social Teaching" (Washington, DC: USCCB, 1991), section III, C, http://www.usccb.org/issues-and-action/human-life-and-dignity /environment/renewing-the-earth.cfm; Benedict XVI, "If You Want to Cultivate Peace," 2; Francis, *Laudato Si'* 13, 157, 196, 211, 217–19, 229.

> Safeguarding creation requires us to live responsibly within it, rather than manage creation as though we are outside of it. The human family is charged with preserving the beauty, diversity, and integrity of nature, as well as with fostering its productivity. Yet, God alone is sovereign over the whole earth. . . . Like the patriarch Noah, humanity stands responsible for ensuring that all nature can continue to thrive as God intended.[24]

Responsibility for caring for creation also rests on the conviction that the earth is intended for the *benefit of all*. "The environment," writes Benedict XVI, "is God's gift to everyone, and in our use of it we have a responsibility towards the poor, towards future generations and towards humanity as a whole"[25] or, as the Second Vatican Council stated, "God destined the earth and all it contains for all people and nations."[26]

Grounding this care, the Catholic tradition holds the deep-seated belief that *creation is sacramental*. It discloses the divine. The entire universe is God's dwelling,[27] discloses God's presence[28]—it is a caress of God to and for humanity.[29] Hence, in respecting creation, we also respect the Creator; to degrade the environment is an affront to the Creator. In addition, we must recognize that other living things are intrinsically valuable in God's eyes making them worthy of our respect and care.[30]

This sacramental vision emphasizes the *interconnectedness of all creation*. As the US Conference of Catholic Bishops (USCCB) points out in *Renewing the Earth*: "The web of life is one. . . . Our tradition calls us to protect the life and dignity of the human person, and it is increasingly clear that this task cannot be separated from the care and defense of all creation."[31] Our natural ecology and social ecology are inextricably related. Pope Francis repeatedly reaffirms this perspective in *Laudato Si'*: "It cannot be emphasized enough how every-

---

[24] USCCB, "Renewing the Earth," section II, A.

[25] Benedict XVI, *Caritas in Veritate* 48.

[26] Vatican Council II, *Gaudium et Spes* (Pastoral Constitution on the Church in the Modern World) 69. See also Benedict XVI, "If You Want to Cultivate Peace," 7.

[27] USCCB, "Renewing the Earth," section III, A. See also Francis, *Laudato Si'* 88.

[28] Francis, *Laudato Si'* 85.

[29] Ibid. 84.

[30] Ibid., 67–69; "Renewing the Earth," section III, B.

[31] USCCB, "Renewing the Earth," section I, A and B.

thing is interconnected"[32] which leads to an *integral ecology* and an integrated approach to protecting nature and restoring dignity to the excluded.[33] "Nature," says Francis, "cannot be regarded as something separate from ourselves or as a mere setting in which we live. We are part of nature, included in it and thus in constant interaction with it."[34]

Solidarity

Sacramental interconnectedness moves to action in *solidarity*. Pope John Paul II, for whom solidarity is a key concept, states that "the ecological crisis reveals the *urgent moral need for a new solidarity*."[35] In his encyclical *Sollicitudo Rei Socialis,* John Paul II defines solidarity as a "persevering determination to commit oneself to the common good; that is to say to the good of all and of each individual, because we are all really responsible for all."[36] It entails a willingness "to 'lose oneself' for the sake of others instead of exploiting [them]."[37] Clearly, this means sacrificing oneself for the good of others and for our common home. Pope Benedict XVI, speaks of an *intergenerational* solidarity with future generations; and *intergenerational* solidarity with the current generation wherever they may be.[38] Fundamentally social, human beings are inherently bound to others in a network of relationships that bring with them responsibilities toward these others.

The Common Good

Solidarity, as John Paul II notes above, implies a commitment to the common good, a commitment clearly articulated in recent documents on care for the environment.[39] As Pope Francis explains in *Laudato Si*: "Human ecology is inseparable from the notion of the

---

[32] Francis, *Laudato Si'* 70, 91, 119, 138, 139.
[33] Ibid., 137 and 139.
[34] Ibid., 139.
[35] John Paul II, "Peace with God the Creator," 10.
[36] John Paul II, *Sollicitudo Rei Socialis* 38.
[37] Ibid.
[38] Benedict XVI, "If You Want to Cultivate Peace," 8. See also Francis, *Laudato Si'* 156, 159.
[39] USCCB, "Renewing the Earth," section III, C; Francis, *Laudato Si'* 156–58.

common good, a central and unifying principle of social ethics. The common good is 'the sum of those conditions of social life which allow social groups and their individual members relatively thorough and ready access to their own fulfillment.' "[40] In the present state of global society, continues Francis, the common good summons us to solidarity and a preferential option for the poorest. The USCCB builds on the common good and extends it globally and environmentally. They state in *Renewing the Earth*:

> Ecological concern has now heightened our awareness of just how interdependent our world is. Some of the gravest environmental problems are clearly global. In this shrinking world, everyone is affected and everyone is responsible. . . . The universal common good can serve as a foundation for a global environmental ethic.[41]

Moral theologian Christopher Vogt highlights how the *Compendium of the Social Doctrine of the Church* construes the common good environmentally:

> A crucial step has been the explicit recognition in Catholic social teaching that a safe and healthy natural environment is an important component of the common good. Every person has a right to live in a place in which the environment has not been degraded . . . In addition, every individual and every society has an obligation to promote and protect the vibrant health of the natural environment. This responsibility stems from humans' duty to protect and build up the common good.[42]

Integral Human Development

The development of the common good is integral to human development, which runs implicitly and explicitly throughout papal and episcopal teaching on the environment. John Paul II provides

---

[40] Francis, *Laudato Si'* 156, 158.

[41] USCCB, "Renewing the Earth," section III, C.

[42] Christopher Vogt, "Catholic Social Teaching and Creation," in Tobias Winright, ed., *Green Discipleship*, 226.

the most sustained discussion in *Sollicitudo Rei Socialis* where he points out that true human happiness and flourishing are not dependent on having things, relentless acquisition of goods, and endless expansion of economic growth, but rather on the pursuit of authentic goods such as becoming a virtuous person and developing one's relationships with God and others.[43]

This concept leads to an *ethic of sufficiency*. Again, Christopher Vogt's insight is worth noting: "People should . . . seek to acquire what they need to live a good, dignified life, but not seek to have more than they legitimately need. They should direct the surplus toward the common good and toward ensuring that others have a sufficient share of material goods to live a dignified life."[44] For the USCCB, authentic development and its implications—moderation and even austerity in using material resources—has practical ramifications.[45] It calls for balancing human progress with respect for nature; invites a view of the good society and human well-being not solely based on material goods; requires affluent nations to reduce overconsumption of natural resources; and encourages the use of technological developments for the benefit of people and the land.[46]

For Benedict XVI, the ecological crisis provides an opportunity to reimagine global development integrally.[47] It begins with examining our lifestyles "and the prevailing models of consumption and production, which are often unsustainable from a social, environmental and even economic point of view."[48] He continues, "We can no longer do without a real change of outlook which will result in *new life-styles*, in which the quest for truth, beauty, goodness and communion with others for the sake of common growth are the factors which determine consumer choices, savings and investments."[49] The new lifestyles, however, require a different perspective. Integral human development cannot be considered adequately without first reflecting on those left out most often.

---

[43] John Paul II, *Sollicitudo Rei Socialis* 27–29.

[44] Vogt, "Catholic Social Teaching and Creation," 234.

[45] USCCB, "Renewing the Earth," sections III, G and V, A.

[46] Ibid., section III, G.

[47] Benedict XVI, "If You Want to Cultivate Peace," 9, 5.

[48] Ibid., 11, 10.

[49] Ibid. See also Francis, *Laudato Si'* 106–14.

Option for the Poor

The option for the poor is a pillar of Catholic social teaching. Pope John Paul II connects poverty, the poor, and the environment in his 1990 address for the World Day of Peace where he states that a proper ecological balance cannot be achieved without addressing structures of poverty throughout the world. As the poor attempt to survive, he observes, they sometimes exhaust the soil or accelerate uncontrolled deforestation or move into urban areas that do not have the infrastructure to accommodate them. Rather than blaming the poor "to whom the earth is entrusted no less than to others," the key is enabling them to find a way out of poverty. "This will require a courageous reform of structures, as well as new ways of relating among peoples and states."[50]

The USCCB and Pope Francis take a slightly different tack. Both observe that the poor tend to suffer more directly from environmental degradation and have the least access to relief.[51] As Francis points out, in hearing the cry of the earth, we must also hear the cry of the poor for the poor contribute the least to environmental degradation but suffer the most from it and have the least access to relief.[52]

> The human environment and the natural environment deteriorate together; we cannot adequately combat environmental degradation unless we attend to causes related to human and social degradation. In fact, the deterioration of the environment and of society affects the most vulnerable people on the planet: Both everyday experience and scientific research show that the gravest effects of all attacks on the environment are suffered by the poorest.[53]

Later in the document, Francis calls for a preferential option for the poorest.[54] The commitment to the poorest, however, ought not only rely on required regulation in order to effect change within our own institutions.

---

[50] John Paul II, "Peace with God the Creator," 11.
[51] USCCB, "Renewing the Earth," section III, F.
[52] Francis, *Laudato Si'* 48, 49.
[53] Ibid.
[54] Ibid., 158.

Subsidiarity

Another pillar of an environmental worldview is subsidiarity. In the words of Benedict XVI, "We are all responsible for the protection of the environment. This responsibility knows no boundaries. In accordance with the *principle of subsidiarity* it is important for everyone to be committed at his or her proper level."[55] Hence, every level of society, including health care, has a responsibility to promote care of the environment. While starting at the local level is important, it requires a reprioritizing of how things ought to be done.

Conversion

A final core element is the need for conversion, individual and communal, in our thinking, our actions, our lifestyles, and the virtues we practice.[56] John Paul II notes that an education in ecological responsibility "entails a genuine conversion in ways of thought and behavior." While not using the term "conversion," Benedict XVI calls us to change our outlook, to examine and develop new lifestyles, which must include "prudence, the virtue which tells us what needs to be done today in view of what might happen tomorrow."[57] Calling for "new attitudes and new actions," the USCCB sees the virtues of prudence, humility, and temperance as indispensable elements of a new environmental ethic. These attitudes and actions explicitly require conversion: "The environmental crisis of our own day constitutes an exceptional call to conversion. As individuals, as institutions, as a people, we need a change of heart to save the planet for our children and generations yet unborn."[58] Francis in *Laudato Si'* echoes similar themes, calling for a "reconciliation with creation" through an "ecological conversion." Quoting the Australian Catholic Bishops, he writes, " 'To achieve such reconciliation, we must examine our lives and acknowledge the ways in which we have harmed God's

---

[55] Benedict XVI, "If You Want to Cultivate Peace," 11.

[56] See John Paul II, "Peace with God the Creator," 13; USCCB, "Renewing the Earth," section V, A; Francis, *Laudato Si'* 111, 114, 202–21.

[57] Benedict XVI, "If You Want to Cultivate Peace," 9.

[58] USCCB, "Renewing the Earth," section V, C.

creation through our actions and our failure to act. We need to experience a conversion, or change of heart.' "[59]

Each core element of Catholic teaching on environmental responsibility carries implications for Catholic bioethics and how Catholic health care organizations deliver care. It is critical that these implications be drawn out.

Taking Action: What Can Be and Is Being Done?

There is hope. As often happens, Catholic health care is leading Catholic bioethics. Over the past fifteen to twenty years, faith-based and secular health care institutions have begun to examine their environmental footprint and implement new initiatives. These initiatives have not been inspired primarily by our theological traditions. Rather, Catholic health care has been spurred by several pioneering secular organizations that have promoted environmentally responsible health care practices.[60] Leaders include Health Care without Harm, an organization that works to transform health care worldwide so that it reduces its environmental footprint, becomes a community anchor for sustainability, and a leader in the global movement for environmental health and justice. Hospitals for a Healthy Environment, jointly founded by the EPA, AHA, and Health Care without Harm, seeks to help health care facilities reduce their environmental impact while saving money and reducing liabilities. Healthier Hospitals Initiative operates as a permanent program of Practice Greenhealth. It provides free tools and resources that help focus sustainability efforts on the health care sector's biggest areas of opportunity and risk. Finally, Practice Greenhealth, one of the major sources for environmental solutions for the health care sector in view of contributing to

---

[59] Francis, *Laudato Si'* 218; see also 111, 114, 201–21.

[60] Among the major organizations, all of whom have numerous resources on their websites, are Health Care without Harm (1996), www.noharm.org; Hospitals for a Healthy Environment (1998 and the precursor of Practice Greenhealth), www .hercenter.org; Practice Greenhealth (2008), www.practicegreenhealth.org; Healthier Hospitals Initiative (a permanent program of Practice Greenhealth), www.healthier hospitals.org.

safer, greener workplaces and communities.[61] Without a doubt, however, as Catholic organizations have begun to adopt various initiatives that appeal to fundamental commitments of Catholic health care. The mission and values of the organization build upon the insights of CST in order to provide a mission and theological foundation for the programs. Here follow the current possibilities.

Energy Conservation

By using less energy, using it more efficiently and obtaining at least some if not all of it from cleaner and renewable energy sources, health care can reduce their emissions thereby protecting the environment and lowering the risks of illness from air pollution. In most cases, it also benefits the bottom line. Using LED lighting, for example, or sensors to turn lights on and off, or adjusting the intensity of lighting to the time of day can make a significant difference over time. Swapping out or retrofitting HVAC systems for better sizing or better efficiency along with heat recovery systems can also have positive results.[62]

Waste Management

The goal here is to reduce waste and increase recycling. A "trash audit" is usually a helpful first step to determine what constitutes the waste and where it ends up, followed by an assessment of where waste can be reduced (e.g., reducing paper use and unnecessary packaging), what can be reused and what can be recycled, or shifting to products that can be reused or recycled.[63]

---

[61] See n. 13. The Catholic Health Association of the United States also has numerous resources on its website including guidelines for "how to get started" and accounts of what various Catholic health care entities are doing, https://www.chausa.org /environment/overview. See also two special issues of CHA's *Health Progress* devoted to the environment, vol. 97, no. 3 (May–June 2016) and vol. 84, no 6 (November–December 2003).

[62] See https://practicegreenhealth.org/topics/leaner-energy, and https://noharm -uscanada.org/issues/us-canada/energy-efficiency.

[63] See https://practicegreenhealth.org/topics/less-waste, and https://noharm -uscanada.org/issues/us-canada/waste-management.

Food

Food production, processing, packaging, and distribution have a negative impact on the environment and on human health. This can be lessened by purchasing foods that are grown in an environmentally sound manner and purchasing locally. Offering healthier foods to patients and in cafeterias can be health promoting. Reducing food waste by employing software to help better plan meals and composting food waste are other environmentally sound measures.[64]

Safer Chemicals

Health care may employ more chemicals than any other sector.[65] Many of these chemicals have a deleterious impact on the environment and on human health as previously noted. Much can be done to address this challenge such as shifting to green cleaning products, reducing the use of products with PVC and DEHP, eliminating all products with mercury, and purchasing furniture and carpeting without harmful chemicals.[66]

Sustainable Design in Renovations and New Construction

Design renovations and new construction ensure the use of safe materials, minimize materials waste, recycle scrap materials, optimize energy performance, and reduce harmful chemicals. In furnishing new spaces, choosing environmentally friendly furnishings and equipment has positive effects. Creating healing environments with natural light, quiet spaces, outdoor green spaces, gardens, and such also has beneficial results as does environmentally sensitive landscaping and watering.[67]

---

[64] See https://practicegreenhealth.org/topics/healthier-food, and https://noharm-uscanada.org/healthyfoodinhealthcare.

[65] See https://noharm-global.org/issues/global/chemicals-health-care: "the health care sector is the single largest user of chemicals, spending more than double the amount spent by the second largest consuming industry sector."

[66] See https://practicegreenhealth.org/topics/safer-chemicals; https://noharm-uscanada.org/issues/us-canada/toxic-materials; https://noharm-uscanada.org/issues/us-canada/safer-chemicals.

[67] See https://noharm-uscanada.org/issues/us-canada/green-building-and-energy and https://noharm-uscanada.org/issues/us-canada/environmentally-preferable-purchasing.

Advocacy

Systems should advocate for legislation that promotes environmentally sound practices and particularly attends to the poor and vulnerable who are most often victims of environmental degradation. Pope Francis offers this reminder, "We are faced not with two separate crises, one environmental and the other social, but rather with one complex crisis which is both social and environmental. Strategies for a solution demand an integrated approach to combating poverty, restoring dignity to the excluded, and at the same time protecting nature."[68] For Catholic health care organizations who tend to view these as separate: in fact, as our social tradition says, everything is interconnected—the human and the natural—and the poor and vulnerable are most affected by environmental degradation. Every effort should be made to address them together.[69]

Conclusion: The Work Ahead

Environmental solidarity is a worldview. This worldview can shape who we are and become as individuals and as organizations and what we do. As Pope John Paul II points out, we "[need] carefully coordinated solutions based on a morally coherent world view. . . . For Christians, such a world view is grounded in religious convictions drawn from Revelation"[70] and as expressed in our social tradition. The CEO in the opening narrative and others like him need to understand that from a faith perspective environmentally responsible health care is not optional. "Christians, in particular, realize that their responsibility within creation and their duty towards nature and the Creator are an essential part of their faith."[71] Hence, leaders in Catholic health care have an obligation to inform themselves about environmentally responsible health care delivery and ensure that their organizations embrace it and make it a part of their culture.[72]

---

[68] Francis, *Laudato Si'* 139.

[69] See https://www.chausa.org/docs/default-source/general-files/connecting-health-care-with-public-and-environmental-health-pdf.pdf?sfvrsn=0.

[70] John Paul II, "Peace with God the Creator," 2.

[71] Ibid., 15.

[72] The Catholic Health Association can be an extremely helpful resource here as can Catholic health care organizations that have already made significant strides in becoming more environmentally conscious. Many of these organizations and their

Attention to environmental responsibility should also be an essential element in Catholic bioethics for which there is yet much work to be done in developing a Catholic *environmental* bioethics.

Becoming more environmentally responsible in health care delivery requires not only a conversion of hearts and minds but a conversion of organizational culture. In the words of Pope Francis, "It is we humans above all who need to change. . . A great cultural, spiritual and educational challenge stands before us, and it will demand that we set out on the long path of renewal. . . Today, in a word, the issue of environmental degradation challenges us to examine our lifestyle."[73] What is the "lifestyle" of our organizations? We must examine our interactions with the environment, seeking to change our minds and hearts, as individuals and as organizations. Environmental mindfulness and practice are not add-ons, a flavor of the month. Rather, they need to become "this is how we do things around here." Environmental responsibility must become embedded in the culture, reflecting the identity of the organization and its employees. There is yet much work to be done in developing Catholic *environmentally sustainable* health care institutions.

---

initiatives are listed on the CHA website: https://www.chausa.org/environment/resources/ministry-policies-and-practices.

[73] Ibid., 202, 206.

Chapter 14

DACA and Institutional Solidarity

Mark Kuczewski

In May of 2011, Professor Herbert Medina of Loyola Marymount University in Los Angeles sent an email message to Loyola University Chicago Stritch School of Medicine describing Rosa, who wished to become a doctor, as "the best student he'd ever had," with a near-perfect grade point average, a double major in biology and Spanish. However, he noted that she was undocumented and that if she were to become a physician, it would probably require the shepherding of her application and support throughout her medical education.

Professor Medina's email prompted me to investigate the structural barriers Rosa would face in trying to attend medical school. An undocumented immigrant would pose a financial aid challenge for the school owing to her being ineligible for federal student loans. Most medical students graduate with more than $150,000 of such debt, and undocumented students would likely have higher than average needs as little to no financial contribution could be expected from many families. More devastating, a student such as Rosa would not be able to work lawfully. This would prevent her from going on to residency, the phase of training that follows medical school. While residency involves training, it is also a job that issues a paycheck and we could see no path to work authorization. To invest in Rosa's medical education would be to use a significant amount of resources to create a doctor who could not treat patients, which is what Rosa aspired to do.

On the one hand, it should be obvious why we were interested in having Rosa apply. We are a medical school and that means we want the best and the brightest applicants we can find. We do not wish to turn away a great student because of contrived reasons. Similarly, a medical school's mission includes producing physicians who are equipped to treat the diverse population comprising our nation's patients. Rosa is bilingual and bicultural; she can be a significant asset in serving underserved patient populations. She also clearly had an ability to navigate obstacles and remain determined in spite of difficulties, a characteristic that educators like to refer to as "grit." What medical school would not want her? On the other hand, what medical school would be willing to take the financial and perhaps legal risks to admit her? Accepting an undocumented medical student was uncharted territory.

❖ ❖ ❖ ❖ ❖

Loyola heard Rosa's story differently. Rosa's story cried out for justice. As a Catholic and Jesuit University our mission demands more. She had done nothing but worked hard her whole life, determined to succeed in serving others as a healer. Unjust and unreformed immigration policies have failed to provide the conditions for her to reach this potential, failing to respect her worth and her dignity. Thus, my initial inquiry on behalf of Rosa revealed an immigration structure created to isolate, marginalize, and demean migrants as unworthy to participate as equal members in our community.

Drawing on Ron Hamel's language in the previous chapter, addressing the challenges raised by undocumented individuals requires conversion. We need to be converted away from a status quo that settles for unjust immigration policies, that remains silent when political figures malign and alienate members of our community that are American in every way. We need to be converted toward recognizing undocumented persons—in this case, DACA (Deferred Action for Childhood Arrival) students—as members of our community, a *metanoia* that opens our eyes and hearts to the injustice and arbitrary nature of the US immigration system.

This process of recognizing and including persons like Rosa does not come without a cost. The vitriolic rhetoric in the US on immigration opens individuals and institutions who support marginalized communities to a steady flow of criticism, isolation, and rejection. Yet to be a Catholic and Christian university—or a Catholic health system—is to stand on the side of communities pushed to the margin, struggle against the structural sin that marginalized them, and take action rooted in solidarity with them. This is our mission. This chapter tells the story of one Catholic institution that has taken such action. The action has come with costs, but true to the gospel, it has, more importantly, borne fruit one hundred-fold that has rippled with grace throughout our lives, our institution, our community, and the nation.

Undocumented Youth:
From Dreamers to DACA Recipients

Undocumented young people are sometimes referred to as "Dreamers" after the never-passed piece of legislation that would provide them with a path to citizenship, the DREAM Act (Development, Relief and Education of Alien Minors). The criteria under which one would qualify under this legislation required that the individual had arrived in the United States before the age of 16, lived here continuously for more than five years, committed no major criminal offenses, and attained a high school diploma or the equivalent or have a record of military service. This legislation was first introduced in 2001 and has come close to passage on a number of occasions. The failure of the DREAM Act meant that a generation of undocumented youth grew up without access to driver's licenses, federal student loans, in-state tuition, and the ability to work lawfully. Harvard sociologist Roberto Gonzales characterizes being undocumented as a "master status" that affects virtually every aspect of one's life.[1]

---

[1] Roberto G. Gonzales and Edelina M. Burciaga, "Segmented Pathways of Illegality: Reconciling the Coexistence of Master and Auxiliary Statuses in the Experiences of 1.5-Generation Undocumented Young Adults," *Ethnicities* 18, no. 2 (2018), 180. Gonzales and Burciaga say, "Individuals possess a variety of status characteristics that shape their social mobility, personal identity, and treatment by others. However, some characteristics are more prominent than others, and override other traits. The most important feature of a master status is that it overwhelms all of the individuals' other status characteristics and becomes the predominant attribute in his or her personal identity and experience."

As Rosa's story above makes clear, the burden imposed by this master status has been significant. Many of these barriers, however, were removed when President Barack Obama announced that the eligibility criteria from the proposed DREAM Act would form the basis for the DACA program. Undocumented youth who qualify for DACA receive a two-year stay of any action on their immigration status and most importantly, receive an Employment Authorization Document (EAD), that is, a work permit. With the EAD in hand, DACA recipients can also apply for a Social Security number. DACA recipients can apply for renewal every two years as long as the program continues. However, DACA recipients remain ineligible for virtually all federal benefits such as federal student loans.

The Stritch School of Medicine saw this opportunity virtually immediately. With a renewable work permit, a DACA recipient who graduated from medical school would be eligible to seek a residency position and obtain a license to practice medicine in many states. As a result, our institution amended its eligibility requirements to enable DACA recipients to apply and compete on a level playing field for admission. We attached a webpage to the admissions site that declared "Dreamers of DACA Status Welcome." Of course, the financial aid barrier was still formidable. By openly proclaiming the intent to enable these students to attend medical school, the school was able to find partnerships with various institutions such as the state's infrastructure bank (Illinois Finance Authority), a major Catholic health system (Trinity Health), and to create loan programs for students who successfully competed for admission. Because of this attention to the necessary financial aid, the Loyola University Chicago Stritch School of Medicine has, to this point, the only genuine community of DACA recipients in one medical school in the US. In 2018, Loyola University Chicago has thirty-two such students, which is more than one-third of all DACA recipients in medical schools in the United States.

What Does Social Justice Mean in the Context of DACA?

In the more than five years of DACA's existence, DACA recipients not only made advances in entering medical school but made across-the-board gains in standard of living. The average hourly wages of DACA recipients increased significantly, and they reported finding employment more closely related to their education and skills.[2] Despite lack of access to federal student loans, DACA recipients made great strides in college attendance, entering at a rate close to their citizen peers.[3] This success in a short timeframe is striking. Of course, being able to live free of fear of imminent deportation and being able to work lawfully should be expected to help raise one's quality of life! Socioeconomic gains are important for the DACA recipients themselves. Combined, the freedom to come out of the shadows, have access to education, and an income all indicate the way in which DACA recipients have become woven more securely into the fabric of the community.

The ways in which DACA improved the lives of its recipients highlights the degree to which the economic poverty of undocumented immigrants is a function of their social marginalization. By being defined as an outcast class, that is, "illegal" aliens, they were segregated from basic economic and educational opportunities. With the implementation of DACA, these persons were able to enter much of mainstream American society and become known by more Americans. As a result, support against deporting them grew from approximately 57 percent in the months after the program was created in 2012, to 80 to 90 percent in 2017.[4] Unfortunately, despite public support and a desire for these individuals to be recognized as members of our community, unjust discrimination toward this community persists.

DACA was rescinded on September 5, 2017, and is closed to new enrollment. Fortunately, two district courts have temporarily held the program open for renewals thereby preventing current DACA recipients from expiring out of the program. However, this situation is inherently unstable as the court orders are based on procedural grounds and it is expected that President Trump will be allowed to

---

[2] Tom K. Wong, et al., "DACA Recipients' Economic and Educational Gains Continue to Grow," Center for American Progress, August 28, 2017, https://www.american progress.org/issues/immigration/news/2017/08/28/437956/dacarecipients -economic-educational-gains-continue-grow/.

[3] Randy Capps, Michael Fix, and Jie Zong, "The Education and Work Profiles of the DACA Population," Issue Brief, Migration Policy Institute, August 2017, http://www.migrationpolicy.org/research/education-and-work-profiles-daca-population.

[4] Scott Clement and David Nakamura, "Survey Finds Strong Support for 'Dreamers,'" *The Washington Post*, September 25, 2017.

close the program entirely at some point in the foreseeable future.[5] Yet, the eyes of the public have been open to the possibilities of what DACA recipients can contribute to the community. Perhaps more significantly, DACA recipients themselves have been empowered by a brief break from living in fear of deportation and have united to advocate for themselves and with their allies.

In the five years of DACA's existence, undocumented youth became their own advocates on a national level and within their own professional communities. The medical students of the Loyola University Chicago Stritch School of Medicine became known for their desire to become physicians for underserved communities and for the skills they bring to the medical encounter. Furthermore, with the rescinding of DACA, some of these students became direct advocates working with congressional representatives to advance legislation. Similarly, as constituents of professional organizations, they have been able to bring along these powerful organizations as advocates in the public domain. Statements have been issued by the American Medical Association and the American Association of Medical Colleges and numerous specialty and health-related organizations.[6] Some of their strongest advocates have been their peers, who have come to know their story and have taken up their cause.

Combating the Status Quo

The most common characterization of undocumented immigrants by reactionary politicians is that of criminals. This reached its zenith in the candidacy and presidency of Donald Trump who launched his campaign with the infamous lines, "When Mexico sends its people, they're not sending their best. They're not sending you. They're send-

[5] Maria Sacchetti, "With Three Months Left in Medical School, Her Career May Be Slipping Away," *The Washington Post*, February 22, 2018, https://www.washington post.com/local/immigration/with-three-months-left-in-medical-school-her-career-may-be-slipping-away/2018/02/22/24a7a780-10f3-11e8-9570-29c9830535e5_story.html?utm_term=.d298b7e7755.

[6] Kevin B. O'Reilly, "'Dreamers' Bolster Physician Workforce, Should Be Allowed to Stay," *AMA Wire*, September 6, 2017, https://wire.ama-assn.org/ama-news/dreamers-bolster-physician-workforce-should-be-allowed-stay; AAMC News, "AAMC Statement on Announcement to Rescind DACA Executive Action: Association Calls on Congress to Pass Legislation to Protect Individuals with DACA Status," https://news.aamc.org/press-releases/article/daca_rescind_09052017/.

ing people that have lots of problems, and they're bringing those problems with us. They're bringing drugs. They're bringing crime. They're rapists. And some, I assume, are good people."[7] The Chief of Staff to the President of the United States, General John Kelly, later added that

> the vast majority of the people that move illegally into [the] United States are not bad people. They're not criminals. They're not MS-13. Some of them are not. But they're also not people that would easily assimilate into the United States into our modern society. They're overwhelmingly rural people in the countries they come from—fourth, fifth, sixth grade educations are kind of the norm. They don't speak English, obviously that's a big thing. They don't speak English. They don't integrate well, they don't have skills.[8]

However, neither Kelly's nor Trump's characterizations are true. On the contrary, significant data shows that the current wave of immigrants are very much like previous waves in that they tend to contribute much to society and take little.[9] Characterizing them as predominantly criminals or terrorists amounts to little more than bearing false witness against one's neighbor. Studies show that criminal activity among immigrants is as low or lower than the general population; terrorist-related violence by immigrants is extremely low and policies to keep any such danger in check do more harm than good by addressing the issue as if it were related to immigration in general.[10] Furthermore, there is absolutely no reason to think that

[7] "Donald Trump Announces a Presidential Bid," *Washington Post,* June 16, 2015, https://www.washingtonpost.com/news/post-politics/wp/2015/06/16/full-text-donald-trump-announces-a-presidential-bid/?utm_term=.3e74555443a8.

[8] *NPR,* "Transcript: White House Chief of Staff John Kelly's Interview with NPR," May 11, 2018, https://www.npr.org/2018/05/11/610116389/transcript-white-house -chief-of-staff-john-kellys-interview-with-npr.

[9] John Bellows, "The Many Contributions of Immigrants to the American Economy," *Treasury Notes,* U.S. Department of the Treasury, May 25, 2011, https://www.treasury .gov/connect/blog/Pages/The-Many-Contributions-of-Immigrants-to-the-American -Economy.aspx.

[10] Anna Flagg, "The Myth of the Criminal Immigrant," *New York Times,* March 30, 2018, https://www.nytimes.com/interactive/2018/03/30/upshot/crime-immigration -myth.html.

the current wave of immigrants is assimilating differently from any previous wave.[11]

Nevertheless, when powerful people repeatedly lie or, in the words of the Decalogue, bear false witness against people who have little political and economic power and influence, those lies become solidified in the minds of many. The lies breed xenophobia into the social fabric of the community, and it feeds on the resentment and anger of disenfranchised citizens against these "others" who are "not . . . you" in candidate Trump's characterization. While opinion polls suggest that the vast majority of US citizens desire a legislative solution to accommodate DACA recipients, fanning the flames of anger among a significant minority upon whom some elected representatives rely can prevent legislation from ever reaching a vote in the House of Representatives. Exactly how is it that this limbo persists in the face of reason? And what must the response be as we accompany undocumented youth into this uncertain future?

In the language of progressive social activists, we respond in terms of empowerment and becoming allies. Alternatively, one could make the argument that DACA students' commitment to poor and underserved communities make them an ideal fit for patient needs and diversifying the physician workforce. However, while the Catholic social tradition would not disagree with these sentiments, we are more likely to characterize this process in terms of accompaniment, social justice, and solidarity.

By accompanying these youths on their journey rather than continuing to keep them at a distance, we support their prophetic voices calling for fair treatment. The DACA recipient medical students also highlight the degree to which the denial of justice for particular persons is amplified and harms unidentified and unseen persons. Practically, justice requires us to consider these DACA students as future physicians who can serve numerous patients in underserved communities who may find themselves without a physician in the future;

---

[11] Alex Nowrasteh, "Terrorism and Immigration: A Risk Analysis," *CATO Institute Policy Analysis* 798, September 13, 2016, https://www.cato.org/publications/policy-analysis/terrorism-immigration-risk-analysis#full; *NPR*, "Fact-Checking What John Kelly Said About Immigration," May 13, 2018, https://www.npr.org/2018/05/13/610777795/fact-checking-what-john-kelly-said-about-immigration.

such communities will certainly be deprived of a culturally aware and sensitive physician should these Dreamers not be admitted to medical school or allowed to complete their training and practice as physicians. In order to create this change, however, greater efforts need to be made toward breaking down the structural sin that persists.

Structural Sin and Welcoming Undocumented Youth as "the Stranger"

Justice is denied to these young people and their future patients as a consequence of social sin. Institutional mechanisms that embody and foster continued injustice are easily manipulated for political purposes. In the case of immigrants, the process is a simple one. It always begins with demagoguery and reinforcing false stereotypes of immigrants. They are portrayed as undesirable criminals or un-educated persons unable to assimilate.

As the ongoing drumbeat of false and negative characterizations of our neighbors continues, it seems to give political legitimacy to such prejudices and even to racism. It is a truism that there are two sides to each issue, and if some politicians proclaim a view, that view is assumed to contain some kernel of truth. And as a political issue, it is seen as controversial, something that nonpartisan organizations should probably refrain from engaging. Yet, the US bishops, Pope Francis, and the entire CST encourage exactly the opposite response, having exerted a thorough condemnation of deceitful rhetoric and unjust policies by proclaiming the Gospel narrative.

Jesus consistently kept the company of people who were marginal-ized by the practices, rhetoric, and the standards of the day. We have become somewhat indifferent to this point with the passage of time and familiarity with the Gospel narrative, and we have lost its truly radical and demanding stance. We tend to take it as obvious that the so-called reputable people of that era were hypocrites and Jesus was spending time with the genuinely good people. And it is an easy extrapolation to infer that in this common era, Jesus would dwell with reputable Christians who are generally upstanding law-abiding citizens. We assume that as contemporary, Christian-influenced in-stitutions we are now better at recognizing the righteous and the saints, and that Jesus would avoid those who were actual sinners. Our age is little different than previous eras in assuming that economic and social success must be a function of merit, especially when we ourselves occupy positions of privilege. And there is a tendency to reassure ourselves regarding the invulnerability of our privilege through ascribing blame to those who fail to attain the same goods.

By contrast, CST counsels a "preferential option for the poor" as a counterweight to this dynamic of social sin. While Jesus came for all, he clearly expressed a preference regarding with whom he spent time and made a priority. Gustavo Gutierrez reminds us that the option for the poor arises out of our faith in Jesus Christ, and "following Jesus is a response to the question about the meaning of human existence; it is a global vision of our life, but it also affects life's small and everyday aspects."[12] As Catholics, we are to be in solidarity with the poor, with those who are marginalized and outcast by society in all its hypocrisy and political opportunism.

As the immigration issue metastasizes, Catholic institutions are challenged to avoid becoming indifferent to the plight of the poor and marginalized. The struggle for justice for Dreamers has been in the public eye since at least the introduction of the Dream Act in 2001. It is easy to become weary of the fight and to become discouraged as even the progress made by the creation of DACA is placed on a path to extinction. It is easy to settle for the status quo. This temptation is especially true since DACA was rescinded. The uncertainty generated by the Trump administration has in many ways frozen the momentum to create structures of solidarity such as new student loan opportunities at the Stritch School of Medicine. However, the attention brought by the jeopardy these youth have been placed in by DACA's rescinding has not only altered public opinion but also brought many more allies to the aid of these young people.

For instance, Loyola University Chicago sought to support its fourth-year DACA recipients in the residency match process (the system of reciprocal ranking of preference by students and residency program directors through which graduating medical students apply to and eventually are assigned to a residency program). However, it

---

[12] Gustavo Gutiérrez, "The Option for the Poor Arises from Faith in Christ," *Theological Studies* 70, no. 2 (2009): 320.

seemed unlikely that any residency programs would be interested in matching with DACA recipients given that residency programs are commonly three to five years in duration and there is no evident way for the students to renew their work permits when they expire in two years. Because of the risk factor of a training program losing their resident after two years, our dean of student affairs prepared the students for the likelihood that they would receive no offers to interview. However, they all received a significant number of interviews and went on to secure residency positions. This outcome was aided by the court decisions that presently enable ongoing renewal of the work permits and also guidance issued by the National Residency Match Program (NRMP).[13] One remarkable aspect of this effort is that the willingness of Loyola to support these students led other secular organizations such as the NRMP and particular residency program directors to hear the same prophetic cry for justice. Standing on the side of justice and in solidarity with those made vulnerable by structural sin creates alternative structures that build networks for change and social justice, that is, a network that participates now in the reign of God in history.

Conclusion:
Standing on the Right Side of (Salvation) History

For Christians, the story of Jesus is the story of salvation, God's entering into and redeeming human history. The gospel accounts tell us how God acts, what is of value, and exemplifies the life Christians aspire to lead by following the actions of Jesus. Jesuit Martyr Ignacio Ellacuría, assassinated in El Salvador for championing truth, justice, and peacemaking, declares that "salvation itself, in deeds and words, is a denunciation of sin and a struggle against it. It is not only forgiveness and understanding; it is also effective action and, of course, a decision to act."[14] The temptation, however, is always to not act.

---

[13] National Resident Matching Program, "Statement on Presidential Proclamation 9645 and Deferred Action for Childhood Arrivals (DACA)," December 11, 2017, http://www.nrmp.org/nrmp-statement-visa-restrictions-daca-program/.

[14] Michael Edward Lee and Kevin F. Burke, eds., *Ignacio Ellacuría: Essays on History, Liberation, and Salvation* (Maryknoll, NY: Orbis Books, 2013), 181.

I offer two concluding points to assist those called to struggle against the temptation to stand idle.

First, Catholic institutions are called to constantly renew their commitment and efforts to accompany immigrants in their journey to full participation in society.[15] The United States has failed for many years to rectify the injustices that have accumulated from its antiquated immigration laws. It is easy to become worn down by the effort required to support affected individuals in achieving their potential. Building alternative systems is not easy and as we know from previous civil rights struggles, separate is never truly equal. Catholic educational and social institutions cannot weary of the struggle for justice and have to be energetic and creative in our efforts of accompaniment. We must not let the duration of the struggle allow us to slip into complacency and indifference. When problems are large and have no foreseeable end in sight, it is easy to simply dismiss them.

This temptation can be even stronger as the accusations and lies hurled at our immigrant neighbors become more entrenched among many citizens. Our institutions will be accused of being too "political" and we will be accused of being more concerned about lawbreakers and criminals than law-abiding citizens. Pope Francis has cautioned us about the globalization of indifference, and as Christians, the answer to his haunting question, "Who will cry for them?" must be "us."[16]

Second, the good news includes that the outcomes that flow from this commitment are likely to promote justice in the fullest sense of that term. That is, as these marginalized and liberated persons become more integrated into the opportunities afforded other citizens, they gain access to venues in which they may represent themselves, and their cry for fairness is heard by an ever-increasing number of people and institutions. This is the counterweight to the metastasiz-

[15] For Catholic health care systems interested in resources for accompanying undocumented patients, we have compiled a comprehensive list of tools and resources in English and Spanish at our website, Treating Fear: Sanctuary Doctoring, http://luc.edu/sanctuarydoctor.

[16] Pope Francis, "Homily of Holy Father Francis, Visit to Lampedusa," July 8, 2013, https://w2.vatican.va/content/francesco/en/homilies/2013/documents/papa-francesco_20130708_omelia-lampedusa.html.

ing of bigotry. Because this role as empowering the prophetic cry of the marginalized is so powerful, Catholic institutions should continually reflect on how their position and resources enable them to provide such a launching pad to being a corrective to social injustices.

In sum, we have a reached a paradoxical time in regard to immigration issues in the United States and Catholic social teaching calls us to be vigilant and determined in our efforts to accompany migrants who seek justice. The anti-immigrant sentiment that has gripped sizable portions of our population has been able to prevent legislative progress for many years. On the other hand, we have seen how incremental acts of empowerment such as the DACA program and the collaborative efforts between political, educational, and health care institutions can foster the ability of this marginalized population to issue a prophetic call for justice to institutions and the broader citizenry. Catholic health care institutions should take the lead. The kingdom of God is among you. Go forth and witness to the Good News.

Chapter 15

Reframing Outsourcing

M. Therese Lysaught and Robert J. DeVita

A few years ago, one of us (DeVita) was tasked, along with a chief medical officer (CMO), to create a "startup" hospitalist service for inpatient medicine at five urban hospitals. Facing the need to meet a strategic deadline for "go live," we chose to use a clinical outsourcing provider. Having launched hospitalist services in other organizations, we knew from experience that as leaders we should provide contextual depth about "soft stuff" including organizational mission, values, and administrative practices. An in-depth orientation and on-boarding about the "soft stuff" would be critical for the clinicians we employed via the outsourcing supplier to be successful. We also discovered that a previous nascent attempt at developing a hospitalist service for inpatient medicine at the same hospitals had failed, primarily due to a lack of alignment with the organization's mission, values, and practices, and an unwillingness by too many of the contract clinicians to take personal responsibility for care. These subtle shortcomings undermined another dimension of care—the successful development of a cohesive care team. Simultaneously, we pursued a parallel strategy of recruiting full-time medical staff who had hospitalist experience and were aligned with our organizational mission, values, and practices. To our surprise, staffing handoffs between contracted and recruited hospitalists became another opportunity for disruption in care coordination. Managing personal disagreements, petty jealousies, and rumor mongering became a full-time job as clinicians employed by the organization began replacing those supplied by the outsourcing contract. Outsourcing decisions can affect not only the in-house ethos of an organization but can directly impact the core service of patient care.

In Britain, a pioneer in outsourcing for cost-savings and efficiency, the National Health System has recently come under fire from the British government itself for situations encountered at Millbrow Care Home, an assisted-living center. As the *New York Times* reports, frail, elderly, and ill residents were being neglected: "For over a year, they had been deprived of food and drink for hours on end. They were not being given the medication they had been prescribed. There were outbreaks of vomiting and diarrhea, and outdated food in the kitchen. No one was in charge of preventing the spread of infections, and managers rarely made an appearance." Management of Millbrow had been outsourced to "a private enterprise, Four Seasons Health Care, Britain's second-largest provider, which in turn was owned by Terra Firma, one of the world's largest private equity groups."[1] Apart from egregious failures regarding patient care, the outsourced services ended up costing far more than if they had been kept in-house. In this instance, outsourcing violated the fundamental principle of medical ethics—"first do no harm"—*and* cost more.

Finally, the impacts of outsourcing can ripple into local communities. Recently, Ascension Wisconsin announced plans to reconfigure a local hospital in a low-income neighborhood of Milwaukee, St. Joseph's Hospital.[2] Ascension acquired St. Joseph's from the former Wheaton Franciscan Health System as part of a merger in 2016. An anchor of the community since its founding over 130 years ago, St. Joseph's presents a challenging "payer-mix"—51 percent of patients on Medicaid, 5 percent uninsured—which resulted in an

---

[1] Kimiko de Freytas-Tamura, "Britain Was a Pioneer in Outsourcing Services: Now, the Model is 'Broken,'" *New York Times*, January 31, 2018.

[2] Guy Boulton, "Ascension Wisconsin Cutting Services at St. Joseph Hospital," *Milwaukee Journal Sentinel*, April 5, 2018, https://www.jsonline.com/story/money/business/health-care/2018/04/05/ascension-wisconsin-reduce-services-st-joseph-hospital-part-broader-long-term-plan/488523002/. While the St. Joseph situation may not technically be an instance of outsourcing, it illustrates the ways in which outsourcing, or its correlates, pervades health care practice (e.g., in transferring certain services from one Ascension facility to another), and how other initiatives, such as hospital mergers, raise similar issues (by, e.g., removing persons and skill sets from local communities and relocating them elsewhere, either to system offices or other geographical sites).

operating shortfall of almost $82 million from 2012 to 2016. Consequently, having already begun to relocate various services to other sites over the past year,[3] Ascension announced a plan to further reduce services at St. Joseph's to ED, obstetrics, and neonatal care, while inviting (outsourcing) local organizations and agencies to use remaining space at the hospital campus as a base to help address the health and social needs of the surrounding neighborhoods. Community backlash was swift and furious.[4] Not only would it leave no general acute care hospital north of downtown Milwaukee in an area plagued by widespread health disparities; it meant that patients, many of whom use public transportation, would have to travel farther for medical treatment; and it would pull jobs and economic resources out of an already imperiled part of the city. Community leaders have chastised the health system: " 'It's just not right. . . . It's just not what nonprofit organizations with a mission are supposed to do'; 'At the end of the day, the organization purportedly is a nonprofit organization, which as part of its mission includes special attention to those who are poor and vulnerable.' " In response to the PR firestorm, Ascension has temporarily put its plans for St. Joseph's on hold.[5]

❖ ❖ ❖ ❖ ❖

Outsourcing is a legitimate business strategy. A subset of "sourcing"—the business practice that determines sources of supply, labor, and services for an organization—"outsourcing" refers to a decision to take an activity that was previously produced within the boundaries of the firm and to have it sourced (supplied) from outside the firm. Over the past forty years, outsourcing has come to permeate

[3] Rich Kirchen, "Ascension Implements Downsizing at Safety-Net Hospital St. Joseph," *Milwaukee Business Journal*, April 5, 2018, https://www.bizjournals.com/milwaukee/news/2018/04/05/ascension-implements-downsizing-at-safety-net.html.

[4] Guy Boulton, "Ascension Faces Mounting Criticism Over Plan to Cut Services at St. Joseph Hospital," *Milwaukee Journal Sentinel*, April 16, 2018, https://www.jsonline.com/story/money/business/health-care/2018/04/16/ascension-faces-mounting-criticism-over-plan-cut-services-st-joseph-hospital/516087002/.

[5] Guy Boulton and Sarah Hauer, "Ascension Wisconsin Puts its Plan to Stop Services at St. Joseph Hospital on Hold," *Milwaukee Journal Sentinel*, April 18, 2018, https://www.jsonline.com/story/money/business/2018/04/18/ascension-wisconsin-puts-plan-stop-services-st-joseph-hospital-hold/529964002/.

almost every aspect of Catholic health care: supply chain, general consulting, clinical locums tenens/traveling physicians, IT, HR, finance and accounting, revenue cycle, facilities, economic forecasting, actuarial science, predictive analytics, and more. Four primary motivations fuel decisions to outsource: cost-savings; focusing on core competencies or essential services; quality issues, particularly around staffing issues in underserved markets; and freeing capital for investment.

These three stories illustrate ethical pitfalls of outsourcing that may not have been fully considered when deciding to outsource. While outsourcing is framed primarily as a business decision, too little attention has been paid to the broader ethical contours of the practice, particularly from the perspective of Catholic mission and identity. In this chapter, we sketch the landscape of outsourcing and summarize the conventional ethical wisdom on the practice as it has emerged in the health care management literature. Given that the topic has been relatively invisible to Catholic bioethics, we then explore insights Catholic social thought (CST) might bring. CST moves beyond a simple cost/benefit analysis and provides an alternative lens—comprised of commitments to integral human development, the value of work, and the principles of gratuitousness and restoration—that help illuminate the practice from the perspective of hospital associates and local communities. This framework, informed by two leadership models, shapes practical recommendations for discerning and managing the ethical ambiguities inherent in this pervasive practice.

Outsourcing: Definitions and Landscape

Outsourcing in health care is a subset of broader trends in outsourcing across industries. In 2016, the life sciences and health care comprised 11 percent of the global outsourcing market, with an estimated 70 percent of US health care participating.[6] Outsourcing can be done domestically or globally (referred to as *offshore outsourcing*).

Although outsourcing in health care was first used primarily to source utility functions (e.g., dietary, housekeeping, and security), it

---

[6] Deloitte, *2012 Global Outsourcing and Insourcing Survey* (Deloitte Consulting, 2012).

has expanded to encompass informational technology, business processing and medical services, as well as executive positions and management consulting.[7] The services most frequently outsourced are necessary but nonclinical or non-"core" services (*utility outsourcing*). These include linen and laundry, housekeeping, clinical and diagnostic equipment maintenance, food service, pest control, waste management, patient satisfaction efforts, grounds keeping, and facilities maintenance. The second largest area is *information technology outsourcing* (ITO). This includes computerized physician order entry (CPOE), electronic medical records (EMRs), inbound voice response systems (IVRs), network and data management, automated claims processing, regulated compliance monitoring, application maintenance, system integration, application development, product re-engineering and maintenance, HIPAA consulting, and e-business initiatives. *Business process outsourcing* (BPO) ranks behind ITO overall and for offshore outsourcing. In health care, these services include physician practice management, back end revenue cycle functions (coding, billing, medical transcription), insurance claims processing, collections/receivables management, front end revenue cycle functions (scheduling and registration, patient admission, insurance verification), medical records storage, patient records transcription, and more.

Unique to health care is *medical outsourcing*. Here, as our opening vignette illustrated, health care providers have begun engaging third parties—either domestic or global—to provide medical services. Once referred to as *locum tenens*, medical outsourcing now includes a range of clinical and diagnostic services: telemedicine (electronic delivery of medical services such as radiograph readings, diagnostic test interpretations, videoconference consultations, and tele-ICUs); clinical microbiology and other laboratory services;[8] specialized interventions, such as cataract surgery; emergency department management; and the offshore outsourcing of medical and surgical care to non-US contexts.

---

[7] Sarah Hazelwood, et al., "Possibilities and Pitfalls of Outsourcing," *Healthcare Financial Management* 59, no. 10 (2005): 44.

[8] G. W. Procop, W. Winn, and Microbiology Resource Committee, College of American Pathologists, "Outsourcing Microbiology and Offsite Laboratories: Implications on Patient Care, Cost Savings, and Graduate Medical Education," *Archives of Pathology and Laboratory Medicine* 127, no. 5 (2003): 623–24.

As of 2010, the medical outsourcing market was estimated to be approximately $80 billion, growing at a rate of 12 percent per year.[9] Health plans, hospitals, or health systems may also contract with offshore hospitals to provide medical care for US patients or may purchase and manage hospitals in offshore settings for the same purpose.

The (Bio)ethics of Outsourcing

One will not find an extended analysis of outsourcing in the bioethics or Catholic bioethics literature. However, bioethical frameworks—specifically, a utilitarianism combined with bioethics' four principles (autonomy, nonmaleficence, beneficence, and justice)—have been used by analysts in health care management and medical journals to identify outsourcing's ethical contours.

While outsourcing's potential benefits, identified in the introduction, comprise a short list, the health care management literature has identified a number of potential risks or costs. Some of these are simply pragmatic: liability, management styles inconsistent with system ethos, vendor quality, cultural barriers, potential political instability, time zone management, lack of consistency in international laws and regulations, labor pool costs, and reimbursement questions. At the same time, more substantive ethical concerns surround patient and stakeholder issues.

As the Millbrow example illustrates, outsourcing can negatively impact patient care in significant ways. The primary concerns regarding potential costs or risks to patients in the literature center on questions of informed consent, confidentiality and security of information, and potentially negative impacts of patient-third party interactions. Patients rarely know which system services are outsourced. HIPPA does not require hospitals or other primary care providers to obtain consent to disclose private health information for routine "treatment, payment, and health care operations."[10] Consent forms regarding disclosure usually remain quite nonspecific. Similarly, patient consent

---

[9] J. B. Boyd, M. H. McGrath, and J. Maa, "Emerging Trends in the Outsourcing of Medical and Surgical Care," *Archives of Surgery* 146, no. 1 (2011): 107.

[10] Sanjiv N. Singh and Robert M. Wachter, "Perspectives on Medical Outsourcing and Telemedicine—Rough Edges in a Flat World?" *NEJM* 358, no. 15 (2018): 1624.

is not ordinarily sought for medical outsourcing, e.g., "teleradiology, or even intensive care unit or consultation services," whether domestic or global.[11] Ought patients be informed that their medical or billing records are being outsourced beyond the confines of the health system? ITO, BPO, and medical outsourcing raise issues of confidentiality and security of patient medical and financial information. While confidentiality and information security concerns are most often raised with regard to offshore outsourcing, 40 percent of federal health insurance contractors and state health agencies who outsourced domestically in 2006 reported breaches in personal health information privacy.[12] A primary question in outsourcing discernment is: "How will outsourcing improve patient service and satisfaction?" All outsourced functions—utility services, IT, BPO, and medical—interface with patients at various points. How can a system ensure that a vendor and its employees interact with patients in ways that reflect a hospital's overall mission, values, and policies?

Stakeholders may likewise be negatively impacted by outsourcing, particularly employees and local communities. "Stakeholder issues" include employee morale, general negative economic and relational impacts on local communities due to layoffs and downsizing, and, specifically, reducing or removing essential medical services from local communities. From an economic standpoint, these present negative and non-quantifiable externalities. Outsourcing decisions significantly impact not only employees involved but the entire organization. How affected employees are treated will be known to remaining employees. How does one measure the negative impact of the lack of mission alignment and clinician engagement captured in our opening vignette? Are the potential financial savings sufficient to offset the disruptions in patient care and clinic ethos we encountered?

As the St. Joseph's situation makes clear, hospitals are frequently an area's largest employer and serve as neighborhood anchors, especially in central cities. Thus, a key question is: How will outsourcing benefit or impact the broader community? Outsourcing certainly can have a negative economic impact by eliminating jobs from local

---

[11] Singh and Wachter, "Perspectives," 1624.
[12] Ibid., 1623.

communities, eroding the tax base, and destabilizing families and community relationships. Additionally, might certain forms of outsourcing remove expertise or essential services? Stakeholders are not only local. Offshoring also raises questions regarding the justice of labor arrangements globally. Questions can be raised regarding not only immediate impacts of outsourcing decisions (e.g., job loss in a particular community) but also the ways Catholic institutions participate in or contribute to larger negative macroeconomic trends that may be at odds with Catholic sensibilities.

"The Priority of Persons over Profit": Outsourcing and the Catholic Social Tradition

Catholic bioethics has yet to engage the issue of outsourcing. Yet occasional comments scattered throughout recent papal encyclicals, undergirded by the broader wisdom of CST, and recent reflection on the practice by theologian Albino Barrera enable us to begin to build a framework for discernment around these issues.

Benedict XVI's final encyclical, *Caritas in Veritate,* appears to be the first papal or Vatican document to address outsourcing directly.[13] While not discussed at length, his comments are pertinent, largely raising concerns about outsourcing's negative effects. He begins by identifying the relationship between outsourcing and global economic policies:

> The global market has stimulated first and foremost, on the part of rich countries, a search for areas in which to outsource production at low cost with a view to reducing the prices of many goods, increasing the purchasing power and thus accelerating the rate of development in terms of greater availability of consumer goods for the domestic market. Consequently, the market has prompted new forms of competition between States as they seek to attract foreign businesses to set up production centers, by means of a variety of instruments, including favorable fiscal regimes and deregulation of the labor market. These processes have led to a *downsizing of social security systems* as the price to be paid for seeking greater competitive advantage in the global

---

[13] Benedict XVI, *Caritas in Veritate* (2009).

market, with consequent grave danger for the rights of workers, for fundamental human rights and for the solidarity associated with the traditional forms of the social State.[14]

Equally, Benedict identifies ways outsourcing impacts domestic colleagues, identifying a broad array of stakeholders:

> Moreover, the so-called outsourcing of production can weaken the company's sense of responsibility towards the stakeholders—namely, the workers, the suppliers, the consumers, the natural environment and broader society—in favor of the shareholders, who are not tied to a specific geographical area and who therefore enjoy extraordinary mobility. . . . There is nevertheless a growing conviction that *business management cannot concern itself only with the interests of the proprietors, but must also assume responsibility for all the other stakeholders who contribute to the life of the business*—the workers, the clients, the suppliers of various elements of production, the community of reference.[15]

Thirdly, he acknowledges positive ways outsourcing can impact resource-challenged areas, recognizing that to realize such gains requires outsourcers to participate in responsible, intentional ways in local communities:

> It is true that the export of investments and skills can benefit the populations of the receiving country. Labor and technical knowledge are a universal good. Yet it is not right to export those things merely for the sake of obtaining advantageous conditions . . . without making a real contribution to local society by helping to bring about a robust productive and social system.[16]

In other words, morally justified outsourcing must recognize that it is predicated upon a system that has already increased hardships on the poor; must consistently attend to outsourcing's impacts on domestic and global stakeholders; and requires the *out*sourcer to be *in*volved in the local and offshore contexts.

---

[14] Ibid. 25.
[15] Ibid. 38.
[16] Ibid.

Benedict's position is premised on three key principles from the Catholic social tradition: the concept of integral human development, the dignity and priority of labor, and the principle of gratuitousness. *Integral human development* broadens the focus on development beyond simple economic questions. Economic progress must be sought in conjunction with and subordinated to other goods critical for the full flourishing of human persons in community—physical, spiritual, emotional, psychological, social, and familial goods. The *dignity and priority of labor* has been at the heart of the church's attention to "the social question" from the very beginning.[17] It is a central and primary activity by which persons advance toward full human flourishing. John Paul II repeatedly affirms the church's position from *Rerum Novarum* forward, namely, "the priority of labor over capital": "In view of this situation we must first of all recall a principle that has always been taught by the Church: the principle of the priority of labor over capital." Or, as he will say elsewhere repeatedly: "the priority of persons over profit."[18] Thirdly, Benedict XVI adds a new principle to the canon, noting that "economic, social, and political development, if it is to be authentically human, needs to make room for the *principle of gratuitousness* as an expression of fraternity."[19] For Benedict, the principle of gratuitousness ought to shape economic, social, and political practices: "in *commercial relationships* the *principle of gratuitousness* and the logic of gift as an expression of fraternity can and must *find their place within normal economic activity*. This is a human demand at the present time, but it is also demanded by economic logic. It is a demand of both charity and of truth."[20]

Theologian and economist Albino Barrera, OP, brings these principles into conversation with scripture to develop what he calls "the principle of restoration." When a decision to outsource is made, costs and benefits are asymmetrically distributed. The health system and those who gain jobs reap the benefits (at least on paper), but displaced workers bear the costs, costs that often occur suddenly and are extraordinarily heavy for individuals. While a health system may

---

[17] John Paul II, *Laborem Exercens* 12.
[18] Ibid. 11–15.
[19] Benedict XVI, *Caritas in Veritate* 34.
[20] Ibid. 36.

weather and recover from a painful downsizing, individual workers may never again regain the same economic status they had prior to job loss—if in fact they can find new employment. They may need to leave their communities, uproot their children, move away from long-cultivated networks of friends, family, and other social supports. Often, these workers are "the very people who are least able to bear" the costs.[21] Those whose jobs typically are outsourced—the lowest paid workers—usually have the lowest asset reserves, educational levels, and the fewest alternative options.

In economic terms, these costs borne by displaced workers are referred to as "adverse" or "negative pecuniary externalities" of the process of market exchange. These are often simply considered to be "the cost of doing business."[22] Given the dignity and priority of labor, however, Barrera asks, is there "an obligation to partially reverse the redistribution of burdens and benefits across market participants caused by price adjustments in the normal course of market operations"?[23] The Catholic tradition unequivocally answers, "yes." For Barrera and the Catholic social tradition, costs ought to be born, or at least shared, by those "who reap the benefits of international trade."[24] Having the right to undertake an action like outsourcing entails correlative obligations or duties, particularly duties toward those who bear the costs: "the beneficiaries of this market exchange must help displaced workers make the transition to a new place in the economy."[25]

At the same time, outsourced jobs and services could, at least in theory, be "a potent vehicle for poverty alleviation because of its enormous positive externalities of job creation and technology transfer in poor nations."[26] Outsourcing can, in theory, bring much needed capital to resource-poor contexts, integrate impoverished persons into the global marketplace, assist vulnerable persons, and in many

---

[21] Albino Barrera, "Unintended Consequences and the Principle of Restoration Retrieved," *Journal of Catholic Social Thought* 2, no. 1 (2005): 89.

[22] Ibid.

[23] Barrera, "Outsourcing," 2.

[24] Albino Barrera, "Fair Exchange: Who Benefits from Outsourcing?" *Christian Century* (September 21, 2004): 25.

[25] Ibid.

[26] Barrera, "Outsourcing," 1.

ways help them to "leapfrog the traditional process of industrial development."[27] Outsourcing could, therefore, be a concrete, practical way of practicing the preferential option for the poor. Thus, Barrera asks, "Is there, in fact, an obligation to engage in this business practice?"[28]

The answer here is a qualified "yes." While there is potentially strong support in the Catholic social tradition for economic partnerships that will address poverty, how such practices are implemented is key. For John Paul II, such ventures may well be a form of solidarity, a primary obligation which falls on those with economic means.[29] Pope Benedict echoes his predecessor but emphasizes that "Much depends on the way programs are managed in practice." They must "improve the actual living conditions of the people in a given region." There are "no universally valid solutions," but are highly context-dependent. And the human person must be central to these endeavors.[30]

Execution is the Chariot of Genius: Managing Outsourcing in Light of CST

"Much depends on the way programs are managed in practice." As is the case with many questions in bioethics and the social tradition, the answer with regard to outsourcing is not a simple "yes" or "no" but rather, how? Or, in the words of the English poet and philosopher William Blake: "Execution is the chariot of genius."

While the prospect of outsourcing a particular service might make sense on paper, the ethical downsides could outweigh the benefits. Catholic bioethics informed by CST provide health care leaders with the tools to stop and ask: How will this move impact patient care? How will it affect our employees? And what effects will it have in local communities? Experience and data are beginning to suggest that outsourcing particular services might present short-term financial gain but in the longer term result in significantly higher costs,

---

[27] Barrera, "Fair Exchange," 23.
[28] Barrera, "Outsourcing," 1.
[29] John Paul III, *Sollicitudo Rei Socialis* 39, 42.
[30] Benedict XVI, *Caritas in Veritate* 47.

particularly due to poor vendor performance, undermining of employee morale, or botched community relations.

Beyond the standard framework of utility and the four principles of bioethics utilized by the health care management literature, CST provides a deeper matrix for assessment. Due to its engagement with outsourcing as a general practice (not specifically focused on health care), CST turns our attention primarily to the ways in which outsourcing affects employees and communities. Is our organization, we must ask, committed to the integral development of our employees? Does our organization understand the deep importance of work—including the types of work we offer and how this work is structured—to the flourishing of those who staff our institutions at all levels? These are questions that must be asked at all times, well upstream of a proposal to outsource. How are these questions manifested on a day-to-day basis? Commitment to persons over profits, more often than not, counter-intuitively translates into greater profits, as a fringe benefit of caring for associates. Understanding this requires a longer-term view of institutional effectiveness than taken by many financial practices. Yet in the short term, such commitments make a difference. Recently, St. Vincent Health System in Indianapolis announced layoffs related to a decision to outsource revenue cycle management. Echoing the principle of restoration, St. Vincent's articulated an intention to assist associates to remain at their local facilities or to be moved to a shared service site, with relocation or transportation assistance.[31]

Equally, outsourcing requires that Catholic health systems take time to consider the relationships between their hospitals and their local communities. St. Joseph Hospital was founded in 1882 as a collaborative effort between Franciscan Sisters and the leadership of Milwaukee. City leaders raised the funds for the initial hospital. As it grew, expanded, and flourished, St. Joseph became known as "The Baby Hospital," fostering deep connections with generations of women and their families.[32] With the economic collapse of inner cities

---

[31] John Martin, "St. Vincent Health System Outsourcing to Have Local Impact," *Courier and Press*, April 28, 2017, https://www.courierpress.com/story/money/2017/04/28/st-vincent-health-system-outsourcing-have-local-impact/101052180/.

[32] "About St. Joseph," https://www.mywheaton.org/st-joseph/about/.

in the late 1960s, St. Joseph became a symbol, refuge, and partner for those otherwise abandoned by US culture. In other words, for 130 years, St. Joseph has been working in solidarity with its local community. Losses to these communities—as well as to our associates who live in them—cannot be understood simply as negative externalities, to be borne by the poor or those lower down the org chart. The social capital embedded in these communities exceeds that which can be captured in a financial statement. If the health system—and particularly senior leaders—will reap financial benefits, the principle of restoration calls them to wrestle seriously with how to at least partially reverse the distribution of the burdens and benefits of a decision—to wrestle, in other words, with what the obligation of solidarity continues to require. With Pope Benedict, they must ask: How will this decision improve the actual living conditions of the people in this particular area?

In addition to the local community, concerns about patient care must remain central. As our narrative illustrates, outsourcing can create a weakened sense of organizational and personal responsibility on the part of the outsourcing supplier. If the outsourced activity is considered a "core business," such a weakness could lead to real harm. Especially in the case of medical outsourcing, physicians, RNs, therapists, and techs are about as core to the business of health care organizations—specifically, patient care—as one can be. Experience shows that it does not matter whether the clinician is technically qualified (e.g., is board certified, has deep practice experience, and no malpractice issues); these are "necessary but insufficient" qualifications. While the practice of outsourcing medical services does not necessarily lead to direct harm to patients, given the potential for clinicians to lose sight of whom they are serving in light of the organization's mission and values as they move from site to site, location to location, patients ought—at minimum—be informed of the multiple providers involved in their care.

Conclusion: Market or Mission?

In most health care organizations, decisions to outsource are taken by senior leadership. As such, problems arise when the organization fails to attend to the above commitments, does a poor job of managing the contractual relationship with the vendor, or fails to assess "mission fit" from the outset. Two leadership insights can help forestall the latter two issues. First, outsourcing companies and their staff must be thoroughly vetted to assure they possess not only the "hard stuff"—i.e., technical competency—but equally, the "soft stuff" meaning competencies such as empathy, values alignment, self-awareness, and emotional intelligence. Outsourcing decision-making is best informed by applying a decision-making model which incorporates these three dimensions of a business decision—what DeVita has named the Iron Triangle: the financial, legal, and ethical dimensions, which should incorporate the insights from CST. These three dimensions are equal in importance for decision-making practice and this equality should be, like iron, immutable and inflexible. If decision-makers ignore one dimension, they do so at great risk to the organization.

Secondly, it is critical to build effective relationships with the outsourcing company's leadership team at both a business and the personal level. DeVita names this process E3: encounter, engage, and execute. Simple but not easy, leadership is rooted in relationships that begin with an encounter—knowing who you are working with. Engagement entails creating mutual understanding of the others' intentions, motivations, values, and behaviors which, like all relationships requires time, honesty, and frequent, formal check-ins along the way to maintain and manage the relationship. Such a process enables an organization to maintain a bright line of sight between the outsourcing vendor, the agreement, and the contracting organization's strategic aims including its mission, vision, and values, forestalling disasters such as those encountered at Millbrow.

In the end, outsourcing remains, from an ethical perspective, a legitimate business strategy. However, for Catholic health care the market-based decision to outsource must be grounded in the institution's mission, which is not market based. At all points, Catholic bioethics should raise as a constant refrain the commitment that lies at the heart of Catholic identity, that is, the principle of gratuitousness. St. Joseph's, as we saw, arose out of gift—the gift of the Wheaton Franciscan Sisters who worked tirelessly for decades for little or no compensation and the generous charity of the people of Milwaukee. Indeed, the reality that is Catholic health care was built out of centuries of gift. Catholic health systems are called to witness to the ways in which the logic of gift can transform secular economic, social, and political practices, enabling Catholic health care to develop and provide new models for improving health care delivery—and the health and well-being of persons and communities—in the twenty-first century.

Chapter 16

Catholic Health Care and Population Health: Insights from Catholic Social Thought

Michael Panicola and Rachelle Barina

We open with a fictional but real-world anecdote that represents everyday conversations, pressures, and tensions surfaced in senior leadership meetings at many health systems across the United States.

"Good afternoon," said Bruce Jacobs, the longstanding CEO of Goodview Health System (GHS) to his senior staff. "Today we are meeting to review capital requests for next year and make decisions about how to spend the $200 million of available capital. Our first presenter is Dr. Clara Martinez, an employed family medicine physician who has worked for GHS for over ten years. From the pre-meeting materials, you can see that Dr. Martinez is requesting $20 million to build a comprehensive care management program for individuals, many of whom will be low-income, with complex medical and social needs. Dr. Martinez will briefly summarize her proposal. After she is excused, we will discuss the proposal and eventually share our decisions with all presenters after vetting our recommendations with the board. The floor is yours, Dr. Martinez."

"Thank you, Bruce," said Dr. Martinez. "Since my time is short and you've already read the proposal, I will simply highlight two points and conclude by sharing a story about a patient of mine. First, this program intends to address critical community needs. It aligns with our mission of transforming the health of communities, with particular concern for the poor or marginalized. Our community health needs assessment validated what we have known for years: chronic disease is highly prevalent throughout our communities, especially for preventable and manageable conditions such as heart disease, type 2 diabetes, and obesity as well as issues in behavioral health. Because poverty is prevalent and our state did not expand Medicaid, more than 30 percent of our patients are uninsured or underinsured. And, our community health ecosystem lacks coordination between health care providers and social service agencies. By improving access and coordinating services, this program will help address many of the complex problems faced by our neediest patients.

"Second, and I want to be upfront about this—the program I am proposing will generate, at best, very little profit under the current fee-for-service reimbursement system. We will serve many low-income patients, and if we are successful, we will decrease emergency department utilization and hospital admissions by working with patients before they experience medical crises. We will focus on preventive and primary care, behavioral health, chronic disease management, and palliative care, delivered in outpatient or home settings. We are also working to obtain grant funding to offset costs of the program, but the reality is we will not be a major contributor to GHS's bottom line right now."

"So, with that said," Dr. Martinez continued, "let me tell you about Charles Junior because he is the type of person we expect to serve through this program. I came to know Charles when he was 46-years-old. At the time, Charles, an African American man, had a good paying steel mill job and was living with his wife of twenty-three years and two children. He was in relatively good health. On his first visit, we diagnosed him with type 2 diabetes and mild hypertension. We got him started on a nutrition and fitness program as well as prescribed medications to control the diabetes. For the first year-and-a-half, Charles was very compliant and did well. But he had a major setback when the steel mill closed. His wife still had a modest income, but she did not receive health insurance through her employer and as a family they made too much to qualify for Medicaid. Charles searched for a new job but found only periodic construction work.

"At first, Charles continued to make his regular check-ups, but things began to fall apart. Charles and his family were evicted, and his wife left him. We connected him with social services. But, he began missing appointments. We called him and found his phone was disconnected. I didn't see or hear from Charles for nearly two years—until I got a call from a surgeon seeking a medical history for Charles who needed a below-the-knee amputation due to infectious foot ulcers caused by diabetic neuropathy. I visited Charles in the hospital after surgery and told him I would like to resume caring for him and would do this free of charge. He agreed, and I scheduled an appointment for him, but he never showed.

"Last year, I learned from a colleague that Charles had died following an apparent suicide attempt. For the first few months following the news, I vacillated between blaming myself and blaming the system. We could have managed his health more effectively, perhaps preventing his amputation and helping him cope with his various challenges. So we decided to propose a program that will help others like Charles. This comprehensive care management program addresses the needs in our communities and paves the way for a better care delivery model. I hope you will fund it and I'm happy to answer questions."

"Thank you. Any questions for Dr. Martinez?" Bruce asked. The room was silent. "Alright, in that case, I'd just like to commend you for your compassion and commitment to Charles and all your patients. We will move now to the closed-door session and deliberate as a team." Dr. Martinez thanked the group again as she left.

Bruce invited comments about the proposal, and the chief strategist was first to comment. "It's certainly a laudable program—that's unquestionable. But given our recent operating performance, we have very little capital and can't spend 10 percent of our total amount on something that might have a negative return on investment during the next few years." The chief information officer concurred, adding, "We have at least $125 million simply in hospital maintenance requests and there are other proposals, like hospital renovations and technology purchases, with a ROI in double-digits. We should provide whatever support we can to help Dr. Martinez obtain a grant for her program but not commit our capital dollars."

After a moment of silence, the chief medical officer spoke up: "I agree there are multiple competing programs vying for finite capital dollars. An argument can be made for each one. But this one, particularly, is uniquely aligned with our mission and it is in the best interest of our patients. If we continue to pass on these types of programs because of the short-term ROI, can we honestly maintain we are living our mission and serving the best interests of our patients and communities?"

❖ ❖ ❖ ❖ ❖

In the political, social, and financial context of the United States, debates about health care are occurring on a widespread scale and amongst parties with significant influence. As we have seen in the previous three chapters, stakeholders who have competing interests and widespread concern about health care are not always accompanied by compromise and consensus about a way forward. In this chapter, we explore the opportunity within the United States to increase focus on improving health and promoting healthy communities. We suggest that the drive for change must be grounded not in a capitalist approach but in a broader foundation of health and wellness which aligns with a Catholic vision. This vision calls health care systems to address social determinants of health and calls individuals and health systems to advocate for national policy that will be in the service of improving health across populations.

Problems Plaguing US Health Care

The above scenario, which plays out routinely in boardrooms, is a microcosm of what is wrong with US health care. Despite knowing that programs such as the one proposed by Dr. Martinez will address urgent community needs and lead to better health outcomes for complex patients who churn through the health system, Faustian-like choices are often made that perpetuate the access, cost, and quality problems plaguing US health care. One major reason for this is that the US health system continues to revolve around hospitals, with acute and specialty care receiving the highest levels of reimbursement and absorbing the bulk of the overall budget. Of the estimated $3.5 trillion the US spent on health care in 2017, hospital services accounted for more than 30 percent, and physician/clinical services 20 percent, a substantial portion of which were related to specialty care.[1] In the zero-sum game of health care, this means that other services such as prevention, primary care, chronic disease management, and social services, which can have a far greater and more sustained impact on health, are overlooked and underfunded. To further complicate matters, health care in the US is still largely reimbursed on a fee-for-service basis, which compels health care executives to maximize high-margin acute/specialty services and incentivizes clinicians to provide "non-value added or even inappropriate care, driving up health care costs without benefit and potentially harming patients."[2] The program proposed by Dr. Martinez provides a case in point.

To be fair, a shift is occurring as payers are increasingly tying reimbursement to health outcomes and consumer decisions are increasingly driven by cost considerations. However, the pace of change has been slow and sustaining the inherently flawed acute/specialty care infrastructure that provides questionable value beyond rescue medicine is often the lens through which major decisions are made from system design and capital investments to service offerings and clinical care.[3] Financing and maintaining the current system has come at a hefty price as the US spends more than any other nation on health care. In total, health care comprises a whopping 18 percent of the US gross domestic product (GDP), or nearly one out of every five dollars spent as a nation, which is over 5 percent more than the next highest spending country, Switzerland, at 12.4 percent of GDP.

Yet for all the money poured into the health system, the US lags behind other countries on critical health indicators. In their study of US health care spending vis-à-vis ten other high-income nations, Irene Papanicolas and colleagues[4] illustrate the significant challenges

---

[1] Center for Medicare and Medicaid Services (CMS), "National Health Expenditure Projections 2017–2026," https://www.cms.gov/Research-Statistics-Data-and-Systems/Statistics-Trends-and-Reports/NationalHealthExpendData/Downloads/ForecastSummary.pdf.

[2] Gary S. Kaplan and C. Craig Blackmore, "Time to Sink the Two-Canoe Argument," *NEJM Catalyst*, March 27, 2018, https://catalyst.nejm.org/sink-two-canoe-payment-models/.

[3] For further discussion of this issue, see Michael R. Panicola, "A Cautionary Tale Revisited," *Health Progress* 98 (March–April 2017): 48–51.

[4] Irene Papanicolas, Liana R. Woskie, and Ashish K. Jha, "Health Care Spending in the United States and Other High-Income Countries," *JAMA* 319 (March 13, 2018): 1024–39.

facing the US health care system. The US has a 10 percent uninsured rate (over 30 million people), the highest percentage of all countries studied, which had a mean of 1 percent uninsured. As detailed in Vigen's chapter, the US also has the highest infant mortality rate at 5.8 deaths per 1,000 live births among all the study countries (mean, 3.6 deaths). This rate remains stubbornly high due to relatively higher US poverty rates, a weaker social safety net, and disparities in care highlighted by the fact that black babies die at a rate of 11.3/1,000 live births compared to 4.9 for white babies.[5] Moreover, while the US spends the most on health care, it maintains the lowest life expectancy at 78.8 years among all the study countries (mean, 81.7 years) and the earliest average age of health decline. Finally, the US has the highest percentage of overweight or obese adults at 70.1 percent (mean of 55.6 percent for countries studied), which is a grave concern considering the link between obesity and major chronic conditions or death.[6]

While data tends to provide distance from the reality of tragedy, these are more than numbers—they are people who are sick, suffering, and dying. The US can better address these negative health outcomes, and Catholic health care has a moral imperative to shift trends of overinvesting in hospitals and high-margin specialty care, waiting for people to get sick, and providing episodic, reactive treatment to individuals in medical crisis. A mindset rooted in something deeper and more enduring than capitalist impulses is needed. A vision of health and health care, rooted in the Catholic social tradition (CST), provides a foundation and offers insight into health care delivery and national health policy.

A Catholic Vision of Health and Health Care

One's ability to flourish as a human person and contribute to the common good is greatly affected by health. However, the tendency for most people, especially in cultures where Western medicine has

---

[5] Linda Villarosa, "Why American's Black Babies and Mothers are in a Life-or-Death Crisis," *New York Times Magazine*, April 11, 2018, https://www.nytimes.com/2018/04/11/magazine/black-mothers-babies-death-maternal-mortality.html.

[6] David Blumenthal and Shanoor Seervai, "Rising Obesity in the United States Is a Public Health Crisis," in *To the Point* (The Commonwealth Fund, April 23, 2018).

had a strong influence, is to think about health relatively narrowly in an overly reductionist way, limited to the absence of physical illness. CST, building on the Gospels, affirms a broader view of health as wholeness—"not only physical, but also spiritual and psychological wholeness; not only individual, but also social and institutional wholeness."[7] Wholeness is not simply being free from sickness but an overall experience of well-being including the wider circumstances, communal life, and social conditions in which the person lives. This vision moves beyond a narrow clinical vision of health and into communities and the complexities of people's lives.

Implicit in this multifaceted understanding of health is the recognition that factors beyond one's physical make-up (biology, genetics, condition) and the availability of medical services impact one's ability to lead a healthy life. In fact, research indicates that 60 percent of health outcomes and premature deaths in the US are rooted in other factors.[8] One such factor is personal behavior, which includes lifestyle and coping skills (diet, exercise, alcohol and drug use, smoking, etc.). Yet, health problems are not caused solely by choice or behavior. Closely associated with and often a major driver of individual health choices are social, economic, and environmental factors over which people have little control, which affect health either positively or negatively. Commonly referred to as "social determinants of health," these are the structural factors and "conditions in which people are born, grow, live, work and age,"[9] including among other things: education, housing, food, employment and working conditions; income, wealth distribution, and social status; transportation, social support and safety networks; social inclusion, public safety, exposure to crime, violence, and social disorder; socioeconomic conditions; residential segregation; natural environment and climate change;

---

[7] United States Conference of Catholic Bishops, *Health and Health Care: A Pastoral Letter of the American Catholic Bishops* (November 19, 1981), 4.

[8] See, for instance, Harry J. Heiman and Samantha Artiga, "Beyond Health Care: The Role of Social Determinants in Promoting Health and Health Equity," *Kaiser Family Foundation* (November 4, 2015); and Steven A. Schroeder, "We Can Do Better: Improving the Health of the American People," *New England Journal of Medicine* 357 (September 20, 2007): 1221–28.

[9] Michael Marmot, et al., "Closing the Gap in a Generation: Health Equity through Action on the Social Determinants of Health," *The Lancet* 372, no. 9650 (November 8, 2008): 1661–69.

exposure to pollutants; and physical barriers, especially for people with disabilities.[10]

Recently, there has been growing attention on how significantly social determinants impact health and the ability to engage in healthy behaviors. Harry Heiman and Samantha Artiga aptly illustrate this complex dynamic:

> Social factors, including education, racial segregation, social supports, and poverty accounted for over a third of total deaths in the United States in a year. In the United States, the likelihood of premature death increases as income goes down. Similarly, lower education levels are directly correlated with lower income, higher likelihood of smoking, and shorter life expectancy. Children born to parents who have not completed high school are more likely to live in an environment that poses barriers to health. Their neighborhoods are more likely to be unsafe, have exposed garbage or litter, and have poor or dilapidated housing and vandalism. They also are less likely to have sidewalks, parks or playgrounds, recreation centers, or a library.[11]

A Catholic vision of health care is driven by the goal of helping people experience well-being and wholeness, and thus must account for the many social determinants impeding health.

Implications for Health Care Delivery

A broader conception of health and its determinants lead to a vastly different view of health care. Rather than simply medical services provided to the physically ill, health care takes on the aim of promoting "health and wholeness in all facets of the human person and human community" with the social, economic, and environmental causes of illness becoming a key focus of concern and action.[12]

---

[10] For a list of and discussion about the social determinants of health, see, among others, the Centers for Disease Control and Prevention, https://www.cdc.gov/social determinants/.

[11] Harry J. Heiman and Samantha Artiga, "Beyond Health Care: The Role of Social Determinants in Promoting Health and Health Equity," *Kaiser Family Foundation* (November 4, 2015).

[12] United States Conference of Catholic Bishops, *Health and Health Care*, 4 and 18.

Importantly, this broader understanding of health care is steadily gaining momentum in the US, occasioned primarily by the urgency of reining in unsustainable costs, especially in the face of an aging population with growing demands for resources. Feeling increasing pressure by payers and consumers alike to provide better care at lower costs, health care providers in the US have started to embrace a more holistic approach to health care, one that more closely approximates the conception articulated herein, known as "population health."[13]

Population health generally refers to the health outcomes and distribution of those outcomes within a population, the social determinants of health that influence the distribution of health outcomes among the population, and the policies and interventions that impact the determinants.[14] When applied to health care delivery, population health is a more comprehensive way of thinking about health care, requiring providers to focus not only on clinical interventions aimed at treating illness, but also on the social, economic, and environmental factors that critically impact the health status and outcomes of their patients. Thus, unlike the traditional medical model, a population health approach necessarily involves health care providers in thoroughly assessing and actively addressing patients' unmet socioeconomic and environmental needs such as food, housing, electricity, heat, transportation, and so on. Meeting these needs is not only essential for achieving better health outcomes but is a key measure of success in population health efforts. As Rebecca Onie and her colleagues note:

> Responding to these social needs used to rely on the beneficence of providers, under the often-fickle headers of "mission" or "community benefit." But if population health is to be more than a Ghost Aim, it has to be part of the definition and system of

[13] Population health is one dimension of the so-called Triple Aim, which includes improving the experience of care and reducing the per capita cost of health care. For a helpful explanation, see Donald M. Berwick, Thomas W. Nolan, and John Whittington, "The Triple Aim: Care, Health and, Cost," *Health Affairs* 27 (May–June 2008): 759–69.

[14] David Kindig and Greg Stoddart "What is Population Health?" *American Journal of Public Health* 93 (March 1, 2003): 380–83; and David Kindig, "Understanding Population Health Terminology," *Milbank Quarterly* 85 (February 2007): 139–61.

care, with clear definitions of success. The objective definition of success is when the patient secures the needed resources. Simply handing a patient a list of community resources or other "points for effort" approaches does not count or win anyone partial credit.[15]

Health care providers need to make assessing and addressing the social determinants of health a standard part of care. Even though they will be limited in how much they can directly impact these broader factors beyond the individual level and outside the clinical setting, providers should also engage in advocacy as well as cross-sector public and private partnerships to address social determinants of health on a community-wide scale. Health care providers, especially health systems like the one described in our opening anecdote, are uniquely positioned, given their standing and resources, to serve as a catalyst in transforming the overall health of communities.

Implications for National Health Policy

The shift from traditional health care delivery to population health with its focus on social determinants has been slow to come by in the US. The fee-for-service reimbursement system with its outsized payments for acute/specialty care still causes providers to focus on sick care, neglecting broader factors that impact health. Too often, health care providers view population health myopically, thinking of it merely as a way to improve care delivery and reduce costs for problematic subsets of patients, namely, those with complex medical needs who absorb a disproportionate share of resources that cut significantly into their bottom line or risk-based insurance contracts. Yet, health care providers are not the sole cause of the problem. In some ways, they are simply reacting in a logical way to how the US health system is structured and financed. For sustained change to occur in health care delivery, national health policy itself has to change. By way of conclusion, we summarize three guiding areas of focus.

---

[15] Rebecca Onie and Thomas H. Lee, "Population Health: The Ghost Aim," *NEJM Catalyst,* December 14, 2016, https://catalyst.nejm.org/population-health-ghost-aim/.

1. *Promoting Health Equity*

Rather than simply striving to provide medical services to all patients in need and expending endless amounts of resources in that quest, the overarching health strategy should be to achieve health equity across the US. Health equity describes a goal where every person has the opportunity to be as healthy as possible. Unfortunately, due to socioeconomic and environmental inequities, largely caused by poverty, structural racism, and discrimination, many people in the US are not able to achieve their full health potential. As a result, avoidable health disparities exist throughout groups and communities in the US and are the primary reason for the access, cost, and quality problems in US health care.[16] With a focus on health equity, measured by the reduction of disparities, finite resources could be deployed in different, more effective ways, targeting the root causes of poor health such as unemployment, housing instability, food insecurity, substandard education, illiteracy, crime and violence, incarceration, exposure to pollutants, and lack of access to health care services. Making health equity a primary objective of US health care should result in a course correction, causing us to rethink how we allocate health care resources and enabling us to better integrate health care with vital public health and social services.[17] Whether this will ultimately prove financially beneficial and to whom benefit will accrue is questionable. At least, however, resources will be going to interventions that have proven to have a far greater impact on health than traditional medical care alone.

[16] Health disparities are differences in the social determinants of health that adversely affect groups of people who systematically experience greater obstacles to health based on their racial or ethnic group: religion, socioeconomic status, gender, age, mental health, cognitive, sensory, or physical disability, sexual orientation or gender identity, geographic location, or other characteristics historically linked to discrimination or exclusion. For a discussion of health equity and disparities, see, among others, the Robert Wood Johnson Foundation's work, https://www.rwjf.org/en/library/research/2017/05/what-is-health-equity-.html.

[17] For a discussion of the importance of social services and their role in achieving long-term health on a national scale, see David H. Freedman, "Health Care's 'Upstream' Conundrum,'" *Politico*, January 10, 2018, https://www.politico.com/agenda/story/2018/01/10/long-term-health-nation-problems-000613.

2. *Universal Health Care*

Though health care services account for only 10 percent of health outcomes, lack of access to such services continues to be one impediment to health in the US. The fact that 30 million Americans lack health insurance and millions more are underinsured, especially with the proliferation of high-deductible health plans, is a moral stain on the nation. The CST unwaveringly holds that a certain level of health care must be provided to all. In his encyclical *Pacem in Terris*, Pope John XXIII listed health care as a basic human right.[18] Similarly, the US bishops stated in their pastoral letter *Health and Health Care*, "This right [to adequate health care] flows from the sanctity of human life and the dignity that belongs to all human persons, who are made in the image of God. It implies that access to that health care which is necessary and suitable for the proper development and maintenance of life must be provided for all people, regardless of economic, social or legal status."[19]

Achieving health equity on a national scale necessitates that the US guarantee adequate health care for all—if not for moral reasons, then for practical ones. As the experience and data from other countries show, when virtually all people of a given region or nation are afforded coverage and have access to basic care across the continuum, insurance risk is spread more evenly, the population is actually healthier, and health care is less costly than is the case under patchwork coverage schemes with gaps in care like that of the US.[20] Claims that the US has universal health care because everyone has access to emergency services are patently false. Emergency rooms do not provide the full spectrum of services people need to maintain health and manage disease, and care provided in an emergency department is the most expensive, least effective location of care. For both moral and practical reasons, a universal and coordinated system of care

---

[18] John XXIII, *Pacem in Terris* 11.

[19] United States Conference of Catholic Bishops, *Health and Health Care*, 18.

[20] For a lengthier discussion of this issue, see Michael R. Panicola, "How Do We Create a High-Value Health Care System?" *National Catholic Reporter*, November 7, 2017, https://www.ncronline.org/news/opinion/how-do-we-create-high-value-health-care-system.

that includes preventive care and chronic disease management is essential.

3. *Delivery System and Payment Reform*

For health and health care to be viewed in a more integrated, comprehensive way, the US will have to fundamentally reform how it structures, delivers, and pays for health care. At the heart of this is the decentralization of health care. Hospitals, which for practical reasons have historically been at the epicenter of the delivery system in the US, have evolved from "charitable almshouses for the poor and destitute who could not afford to receive care at home . . . into large, profitable, expensive, technology-laden institutions."[21] Given their high cost and safety issues, the increase in outpatient access points, and the advent of the electronic health record as well as other consumer-friendly technological advances, hospitals no longer serve the same purpose they once did and have actually exceeded their utility as the integrator of care. As other nations have done, with positive results to show for it, US health care should be centered around primary care that is provided in low-cost, accessible outpatient settings, including the home and through technology, with a focus on health promotion, disease prevention, behavioral health, chronic disease management, palliative, and end-of-life care. Hospitals would still have a place in such a delivery system, but they would be secondary to and complementary of these other services, providing high-acuity, specialty care that cannot safely be provided in lower-cost settings (e.g., trauma, intensive care, select surgeries, and high-risk births). To make this feasible, health expenditure trends that favor acute/specialty services and high-tech diagnostics over comprehensive primary care need to be eliminated and replaced with a reimbursement model that adequately incentivizes and compensates providers for effectively managing the health of populations, including assessing and addressing the social determinants of

---

[21] Jennifer L. Wiler, Nir J. Harish, and Richard D. Zane, "Do Hospitals Still Make Sense? Case for Decentralization of Health Care," *NEJM Catalyst*, December 20, 2017, https://catalyst.nejm.org/hospitals-case-decentralization-health-care/.

health.[22] If behavioral economics has taught us one thing, it is that people have a propensity to do the very thing for which they are rewarded most. Right now the US health system is getting exactly the (poor) results for which it pays—specialist-driven, hospital-focused care that misses important health and welfare needs. Continuing to underfund and underpay for primary care and related services while also failing to reimburse providers for tackling the root causes of poor health will prevent the US from establishing a just, sustainable, and effective health system.

These three points are, of course, macro-level policy interventions and achieving them will take compromise and collaboration between many stakeholders. Catholic ministries have a particular obligation from the social tradition to be catalysts in the transformation of US health care. And they are well-positioned to do so. Catholic health care can work toward these goals not only through strategic and advocacy efforts, but also by collaborating with other Catholic and like-minded educational institutions and social service organizations. No single person or organization can achieve systemic change. However, by heeding the call of the Catholic tradition, Catholic institutions can be leaders with an agenda oriented by the common good, a special concern for the lives of the poor and marginalized, and the goal of improving the health of all.

---

[22] There is evidence within US Medicare Advantage plans indicating that primary care centered approaches supported by appropriate incentives result in better care at lower costs for medically and socially complex patient populations. As an example, see Bob Kocher and Christopher J. Chen, "Opportunities for Risk-Taking Primary Care Providers," *NEJM Catalyst*, May 8, 2018, https://catalyst.nejm.org/opportunities-risk-based-primary-care-providers/.

PART FIVE

Embodying Global Solidarity

"Moving the table" takes us not only into the communities that surround our hospitals and clinics; it takes us across borders. The lens of CST brings into view pressing issues in global health. Why should such questions matter for Catholic health care? Do we not have enough to attend to in our own backyard? The chapters in this section challenge that perspective. Global health is an essential topic for Catholic bioethics for a number of reasons. First, given the structures of global inequity, global health is ultimately concerned with health practices and problems—both national and international—that encompass vulnerable and underserved populations, persons named in directive three of the ERDs. Second, in our globalized world, the boundaries between "national" and "international" become increasingly blurred, as practices such as medical outsourcing, clinical research, medical mission trips, and global epidemics challenge ad hoc national boundaries. Third, as Brian Volck reminds us, the church—as the Body of Christ—is the original transnational organization; it transcends national boundaries. If Catholic health care is a ministry of the church, an activity of the Body of Christ, each of us is connected to the vulnerable who suffer in every corner of the globe.

Together, the chapters in part V remind us of what it means to serve in the global South while being cognizant of the dignity, rights, and interconnectedness of each member of the Body of Christ. Rather than showing up with one's own agenda, our authors encourage an agenda that is rooted in the Catholic tradition of the virtues and the practice of the Eucharist as the foundation for cultivating collaborative relationships with global communities. Beyond mission trips and vaccinations for infectious diseases, these chapters turn our attention to the ethical complexities of caring for patients in a myriad of settings, including pain management and end of life, as well as the thorny issue of responding to humanitarian crises.

Pediatrician Brian Volck opens with a challenge to anyone interested—or not interested—in participating in global health outreach. In chapter 17, "Body Politics: Medicine, the Church, and the Scandal of Borders," he offers a first-hand encounter of his experience of the realities and challenges of global health. Volck describes the global experience of poverty and illness in which 15,000 children die each day. Yet, in the US, he notes, we rarely consider that reality, because those deaths tend to be invisible to us. He argues, however, that for Catholics, these deaths affect us directly. Via baptism, God has "called a globally scattered humanity into the body of Christ"—and we are part of that body. This Body of Christ breaks down the artificial borders that have been constructed to separate one nation from another and reveals that we are all, in the words of St. Paul, "members of one another." Thus, Volck envisions a borderless ethic for global health that takes seriously the Christian call to live as one body.

To function as one body, as Volck argues, requires being in relationship with others and aware of all its various parts. In chapter 18, "Creating Partnerships to Strengthen Global Health Systems," Bruce Compton takes up the growing interest among those who work in Catholic health care in developing international outreach activities. While generated from the right impulses—such as those identified by Volck—too often such ventures have negative outcomes for the recipients. Compton counsels health care associates to take a step back and assess more carefully what it takes to serve in these contexts. He argues that the foundation of any global health venture must be a real bilateral relationship. Such relationships, grounded in deep understanding and awareness of our global partners, requires that we establish authentic partnerships that take years, not weeks or days, to develop. He draws a parallel between the collaborative efforts of the religious sisters who founded Catholic health care in the US and the work needed to create partnerships for global health today. In contrast to *Toxic Charity*, Compton draws on his work at the Catholic Health Association to outline guiding principles and practices for strengthening global health systems and partnerships—principles and practices that resonate with the Catholic virtue tradition.

For the most part, however, US Christians do not understand themselves as deeply interconnected to their brothers and sisters in impoverished global settings. As such, these members of the body suffer greatly, not only from acute infectious diseases but from chronic conditions. Their suffering can be magnified greatly during and at the end of their lives. In chapter 19, "Non-Communicable and Chronic Diseases: Putting Palliative Care on the Global Health Agenda," Alexandre Martins—a nurse, theologian, and Camillan priest—narrates the story of Michelin, a 26-year-old Haitian man who discovers his terminal cancer when he suffers a broken bone after a motorcycle accident. The unjust realities of Michelin's story manifest the layers of structural violence that result in lack of access to needed health care services, preventing many chronic diseases from being diagnosed, much less treated. Thus, while noncommunicable and chronic diseases are treated aggressively in the Global North, particularly with pain medications, such conditions go uncontrolled in the majority of the world, causing senseless suffering at the end of one's life. Martins argues that palliative care is not a privilege for the Global North; lack of palliative care across the globe is a glaring injustice. Justice in global health, he posits, begins by hearing the stories of the poor—by listening to and engaging with them as bilateral partners in order to advocate for and with them.

Those who work in Catholic health care feel compelled not only to participate in global health ventures; they often feel deeply moved to act by humanitarian disasters. In chapter 20, "Humanitarian Ethics: From Dignity and Solidarity to Response and Research," Dónal O'Mathúna describes the all too familiar scene of humanitarian disasters that elicit a rash of donations and a flood of volunteers, injecting new chaos into an already chaotic situation. Rather than immediately responding out of one's excess, humanitarian ethics ask how we can best respond to the immediate needs of those in crisis. Rather than presuming that the crisis is accurately depicted by media sources, O'Mathúna cautions that humanitarian crises often reveal deeper social problems within particular contexts, enmeshed as they are in international injustices. Drawing on the work of Jesuit liberation theologian Jon Sobrino, he asks what role human choice has made in the making of natural disasters. With this frame of reference, he calls on Catholic institutions to ensure that any response to a humanitarian crisis is based on well-researched best practices and is rooted in solidarity and, again, bilateral human relationships that cultivate knowledge of local particularities and extend over time.

Chapter 17

Body Politics:
Medicine, the Church, and the
Scandal of Borders

Brian Volck, MD

The Poor Have Names

Some years ago, my son Peter came home from high school with a challenge from one of his teachers, who told the class, "If you say you care about the poor, what are their names?" Peter looked at me, nodded knowingly, and said, "Roberto."

I knew exactly whom he meant. I met Roberto when he was seven, just barely living with his family in a squalid mountainside hut in southern Honduras. Roberto was developmentally delayed. He never reached the table fast enough to eat what little his family could afford, leaving him severely malnourished. Roberto stank. When his family left the clinic, we sprayed the room down before the local staff was willing to use it again. The dentist pulled all of Roberto's rotting teeth to reduce his risk of overwhelming infection. Roberto needed two delousing treatments to clear him, for the time being, of more vermin than I had ever seen on one body. Roberto hurt from hunger, infection, and the harshness of his circumstances, and he made no polite efforts to hide his anguish. With medicine and food, Roberto grew comfortable enough to smile at his mother and even laugh. We, in turn, grew to love Roberto, hope for his future, and help his family to the extent they accepted our assistance. Yet, for a person like me—

coming from a world of deluxe grocery stores, deodorant, and teeth whiteners—Roberto was not easy to like.

Two years later, my son came with me to Honduras and met the boy I had been telling him about. Peter brought his video camera, a hit with the kids at the clinic and in the villages we visited on foot. At the hillside hut where Roberto lived, Peter filmed as we brought Roberto from his hammock to be weighed, but Peter soon put his camera down and silently watched, an electronic veil no longer sufficient to disguise his distress and sense of conviction. From that moment, Peter could not think of the poor without recalling a disturbing face and a single name.

❖ ❖ ❖ ❖ ❖

Like Peter, part of me wishes I had never met Roberto. He once was invisible, and then he wasn't. When I grow comfortable in my privileged American life, Roberto simultaneously convicts and blesses me with fierce hope for his future. He puts a face and body on otherwise mind-numbing statistics. In 2013, an estimated 767 million people worldwide—more than 10 percent of the global population—lived on less than $1.90 per person per day.[1] Half of them were children. In 2016, 5.6 million children worldwide died before their fifth birthday, mostly in poor, so-called developing countries, and for entirely preventable reasons.[2] That is 15,000 child deaths every day. If there is any good news here it's that, thanks to concerted international effort, these figures are less than half what they were twenty-five years ago.[3] The bad news is twofold. First, global reductions in

---

[1] Data cited in International Bank for Reconstruction and Development, *Taking on Inequality: Poverty and Shared Prosperity, 2016* (Washington, DC: The World Bank, 2016), 3.

[2] Lucia Hug, David Sharrow, and Danzhen You, *Levels and Trends in Child Mortality Report 2017* (New York: United Nations Children's Fund, 2017).

[3] Substantial credit for this improvement is due to coordinated global efforts in pursuit of the United Nations' Millennium Development Goals, "Millennium Development Goals Report," 2015, http://www.un.org/millenniumgoals/2015_MDG_Report/pdf/MDG%202015%20rev%20(July%201).pdf. Now continued and expanded as the Sustainable Development Goals, see "United Nations Sustainable Development Goals," http://www.un.org/sustainabledevelopment/. These programs are resonant—though not fully compatible—with Catholic moral and social teaching.

poverty and child deaths have been geographically uneven, further localizing the greatest economic and health disparities to South Asia and Sub-Saharan Africa. Second, what progress has already been made is threatened by growing mass migrations, war, global climate change, and the resurgence of xenophobic nationalism. The coming decades will determine whether the nation states commonly called "developed" are best measured by their moral habits or by their wealth and consumption.

To catch a glimpse of global health disparity, consider that in 2016, there were 36.7 million people in the world with HIV infection and nearly three quarters of them in Sub-Saharan Africa. In a time when antiretroviral therapy has—for much of the economically developed world—turned HIV from a death sentence into a manageable, if life-threatening, chronic disease, more than a million people still die from AIDS-related causes each year.[4] There are equally sobering statistics about the worldwide burden of malaria, TB, or even pneumonia and diarrhea, all conditions for which effective treatments exist and should be readily available worldwide.

Global health disparities are associated with—and exacerbated by—corresponding wealth disparities. In 2012, (the last year for which comprehensive global wealth transfer data are available) the developing world received $1.3 trillion in aid, investment, and income from the developed world. At the same time, developing countries *returned* $3.3 trillion to the developed countries, some in the form of debt interest payments to large banks or profits taken by

---

See also Pope Francis, "Address to the United Nations General Assembly," September 25, 2015, https://sustainabledevelopment.un.org/content/documents/20225pope-francis-eng-.pdf; and United States Conference of Catholic Bishops, "Background on Sustainable Development Goals," http://www.usccb.org/issues-and-action/human-life-and-dignity/poverty/global/background-on-sustainable-development-goals.cfm. The differences are not limited to what does or does not comprise "reproductive health." The UN programs stress technological remedies to a list of individual socioeconomic targets, while relevant passages of *Laudato Si'* focus on systemic, holistic reformation of human relationships with all creation. See, for example, Jason Hickel, Martin Kirk, Joe Brewer, "The Pope v the UN: Who Will Save the World First?" *The Guardian*, June 23, 2015, https://www.theguardian.com/global-development-professionals-network/2015/jun/23/the-pope-united-nations-encyclical-sdgs.

[4] From World Health Organization, "Global Health Observatory data," http://www.who.int/gho/hiv/en/.

corporate investors, but far more through unrecorded—and often illegal—corporate money transfers.[5]

The immensity and apparent intractability of global inequities drive many good people into cycles of guilt and perceived powerlessness, and ultimately to passive resignation. If it were not for the occasional television commercial soliciting donations for starving children, few outside the disciplines of public health would give them much thought. As to any moral obligations to reach across international borders and class divides and rectify these disparities, standard Anglo-American medical ethics, preoccupied with questions of autonomy and technology, has little to say.[6] When US political discourse rises above explicitly nativist and xenophobic speech, the result is often a few politically expedient band-aids: promises of aid that may or may not pan out, programs begun but never completed, money draining away through the sieves of waste and corruption.

While the Catholic Church is no stranger to waste and corruption, it has compelling theological reasons to find this state of affairs not merely unacceptable, but truly sinful. Central to our understanding of the church is that God calls a globally scattered humanity into the Body of Christ. We are linked through baptism across arbitrarily drawn national borders not only to the world's billion fellow Catholics, but to all Christians. We are likewise related to all humanity, even those "who, without any fault of theirs, have not yet arrived at an explicit knowledge of God, and who, not without grace, strive to lead a good life."[7] Nor is this the concern of a select few within the church, but part of the "Universal Call to Holiness," in which all, regardless of rank or status, must "wholeheartedly devote themselves to the

---

[5] See Global Financial Integrity, "New Report on Unrecorded Capital Flight Finds Developing Countries are Net-Creditors to the Rest of the World," December 5, 2016, http://www.gfintegrity.org/press-release/new-report-on-unrecorded-capital-flight-finds-developing-countries-are-net-creditors-to-the-rest-of-the-world/; and Jason Hickel, "Aid in Reverse: How Poor Countries Develop Rich Countries," *The Guardian*, January 14, 2017, https://www.theguardian.com/global-development-professionals-network/2017/jan/14/aid-in-reverse-how-poor-countries-develop-rich-countries.

[6] See Paul Farmer, *Pathologies of Power: Health, Human Rights, and the New War on the Poor* (Berkeley, CA: University of California Press, 2003), 204; and Paul Farmer and N. Gastineau-Campos, "Rethinking Medical Ethics: A View from Below," *Developing World Bioethics* 4, no. 1 (2004): 17–41.

[7] Vatican Council II, *Lumen Gentium* 16.

glory of God and to the service of their neighbor."[8] For Catholics—most certainly including those in health care—to ignore the welfare of those beyond their national borders is a failure of imagination, nerve, and duty.

Autonomy and Idolatry

I suspect few American Catholics—and those who survey their opinions—think much about medicine and theology outside of high-profile teachings on abortion, physician-assisted suicide, and contraception. Fewer still think theologically about Christian obligations across borders, whether national or ethical. North American Christians have ceded considerable authority to biomedicine, accepting with minimal critique its assumptions, language, and logic. Chief among the claims Christians should question is the primacy of personal autonomy, the belief—especially among the materially comfortable—that we are in control of our own lives.

The United States follows a particularly fanatical form of the cult of the individual, making the isolated patient the basic unit of health. This is curious, since the most significant measurable improvements in health over the last century had more to do with public health interventions—vaccinations, improved sanitation, and so forth—than individual encounters between doctor and patient. Anglo-American medical ethics typically focuses on tough individual cases at the margins of life: embryonic stem cell research, physician-assisted suicide, or how dead a body must be to harvest its organs for transplant. Physician and social critic, Paul Farmer, the founder of Partners in Health and the subject of Tracy Kidder's book, *Mountains Beyond Mountains,* calls these the "quandaries of the fortunate."[9]

Farmer works in Haiti and other parts of the world where extreme poverty, malnutrition, and infectious diseases such as HIV, tuberculosis, and malaria make North America look like another planet. In Farmer's world, infectious disease makes its own preferential option for the poor. Medicine and medical ethics in the US render large parts

[8] Ibid. 40.
[9] Farmer, *Pathologies of Power*, 175.

of the globe invisible—out of sight, out of mind—so that we lack even the vocabulary to talk about the poor with whom we share the earth.

Catholics have done little better—and sometimes worse—than other religious traditions in thinking theologically about borders and health care. Though Catholics are more likely than other Americans to be immigrants or children of immigrants,[10] Catholic organizations that assist immigrants with social integration, "identified the 'receiving community'—i.e., lack of community support, racism, anti-immigrant sentiment, and restrictionist immigration policies—as the largest obstacle they faced."[11] What is absolutely scandalous, however, is the way in which Catholics in the US have permitted economic boundaries and national borders to shape our consciousness. When churches ask, "Is this good for us?" or, "Is this good for America?" instead of "Does this serve the poor, the weak, and the ill in whom Christ is found?" the pressing questions do not concern church-state relations, but idolatry.

Nation-states establish borders. Their governments enforce and guard them. Christians acknowledge the nation-state's legitimate authority but, isolated verses from Romans 13 notwithstanding, we must never confuse the limited authority of the state with that of the God revealed in Christ. To do so makes an idol of the state. Christ commands us to serve the poor, not the deserving poor, not the poor with proper documents, or the poor whose welfare coincides with US geopolitical objectives.

Resources from the Catholic Tradition

Paul Farmer, working against the hellish injustices US-supported Haitian dictators imposed upon the people, found no language sufficient to describe his experience until he encountered Catholic liberation theology. Phrases like "preferential option for the poor" and "structural sin" captured what standard bioethics ignored. The pil-

[10] M. Lipka, "A Closer Look at Catholic America," Pew Research Center, September 14, 2015, http://www.pewresearch.org/fact-tank/2015/09/14/a-closer-look-at-catholic-america.

[11] D. Kerwin and K. Barron, "Building Structures of Solidarity and Instruments of Justice: The Catholic Immigrant Integration Surveys," Center for Migration Studies, March 2017, http://cmsny.org/publications/ciiisurveysreport/.

grimage to justice begins with naming the sin. In responding to health care inequities, Catholics have much to draw on from Scripture, the early church, and Catholic social teaching.

In chapter 11 of the First Letter to the Corinthians, Paul details the social obligations inherent to the celebration of the Eucharist. Paul has heard that some of the Corinthians gathered for the liturgy eat and drink unworthily, by "not discerning the body." The wealthy are not meeting the real needs of the poor who approach the table hungry and thirsty. With this failure, Paul says, the powerful eat and drink condemnation upon themselves. He then describes the church as a body in which every part is essential to the whole. In 12:26, he says: "If one member suffers, all suffer together with it; if one member is honored, all rejoice together." The God revealed in Christ calls us together as a eucharistic Body not because we like each other or are like-minded, but because we need each other.

But the Body does not stop at the walls of the building we call the church. The church goes on down the street, across the county, the state, the country, the world. In the Last Judgment scene in Matthew 25, the Son of Man sits before "the nations," separating sheep from goats, not based on a calculus of success, power, or celebrity, but by what the gathered nations did "to the least of these": the hungry, thirsty, estranged, naked, sick, and imprisoned. Matthew's Jesus is straightforward here: take care of these folks, or you can go to hell. That's why church tradition names these practices (not the ideas of the practices, but the practices themselves), corporal acts of mercy.

In the so-called Good Samaritan parable in Luke 10, a man lies half dead at the side of the road, where a priest and Levite pass him by. A third traveler sees the injured man, stops, provides first aid, takes him to shelter, and pays for his care. The scandal here is that the injured man's neighbor is a Samaritan, whom first-century Palestinian Jews considered an enemy, outside the law, and hostile to God's people. To first-century Jewish ears, a "Good Samaritan" makes as much sense as a "good suicide bomber" or a "good mass shooter" makes to us today. That a Samaritan might observe the law better than those who constantly study it reinforces the universality of the law—the love of neighbor (Lev 19:18) in particular—while extending its obligations past boundaries and borders Jesus' hearers thought uncrossable.

Early Christians took these obligations seriously, and their non-Christian neighbors took note. The anonymous Christian author of the second-century Letter to Diognetus felt it necessary to explain his community's peculiar manners:

> They live in their own countries, but only as aliens; they participate in everything as citizens and endure everything as foreigners. Every foreign country is their fatherland, and every fatherland is foreign. They marry like everyone else, and have children, but they do not expose their offspring. They share their food but not their wives. . . . In a word, what the soul is to the body, Christians are to the world. The soul is dispersed through all the members of the body, and Christians throughout the cities of the world.[12]

In church historian Rowan Greer's assessment, "at one level, the Church grew rapidly more because its common life acted as a magnet attracting people than because the Christians were effective in their public preaching."[13] From the fourth century's early hospitals to the Byzantine and Western medieval *xenodochia*, *xenones*, and hospices (the root from which all these institutional terms derive can mean "guest," "host," "foreigner," and "stranger"), the church prioritized care for the poor, the sick, and the pilgrim.[14] Benedictine practices of hospitality became models for new religious orders founded specifically to care for the sick.[15] Medieval universities created the first western medical schools, and the Catholic Church remains the largest non-governmental health care provider in the world, with more than half its facilities in the "developing" world.[16]

[12] "The Epistle to Diognetus," in *The Apostolic Fathers*, ed. M. Holmes (Grand Rapids, MI: Baker Books, 1992), 541.

[13] Rowan A. Greer, *Broken Lights and Mended Lives* (University Park, PA: Pennsylvania State University Press, 1986), 123.

[14] See T. Miller, *The Birth of the Hospital in the Byzantine Empire* (Baltimore: Johns Hopkins University Press, 1995); and Gary B. Ferngren, *Medicine and Health Care in Early Christianity* (Baltimore: John Hopkins University Press, 2009).

[15] See R. Porter, *The Greatest Benefit to Mankind—A Medical History of Humanity from Antiquity to the Present* (New York: Harper Collins, 1997).

[16] Robert Calderisi, *Earthly Mission: The Catholic Church and World Development* (New Haven, CT: Yale University Press, 2013), 40. Not everyone considers this a good thing. See J. Stone, "Healthcare Denied At 550 Hospitals Because of Catholic Doctrine,"

Catholic social teaching makes clear that concern for global health—among other goods—is not the province of a saintly few, but a required and universal solidarity that may demand real change in how we think and act.

> All must consider it their sacred duty to count social obligations among their chief duties today and observe them as such. For the more closely the world comes together, the more widely do people's obligations transcend particular groups and extend to the whole world. This will be realized only if individuals and groups practice moral and social virtues and foster them in social living.[17]

John Paul II was particularly forceful on this matter:

> Solidarity responds morally to the growing interdependence among all individuals and nations that is the hallmark of globalization. Solidarity is not a feeling of vague compassion or shallow distress at the misfortunes of so many people, both near and far. On the contrary, it is a firm and persevering determination to commit oneself to the common good; that is to say, to the good of each and every individual, because we are all really responsible for all.[18]

Elsewhere, the late pope made clear that a commitment to global solidarity must include redress of health disparities:

> there is an increasingly urgent need to fill the very serious and unacceptable gap that separates the developing world from the developed in terms of the capacity to develop biomedical research for the benefit of health-care assistance and to assist peoples afflicted by chronic poverty and dire epidemics. . . . It is essential to realize that to leave these peoples without the resources of science and culture means to condemn them to

---

Forbes Magazine, May 7, 2016, https://www.forbes.com/sites/judystone/2016/05/07/health-care-denied-at-550-hospitals-because-of-catholic-doctrine/.

[17] Vatican Council II, *Gaudium et Spes* 30.

[18] John Paul II, *Sollicitudo Rei Socialis* 38.

poverty, financial exploitation and the lack of health care structures, and also to commit an injustice and fuel a long term threat for the globalized world.[19]

When read in the light of Christian tradition from the first century to the present, there is nothing revolutionary in the rigorous and universal demands of these recent documents. Any novelties to be found are no more than specific applications to particular modern conditions.

Embodying the Tradition

What, then, are we to do? My experience is that generic Americans— without reference to theology or religion—are individually generous in times of crisis. Show video clips of drowned villages or earthquake-shattered cities and our checkbooks fly open, as described in Dónal O'Mathúna's chapter later in this section. But even before CNN stops covering those villages, we are already busy with other things. What with so many immediate concerns and a thousand other causes jockeying for our attention, our compassion quickly fades.

But when you know someone who is suffering—when it is your brother or the homeless woman you could not avoid on your way to work—forgetting is not so easy. Bodily encounters redefine the borders of our compassion. Which brings us back to Paul's insistence on the Eucharist joining us in the same body with those who suffer. By sharing the Body and Blood of Christ, we lose the privilege of choosing if and when to address the needs of our sisters and brothers in Syria, Haiti, or Harlan County. When members of Christ's Body suffer, my compassion (literally, "suffering with") is no longer optional.

I anticipate two objections to the approach I am taking here. First, none of us is used to talking about health this way. In matters of community health, Christians from the global North usually abandon theology for rights-talk such as, "people have a right to health care."

---

[19] "Address of John Paul II to the Members of the Pontifical Academy for Life," February 24, 2003, 6, http://w2.vatican.va/content/john-paul-ii/en/speeches/2003/february/documents/hf_jp-ii_spe_20030224_pont-acad-life.html.

Surely this claim is in some way true, but I am not sure what it accomplishes, not only because it leaves undefined how much health care we have a right to, but more importantly because it turns the enforcement of such rights over to nation states, like the United States, or Haiti, or North Korea. Long before anyone even heard the word "globalization," the church understood itself as transcending boundaries, just as the demands of the law transcended the boundary between Samaritan and Jew.

What practices might we adopt if we are to start living as a body? First—and this will sound crazy in the face of the world's profound needs—worship regularly and well. When you present yourself for the Eucharist, know what you are getting yourself into. All else flows from this. "Eucharist" in Greek literally means to give thanks, and we cannot begin to be generous until we are thankful for the undeserved graces God has already given us.

In Deuteronomy 8, Moses warns those about to cross the Jordan into "the good land," not to forget the God who led them there, nor imagine they've earned their blessings. As Walter Brueggemann notes, "Israel does not have many resources with which to resist temptation. Their chief one is memory."[20] On the cusp of the Promised Land, the people of Israel remembered their suffering in Egypt, their miraculous emancipation, and God's many wilderness mercies. Genealogically, I am the descendant of German draft dodgers, drunkards, and bigamists who came to America for a shot at prosperity, for which I am grateful. More importantly, though, "A wandering Aramean was my ancestor" (see Deut 26:5), and for that I am eternally grateful.

But remember what demands accompany this gratitude: forgiveness, peace, and service to the Body of Christ. If you are not ready to shoulder these tasks, ask for that grace at communion. The Eucharist is meant to transform us. Jesus was downright promiscuous in sharing meals, breaking bread with tax collectors and prostitutes, but he did so precisely so they could leave as something more than tax collectors or prostitutes.

---

[20] Walter Brueggemann, *Deuteronomy* (Nashville: Abingdon Press, 2001).

Second, as a church community, resist the power of medicine to make the poor and suffering invisible. If church teaching is undeniably clear what technologically driven moral boundaries we should not cross, it is similarly clear about embodying the corporal acts of mercy. Rather than merely stating an opposition to abortion and euthanasia, open your church and your homes to the pregnant teen, the intellectually disabled, the terminally ill. If the developed world values some diversities more than others, as in the effort to eliminate Down syndrome through prenatal identification and selective termination, show the world a better, more inclusive way. When communities share the burdens of the sick among you, including driving people to the doctor or assisting with medications and treatment, the desperate pursuit of individual health loses its urgency. When we consider as a group what treatments really serve the gathered body, we resist the commodified and individualized way medical care is sold. As a group, learn about the needs of the poor and ill among and near you. Support one other in bodily presence and direct service. As a community, let this cost something dearer to you than you would like: your time, your spare room, your schedule.

For the poor of the world, become as aware of their needs as you are of your physical body. Learn as much as you can about one problem or one part of the world: HIV or malnutrition, Guatemala or the inner city, and then ask, "What can I—what can we—do to be present to this?" If you can, participate in a mission service trip with an organization that consults and works with the people they serve. Avoid those that presume to already know what the poor need and how to provide it. If you cannot travel, you can support a medical mission, child, school, or hospital. Do more than send a check. Write a letter, share your commitment with friends, get your church involved.

Workers in Catholic health care should model and advocate for awareness of and service to the stranger and sojourner among you. Leaders in Catholic health care should know and heed the scriptural, theological, and magisterial tradition regarding our interdependence within the Body of Christ and our common duty to the neighbor. Any nominally Catholic health care institution systematically neglecting that duty should be called to account by members of the Body. Active outreach to those in need—locally to begin with and, if and when possible, across borders—should be encouraged.

Conclusion:
It's Your Body. Act That Way

These, of course, are preliminary steps, prelude to a more substantial conversion. For Christians, that conversion begins when we stop acting as if health were something held in isolation, as if extravagant claims to autonomy and individual choice were true, or that the people of God have nothing to say about the practice of medicine. As Wendell Berry so elegantly puts it:

> The grace that is the health of creatures can only be held in common.
> In healing the scattered members come together.
> In health the flesh is graced, the holy enters the world.[21]

"The holy enters the world." Sounds like a birth. I have never given birth myself, but I have been present at quite a few, including those of my sons, and I have noticed they are painful. Modern anesthesia masks this reality, but not completely. Giving birth to faithful practices of health is painful, too, in much the same way that Roberto's refusal to vanish causes me pain.

Roberto died two years after he met my son. I am not sure of the circumstances, but his death did not come as a surprise. Poverty and disease know no mercy. Even so, Roberto's disturbing presence remains. In the communion of saints, that cloud of witnesses it would often be easier to live without, he still shows me what it means to suffer together as a body. When I think of Roberto, the words that come to mind are not, "There, but for the grace of God, go I," but rather, "There *by* the grace of God go I." Roberto not only abides in my memory, he shares my body, sustaining a fierce and undimmed hope. For Peter and me, he is not only the face of the poor. He is the face of Jesus.

---

[21] Wendell Berry, *What Are People For?: Essays* (San Francisco: North Point Press, 1990), 10.

Chapter 18

Creating Partnerships to Strengthen Global Health Systems

Bruce Compton

For centuries, Catholic health care has responded to the call to advocate for and create partnerships to strengthen health systems globally.[1] With the reconfiguration of Catholic health care into systems, combined with the growing awareness and commitment to global health, this call remains a challenging one. I open with two stories that capture some of the complexities.

First, consider Ernest Sirolli. Ernest went to Zambia on a mission to help a local community grow tomatoes. The cooperative locals planted the tomatoes in what looked like a perfect location chosen by the foreigners. The tomato vines grew perfectly, and everything looked great. They left one evening as the tomatoes were starting to ripen, turning nicely red. When they returned the next morning, all the tomatoes were gone. Stunned, they asked the locals "What happened?" The locals responded, "Well, the hippopotamuses came out of the river. The tomatoes were planted in the river bottom, and the hippopotamuses came out and ate all the tomatoes like they always do. That's why we don't plant anything there."[2]

---

[1] For a good overview of the history and scope of Catholic health care's global initiatives, see Robert Calderisi, *Earthly Mission: The Catholic Church and World Development* (New Haven, CT: Yale University Press, 2013).

[2] Ernest Sirolli, "Truly Sustainable Economic Development," *Ted Talks*, September 18, 2012, https://www.youtube.com/watch?v=SpIxZiBpGU0.

Or consider a typical scenario that might happen in a Catholic hospital.[3] Two hospital associates sit at a lunch table. One is talking about a church mission to Guatemala from which she has just returned. She believes their hospital ought to start a medical mission, saying, "All it'll take is our passports and plane tickets." Her lunch partner responds: "Oh, well let me know. I'd love to see Guatemala and my wife could maybe do some shopping down there as well. I'm sure she'd love to see Guatemala."

These stories capture snapshots of just two problems at the heart of many global health initiatives. Too often, such ventures are about us and our solutions. We forget at best to inquire, and ignore at worst, the concerns, ideas, and knowledge of the local communities. A critically important first step in any global initiative is to get to know the local community in a textured, in-depth way. It is critically important to know if there are hippopotamuses, where they are, and what they eat! The only way to do that is to develop relationships and partnerships with the people who have this knowledge—namely, members of the local community.

Developing relationships takes time, immersion, commitment, and the willingness to let questions be defined and solutions to be shaped by those who do not *appear* to have what we count as either knowledge or power. Moreover, while bringing our health care expertise to remote and underserved corners of the globe might sound like a good idea or exciting, it can be a burden and distraction for the local communities. When we do not understand or address adequately all the problems of even our own neighborhoods, how can we begin to take on the responsibility for the immense problems that face the world at large? When we see the face of the homeless family in Haiti suffering from the consequences of Hurricane Matthew, when we see a fledgling health system before the hurricane, dying infants in Africa, mothers without medication for AIDS in Kenya, or the disfigurement of a war survivor somewhere else in the world—a voice deep within us convicts us that these persons, too, are our brothers and sisters,

---

[3] Catholic Health Association, "Video Scenario—Conducting Mission and Immersion Trips," https://www.chausa.org/international-outreach-video-scenarios/video-scenario---conducting-mission-and-immersion-trips/video-scenario---conducting-mission-and-immersion-trips.

and their suffering cries out to God. We feel called to respond to that suffering. However, that response does not start with a plane ticket. It starts from within. We must pause for discernment.

❖ ❖ ❖ ❖ ❖

Often what we see at first glance in the developing world—either in photos or in person—is hard to interpret accurately. While images and stories that come to us through social media may conjure certain feelings, do we really know the history behind the story? Who are the players? Do they really need help? Who took the picture or made the film? What is their agenda, their role, their objective? It is hard to know the answers to these questions based solely on the images.

As it is with images, so it is with the realities of global health and health care. Even for those who move beyond images to visit countries struggling with health injustices, it is difficult to understand the complexities of any particular place or how to accurately interpret what they are experiencing in order to determine the appropriate response. While the global realities of providing health care and the global reach of US Catholic health systems' initiatives to develop partnerships is relatively new, the model for how best to provide that care is not. When religious communities, primarily religious sisters, came to the US over 150 years ago, they were not embarking on a short-term mission. They came for the long-term with a vision of working to create long-term effects. They moved into urban centers or rural outposts and became integral members of those communities. They thought carefully about how they were going to develop structures and an infrastructure to care for those in need. They were not going to do this work, however, without the support and participation of the communities in which they resided.

The approach of the religious sisters began with a discernment and emphasis on working with local communities. This approach lies at the foundation of Catholic health care both locally and globally. To mirror the focus of the religious sisters requires a deeper commitment than what one encounters on a typical one or two-week immersion prominent in global health today. In this chapter, I outline why it is time to pause and carefully assess the way we think about and approach global health. I specifically draw on the work of the Catholic

Health Association (CHA), Catholic social teaching (CST), and the insights of religious communities to develop a model for global health that emphasizes the importance of discernment, preparation, and program design for those engaged in global health initiatives.

Toxic Charity:
Short-Term Medical Mission Trips

A primary way that private US institutions and committed persons have approached global health is through short-term medical mission trips. Over the past two decades the number of short-term international trips for the provision of health services has dramatically increased. According to Harvard medical school study, an estimated 6,000 medical missions are sent from the United States to lower middle-income countries every year with an annual expenditure of at least $250 million.[4] While some would say that these estimates are very low, the statistics communicate the prevalence of these brief experiences in global health. Though these initiatives provide some benefits to participants on both sides of the relationship, they also raise consistent concerns about the value and effectiveness of short term medical mission trips. These include:

- Lack of Preparation, Selection, and Qualities of Volunteers—All must have the ability to work with a team, to train local staff for patient care, knowledge of local customs/culture, and willingness to learn from the local community.

- Absence of Needs Assessments—Just over half of current missions conduct a needs assessment. Too often the needs are being identified by the US partner. Needs assessment must be managed by the international partner or equally co-managed with the US partner.

- No Mutually Developed Goals—Likewise, international partners overwhelmingly indicate their desire to be more involved in the

---

[4] Jesse Maki, Munirih Qualls, Benjamin White, Sharon Kleefield, and Robert Crone, "Health Impact Assessment and Short-term Medical Missions: A Methods Study to Evaluate Quality of Care," *BMC Health Services Research* 8, no. 121 (2008).

process of defining the goals and activities of missions, which are heavily controlled by US partners.

- Length of Trip—One week or less is far from the ideal amount of time for a medical mission.

- Limited Involvement (Role) of the US Partner—Capacity building is equal to or more important than clinical care. Interviewees consistently reiterate the need for training and capacity building.

- Unusable In-kind Donations—The majority of international organizations had received support with medical products, vaccines, and technologies. Most, however, neither have nor know about quality control guidelines for supplies being brought in by volunteers. Thus, donations are inconsistent with the greatest needs and are at times unusable.[5]

Many of these concerns, while problematic, can be improved upon by engaging the local community in planning and education.

As an analogy, we would think it preposterous to simply show up in a community in the US and start giving out shots or pap smears for a week or to suggest that after such an intervention, one could assess the results. One would always want to be sure that there was follow up. Yet too often, we think that by simply going to a particular country and delivering an intervention, we can address these issues. We are presented with troubling images through media, and we think we have technological and medical aptitude available in the US to address many of the health-related issues regardless of context. However, we fail often to consider the potential long-term implications of our brief stays in local communities.

In spite of deep commitments on the part of those engaged in global health work, the results of the significant investment of resources in development and global health initiatives over the past thirty years has been ambiguous. Yet, at the same time, many critics today focus on what is going wrong. Over the past decade, a new

---

[5] Michael D. Rozier, Judith N. Lasker, and Bruce Compton, "Short-term Volunteer Health Trips: Aligning Host Community Preferences and Organizer Practices," *Global Health Action* 10, no. 1 (2017): 8.

genre of books has emerged that highlights the limited effects of a wide-range of charity initiatives that fail to live up to the ideals behind many community services opportunities. The first chapter of Robert Lupton's *Toxic Charity* describes widely popular charity efforts as "The Scandal," which reflects many of the challenges cited above. Chapter two offers a further diagnosis of the problem by highlighting "The Problem with Good Intentions." Similarly, in 2014, Judith Lasker's *Hoping to Help* takes to task the "Tsunami of Volunteers" that descend on places in the midst of crisis (see also Dónal O'Mathúna's chapter 20).[6] In *When Helping Hurts*, Steve Corbett and Brian Fikkert frame the challenge with a story about a faith-filled person who acted without the participation of the local community and his guilt about his failure to understand the local situation and to empower others to participate.[7] Finally, Dambisa Moyo and Niall Ferguson's *Dead Aid* examines the more than one trillion dollars in development-related aid that has been transferred from rich countries to Africa, exploring the question: has this assistance improved the lives of Africans? The answer they arrive at is: no. In fact, across the continent the recipients of much of this aid are "not much better off" as a result of brief encounters with medical volunteers. Some say these encounters leave the community worse than they found it, much worse.[8]

Thus, if our goal is to strengthen health systems internationally, it is not enough to merely show up and perform procedures or to send money, though both of those may be part of the solution. Given that these initiatives entail significant human and economic investment but do not yield the desired outcomes, how do we ensure that "good intentions" are not "toxic"? How do we gain a better understanding of these activities and consider how they can be conducted so as to maximize the benefit for all involved?

---

[6] Robert D. Lupton, *Toxic Charity: How the Church Hurts Those They Help and How to Reverse It* (San Francisco: HarperOne, 2011); and Judith N. Lasker, *Hoping to Help: The Promises and Pitfalls of Global Health Volunteering* (Ithaca, NY: ILR Press, 2016).

[7] Steve Corbett and Brian Fikkert, *When Helping Hurts: How to Alleviate Poverty Without Hurting the Poor and Yourself* (Chicago, IL: Moody Publishers, 2014).

[8] Dambisa Moyo and Niall Ferguson, *Dead Aid: Why Aid is Not Working and How There is a Better Way for Africa* (New York: Farrar, Strauss, and Giroux, 2010).

Guiding Principles and Practices:
Catholic Social Teaching Meets the Virtues

To assist Catholic health systems to strengthen health systems around the world, in 2015 CHA issued a document entitled "Guiding Principles for Conducting International Health Activities."[9] The document identifies six guiding principles for conducting international health activities as well as a series of recommendations for practice. These principles bring to life the richness of Catholic social teaching and tradition—particularly the commitments to the preferential option for the poor, participation, subsidiarity, and solidarity. Equally, they draw on the depth of the Catholic moral tradition, a tradition of the virtues of prudence, authenticity, honesty, patience, excellence, and humility.

The first guiding principle is *prudence*. Prudence, as all Catholic bioethicists should know, is for Thomas Aquinas the chief cardinal virtue.[10] Prudence recommends: "Don't just do it." In the absence of prudence, the enthusiasm to do good can create more harm than good. Lupton argues, motives alone are not sufficient.[11] Certainly, we mean well, our motives are good. But too often, we neglect to conduct careful due diligence to determine the myriad of emotional, economic, and cultural outcomes on the receiving end of our charity. Why do we miss this crucial aspect in evaluating our charitable work? Because he says, as compassionate people, we have been evaluating our charity by the rewards *we* receive through service rather than the benefits received by those served.[12] We have failed to adequately calculate the effects of our service on the lives of those reduced to objects of our pity and patronage. This unidirectional, self-centered approach to charity is equally a failure of true solidarity. With that in mind, we must ensure that when conducting international outreach, we act with prudence and appropriate respect. We should act

---

[9] Catholic Health Association, *Guiding Principles for Conducting International Health Activities* (St. Louis, MO: Catholic Health Association, 2015).

[10] For succinct introductions to prudence, see James F. Keenan, "The Virtue of Prudence," in *The Ethics of Aquinas*, ed. Stephen J. Pope (Washington, DC: Georgetown University Press, 2002), 259–71; and Daniel Westberg, *Right Practical Reason: Aristotle, Action, and Prudence in Aquinas* (New York: Oxford University Press, 1994).

[11] Lupton, *Toxic Charity*, 127.

[12] Ibid., 5.

with prudence in planning, implementing, and evaluating all of our international health activities.

The second principle is *authenticity*. Authenticity highlights the intersection of solidarity and participation. Charles Taylor notes that true authenticity moves us beyond the good relative to ourselves, which as noted above is linked to "toxic charity," and requires dialogue, innovation, but also agreed upon horizons that are significant in understanding oneself. These norms, however, are constantly negotiated.[13] For Taylor, authenticity is that which comes to be discovered in and through relationships. What should be at the core of global health work is an emphasis on creating authentic and collaborative relationships.

Creating partnerships is about retrieving what is important and criticizing practices that do not meet the ideal. In short-term mission work, however, there may be little room for being critical of practices or dialogue with partners. Yet, authentic collaboration requires both knowing yourself and your partner. Successful and authentic work is organized and productive and does not settle for a facile acceptance of "the way things are." Instead, it works with a resolve to do better and move toward a goal with local partners. The principle of authenticity reminds us that we must work with a local partner, strive to understand everyone's motives, and be honest regarding our goals if we are going to do our best work.

Related to authenticity is *honesty*, which provides the critical and necessary foundation of trust. Being honest and communicating truthfully can be difficult because of the power dynamics involved in many of these global health partnerships. On the outside, it is a relationship of unequals. Many Westerners believe they come in to "fix" a problem. However, insofar as these relationships are authentic they have to begin by establishing an open and honest partnership. However, this trust is not a given, but is earned and learned.

Consider, for example, the case of Hurricane Mitch. US mission teams rushed to Honduras to help rebuild homes destroyed by the storm and subsequent landslides. While well meaning, expenditures

---

[13] Charles Taylor, *The Ethics of Authenticity* (Cambridge, MA: Harvard University Press, 1991), 64–72.

for a week of service by church and college groups was grossly out of proportion with what was actually accomplished. In total, such teams spent on average $30,000 per home—for homes that could have been built by local people for $3,000 each. It is difficult, however, in the midst of a humanitarian crisis to communicate honestly when you have great need or to be honest when you are motivated to respond to great needs. Nevertheless, we have to think about the implications. We feel good, but we possibly prevent someone with local skills from making money. We spend ten times more than it would have cost locally. Being honest with our partners, asking them to be honest with us is another way of practicing solidarity and creating an authentic partnership. Creating the space for this type of communication is extremely important for our long-term success. We must ensure honesty in all of our communications in order to build meaningful and lasting partnerships.

Creating this space and engaging in this sort of conversation requires another classical Christian virtue, *patience*. It takes patience to build capacity, not dependency. However, compassionate people desire to see action on behalf of struggling communities, and Americans are results-oriented, evaluating so many aspects of our lives—particularly within Catholic health care—in terms of short-term metrics. But *building* capacity and *strengthening* an infrastructure—from which resources have been extracted through the long history of colonialism, compounded by the destruction wrought by wars or natural disasters, and now exacerbated by structures of neoliberal economics—takes *time*.[14] We must practice patience in getting to know our partner's history, context, and culture, to understand all of their assets and their true needs. We also need to understand our own assets and our true motivations in doing this work. That, too, takes patience. As I have said more than once, we have to honestly evaluate the benefits and the limitations of all of our interventions in order to assist in building capacity for the long term that addresses the true needs of a community. By building capacity, we transform hurt into hope (a theological virtue).

[14] John Paul II, *Sollicitudo Rei Socialis*; and Jim Kim, Joyce V. Millen, and Alec Irwin, *Dying for Growth: Global Inequality and the Health of the Poor* (Common Courage Press, 2002).

The fifth principle is *excellence,* yet excellence cannot be considered only in terms of observable outcomes, nor do they equal best practices. We want to avoid the pitfall of our well-intentioned efforts providing little more than "junk for Jesus!" As we do this work, we have to promote excellence by demanding high standards that result in quality service delivery, that result in strong health systems around the world. This commitment to excellence is equally a commitment to human dignity and the preferential option for the poor. It does not honor human dignity to give expired medications to poor patients or broken medical devices to resource-challenged communities simply because it is "better than nothing" or they would just otherwise go to waste. It also manifests the preferential option for the poor. As Paul Farmer has stated, the poor deserve the highest quality care because they have been given the least because of the structures of poverty and sin.[15] To give less than the most excellent care, attention, or facilities to the poor states clearly that we think they are worth less as persons; in doing so, we continue to undermine their dignity.

Finally, we end with the virtue of *humility.* We all have something to learn, but we often lead with pride, as if we know all that needs to be known and have all the skills necessary. Humility requires an understanding that we are not perfect, that we lack important strengths, that we are flawed and sometimes fail, that we can learn from others. Many programs and ministries actually work at cross-purposes with the goals to meet the needs of the local communities. The transition from betterment to development is really important, and we have to be aware that we do not have all of the answers, and that we need to encourage mutuality and respect. Humility, likewise, points to the way we understand these collaborative relationships. It requires a recognition of the other, allowing local communities to lead. Rather than planting tomatoes for hippos—a bad name for an aid organization—we need to recognize our own limits and the strengths of our partners by asking questions in order to learn how best to work with the community.

[15] Michael Griffin and Jennie Weiss Block, eds., *In the Company of the Poor: Conversations between Dr. Paul Farmer and Fr. Gustavo Gutierrez* (Maryknoll, NY: Orbis Books, 2013).

Despite the United States being technological leaders in health care, we have much to learn about developing collaborative partnerships to meet the health needs of our global partners. We do not want to export our system throughout the world, but we can support others as needed and learn from others. This process requires humility; we do not know it all; we do not understand everything about the places that we are going. Therefore, we need to be prudential in developing authentic partnerships grounded in honest communication that requires a humble assessment of what leads toward an improvement of the global health systems in which we operate.

Practical Recommendations for Establishing Global Health Care Partnerships

What might these principles look like in practice? In this final section, I would like to highlight a few examples of initiatives that have committed for the long-term and seek to create sustainable partnerships. Several large Catholic health systems are taking the time to study and understand the needs in places and to develop long-term partnerships with people on the ground. Different systems employ different approaches. Here, I highlight three, and then link to further examples. In addition, I will point to some examples from my own work in Haiti.

Dedicate institutional resources to establish global health partnerships. Providence-St. Joseph's Health System (PSJH) has developed an entire department dedicated to educating and forming their associates that participate in short-term interventions. They are working with a local medical school in Guatemala on the ground, as well as their medical school in the United States, and they have an educational liaison.[16] Thus, even though PSJH uses the model of short-term mission trips, this partnership enables them to build a relationship over time, patiently, with their colleagues in Guatemala; it provides a structure for them to practice authenticity—to allow their Latin

[16] See Providence Health and Services, "Global Partnerships," https://www.providence.org/about/global-partnerships.

American partners to take the lead in identifying local needs and goals while equally meeting the needs of the PSJH associates.

Utilize a discernment resource that orients, reflects, and processes each phase of short and long-term experiences. CHA has developed a discernment guide that takes people through a step-by-step process of reflection that covers all phases of such trips.[17] It was developed in response to many health professionals being unprepared for the reality of the communities in which they were partnering and a genuine lack of orientation. The discernment guide walks participants from the time of preparation prior to leaving on an international health activity, during the time in-country, at the point of departure from abroad, through and beyond the return. It helps participants assess: Does this work really make sense? What does it really mean? What does it mean for me? What does it mean for the people that I am serving? What does it mean for the greater good that I am hoping to be part of? How does this help in that work? In essence, the guide attempts to foster each of the virtues for establishing collaborative global partners.

Get to know your global partner by establishing open and honest communication about the gifts, talents, needs, and expectations of both partners. The Ascension Global Mission project shifted the paradigm away from short-term mission trips and committed to "an initial five-year period of listening, learning, and working collaboratively with local partners," to more honestly understand the needs and resources of the community in order to determine how best to contribute to community health improvement.[18] Their Guatemalan partners were surprised by this approach, repeatedly asking, "What are you going to give us? What project are you bringing to us?" Their partners were not used to being consulted or having a voice. They expected that Ascension, like other US organizations, was simply bringing a project and the relationship was focused on Ascension's desire to "help," not partner. Equally, Ascension's expectations were challenged. They

---

[17] Catholic Health Association, *A Reflection Guide for International Health Activities* (St. Louis, MO: Catholic Health Association, 2016).

[18] Andrea Findley and Susan Huber, "Ascension Global Mission in Guatemala: Shifting the Paradigm for More Effective Giving," *Health Progress* (January–February 2017).

learned that they needed to not only find in-country partners, but to invest time in listening and learning at the community level much earlier in the process, to develop not only partners but co-leaders, and to enable not only community participation but community *ownership* of initiatives. Replete with words like patience and trust, they learned the importance of humility, mutuality, and respect.

A final example of a collaboration approach has been adopted by Holy Name Hospital in Teaneck, New Jersey. For over twenty years, Holy Name staff had volunteered at Hôpital Sacré Coeur in Milot, Haiti. Their passion for the people of Haiti grew stronger and deeper. So much so, that in 2012, Holy Name Medical Center acquired The CRUDEM Foundation, Inc., a 501(c)(3) non-profit founded in 1995, devoted to providing financial, volunteer, and medical resources to Hôpital Sacré Coeur. Now, The CRUDEM Foundation functions under the Holy Name umbrella of exceptional healthcare facilities and programs. They are working with patients, doctors, administrators, and others to try prudently to understand how to invest the right resources to make this Haitian-operated hospital sustainable, just like the women religious did here in the United States years ago.

Conclusion:
More than Passports and Plane Tickets

As we advocate for and create partnerships to strengthen global health systems, we in Catholic health care know that we are compelled to continue Jesus' mission of love and healing in the ways we can today. US-based Catholic health care organizations are already reaching out to our communities here at home and around the world to establish partnerships that work collaboratively to improve overall health status and their quality of life. This tradition of international ministry is a testament of the commitment of associates from across Catholic health ministry to live up to the gospel mandate to provide compassionate care, with special attention to those most in need. International projects, like those in the United States, call for careful consideration. Through technological advances, the increasing travel infrastructure, and social media, we are making global connections. The principles I have outlined above and the tools described demonstrate that it takes more than passports and plane tickets to do this work well. While bioethics has commented extensively on global health inequalities, it is my hope that this chapter establishes a framework for evaluating ethically the importance of creating global health partners grounded in a relationship of mutual trust.

Chapter 19

Non-Communicable and Chronic Diseases in Developing Countries: Putting Palliative Care on the Global Health Agenda

Alexandre Andrade Martins, MI, PhD

Michelin was a twenty-six-year-old man with cancer in the final stage of his young life. His existential journey was not long, ending precociously after a journey searching for health care assistance until he arrived at our hospital in Mirebalais, where he died peacefully. Michelin, as is typical of people his age, had dreams and plans for his life. Pursuing his dreams in the midst of poverty and lack of opportunities, as is the reality in Haiti, Michelin bought a small motorcycle and became a moto-taxi driver, blending his passion for motorcycles with the possibility to make some money to survive. One day, already feeling weak, Michelin had a motorcycle accident that severely damaged his left leg. Michelin's friends took him to a public hospital in Port-au-Prince, but the doctors were on strike and not available. His friends took him and searched for another place where they could find a doctor. With no success, Michelin returned home to the small village where he lived with his mother. A few days later, someone told Michelin that he could find a doctor at the University Hospital of Mirebalais, an institution supported by the NGO Partners in Health. Fortunately, after this less-than-ideal delay, Michelin received all the needed treatment for his leg. Unfortunately, his doctors also discovered that he had cancer, which had spread into his bones.

I arrived at Mirebalais about a month after Michelin had begun his cancer treatment; he was already in palliative care. My relationship with him and his mother was short, but meaningful. We provided the best care available, and he died with dignity comforted by his mother.

I learned a lot listening to him and his mother, a strong woman who had to travel two hours to be with her son. She was a widow and had no other children. She did not have money to make this trip every day. She basically stayed all the time in the hospital and, often enough, she had to sleep on the ground outside the hospital because she did not have a place to go. After her son died, she said, "I am sad because my son passed away. But I am thankful for all the care you gave to him and for seeing us as human beings who deserve your attention."

❖   ❖   ❖   ❖   ❖

Michelin's case is useful to show elements involved in non-communicable diseases (NCDs) and palliative care in low-income countries. It begins with the structural violence that makes poor people vulnerable and generates lack of health care assistance. Michelin was feeling sick before the accident, but finding a doctor to understand why he was feeling weak never appeared to him as an option. As a result, his undiagnosed cancer went untreated. This increased his risk of having a motorcycle accident. After the accident, another violence occurred: no health care! He was lucky to find the Hospital in Mirebalais, but it was too late.

Health care assistance must not be a matter of luck, rather, it is a matter of human rights and responsibilities. In Mirebalais, he received care, first curative treatment, and then palliative care. He could not be healed, but he could be cared for in a respectful way that preserved his dignity. Unfortunately, palliative care was limited because of the lack of resources needed to care for his mother. Her situation revealed the structural violence of which she was also a victim.

NCDs and chronic diseases are present in the reality of the poor. They make many people suffer and kill many others. Global health must address this disease burden. Michelin's case is an example of the need for palliative care as part of the global health agenda in low- and middle-income countries. This agenda needs an integral and holistic vision of care able to integrate health care and social justice. Here narratives and Catholic social teaching have a strong potential to contribute to the expansion of palliative care in poor areas and actions of care along social justice in global health.

The World Health Organization defines palliative care as:

> An approach that improves the quality of life of patients and their families facing the problems associated with life-threatening illness, through the prevention and relief of suffering by means of early identification and impeccable assessment and treatment of pain and other problems, physical, psychosocial and spiritual.[1]

Initially, palliative care focused only on patients who did not respond to curative therapy, relegating palliative care to the last stage of care. It was also centered on patients, neglecting families and communities. Nowadays, the focus on terminal patients still exists in many countries, making palliative care almost synonymous with hospice care.[2] However, palliative care has been extended to embrace chronic, life-limiting diseases without an immediate prospect of death, such as HIV, cardiovascular diseases, and diabetes; involve families and communities; and consider not only the physical needs of patients, but also their social, emotional, and spiritual needs.[3] In addition, palliative care has been put on the global public health agenda by the recognition of its need in low- and middle-income countries.[4]

---

[1] World Health Organization, "Palliative Care," http://www.who.int/ncds/management/palliative-care/introduction/en/#.

[2] This is the perspective of many regarding palliative care in Brazil where many health care providers and institutions limit palliative care to terminal patients, especially those with cancer, and elderly patients with dementia and degenerative chronic disease. For a presentation on this limited perspective on palliative care, see Ludugério de Souza, et al., "Cuidados Paliativos na Atenção Primária à Saúde: Considerações Éticas," *Revista Bioética* 23, no. 2 (May 2015): 349–59; Leo Pessini, "Vida E Morte Na UTI: A Ética No Fio Da Navalha," *Revista Bioética* 24, no. 1 (2016): 54–63.

[3] Cecilia Sepúlveda, et al., "Palliative Care: The World Health Organization's Global Perspective," *Journal of Pain and Symptom Management* 24, no. 2 (August 2002): 92.

[4] Richard A. Powell, "Putting Palliative Care on The Global Health Agenda," *The Lancet* 16, no. 2 (2015): 131–32. See also the WHO general assembly that addressed the need on palliative care in the global health agenda.

Palliative care is not a privilege of high-income countries but a global health commitment that must be part of the agenda of public health actions and advocacy for health care as a human right.[5] Michelin's case shows the importance of accessing palliative care to promote patients' quality of life and death with dignity. We cannot always heal, but we can always care.

Non-communicable, Chronic, and Terminal Illnesses: The Need for Palliative Care in the World of the Poor

Conventional wisdom holds that the immense majority of the poor die because of communicable diseases, especially tropical diseases. The rich, or those who live in high-income countries, die because of non-communicable diseases (NCDs), primarily cancer and cardiopathies. This conventional wisdom captures only part of the truth about the leading causes of death in low- and middle-income countries. True, communicable diseases are killing people in these nations. HIV/ AIDS and tuberculosis are still the leading causes of death in Sub-Saharan Africa.[6] However, NCDs also kill people in low- and middle-income countries. NCDs are responsible for 38 million deaths each year, cardiovascular diseases being the reason for 17.5 million deaths annually, cancers 8.2 million, respiratory diseases 4 million, and diabetes 1.5 million. The majority of these deaths occur in low- and middle-income nations.[7]

Evidence-based studies have shown that NCDs are a huge burden for the poor. Cardiovascular diseases are the number one cause of death and disability in the world. Close to 80 percent of these deaths occur in low- and middle-income countries.[8] A study in rural Haiti shows that heart failure is the most common cause of hospitalization and that the "majority of cardiovascular disease morbidity is in low-

---

[5] Liz Gwyther, et al., "Advancing Palliative Care as a Human Right," *Journal of Pain and Symptom Management* 38, no. 5 (2009): 767–43.

[6] Eve Namisango, et al., "Possible Direction for Palliative Care Research in Africa," *Palliative Medicine* 30, no. 6 (2016): 517.

[7] Ibid.

[8] Gene F. Kwan, et al., "Descriptive Epidemiology and Short-Term Outcomes of Heart Failure Hospitalisation in Rural Haiti," *Heart* 102, no. 2 (2016): 140.

income and middle-income countries."[9] Health systems fail to reach these people. Available data is only derived from those who arrive at urban hospitals. Therefore, the reality of cardiovascular diseases in low-income countries is worse than the available data shows. Another evidence-based study shows that in the sixteen poorest countries in the world, 34 percent of the combined cardiovascular diseases and congenital heart anomalies accrued in people under 30 years of age.[10] Among other factors for cardiopathies, the most prevalent are increasing "exposure to indoor and outdoor air pollutions, schistosomiasis, tuberculosis and sickle cell disease . . . using solid cooking fuels, over-crowding, poor hygiene and lack of access to basic health care."[11]

Studies also show that cancers have high incidence in low- and middle-income countries. Projections are that by 2025, 75 percent of cancer cases worldwide will occur in developing nations.[12] In most African countries, cancer control is difficult because of low awareness, late-stage treatment, and poor survival.[13] Cancers along with HIV/AIDS are "the two diseases that predominantly contribute to Africa's disease burden for conditions that require palliative care."[14] The world has testified to a shift in the global burden of diseases to NCDs in which cancer claims increasing responsibility for morbidity and mortality in low- and middle-income countries. An estimated 65 percent of cancer deaths occur annually in these countries.[15]

---

[9] Ibid., 145.

[10] Gene F. Kwan, et al., "Endemic Cardiovascular Diseases of the Poorest Billion," *Circulation* 133, no. 24 (2016): 2562–75.

[11] Kwan, et al., "Descriptive Epidemiology and Short-Term Outcomes of Heart Failure Hospitalisation in Rural Haiti," 142; Kwan, et al., "Endemic Cardiovascular Diseases of the Poorest Billion," 2565.

[12] C. Norma Coleman, et al., "Establishing Global Health Cancer Care Partnerships Across Common Ground: Bridging Nuclear Security, Equitable Access, Education, Outreach, And Mentorship," *The Lancet* 4, special issue (2016): 14.

[13] Sten Z. Zelle, et al., "Costs, Effects and Cost-effectiveness of Breast Cancer Control in Ghana," *Tropical Medicine and International Health* 17, no. 8 (2012): 1031–43.

[14] Eve Namisango, et al., "Possible Direction for Palliative Care Research in Africa," 517.

[15] Faluso Ishola and Oluwatosin Omole, "A Vision for Improved Cancer Screening in Nigeria," *The Lancet* 4, no. 6 (2016): e359.

The burden of NCDs in low- and middle-income countries goes beyond cardiopathies and cancers.[16] Therefore, the global health agenda must include a significant effort to address NCDs in low- and middle-income countries, including palliative care initiatives. According to WHO, over 20 million people require palliative care at the end of life every year.[17] About 80 percent of these people live in low- and middle-income countries.[18] "The great majority of adults in need of palliative care died from cardiovascular diseases (38.5 percent), or cancer (34 percent), followed by chronic respiratory diseases (10.3 percent), HIV/AIDS (5.7 percent), and diabetes (4.5 percent)."[19] Among children, interesting data shows that 49 percent of children in need of palliative care are in Africa.[20] In addition, "as populations age and societies industrialize, the number of people who will need palliative care to manage the problems associated with chronic progressive illness, especially cancer, are predicted to increase in low-income and middle-income countries."[21]

Although the burden of life-limiting and life-threatening diseases is higher in these contexts, 80 percent of palliative care is delivered in high-income countries.[22] This corresponds to less than 14 percent of the total global population that needs this kind of care.[23] Research has shown the cost-effectiveness of hospices and palliative services.[24] This evidence has led to a huge investment in these services in high-income countries, where most of the evidence-based research

---

[16] See, for example, this study on chronic kidney disease in Nicaragua, P. A. Clark, J. Chowdhury, B. Chan, and N. Radigan, "Chronic Kidney Disease in Nicaraguan Sugarcane Workers: A Historical, Medical, Environmental Analysis and Ethical Analysis," *The Internet Journal of Third World Medicine* 12, no. 1 (2016): 1–16.

[17] World Health Organization, *Global Atlas of Palliative Care at the End of Life*, 25, http://www.thewhpca.org/resources/global-atlas-on-end-of-life-care.

[18] Ibid., 16, 20.

[19] Ibid., 13.

[20] Ibid., 20.

[21] Richard Harding and Irene J. Higginson, "Inclusion of End-of-Life Care in the Global Health Agenda," *The Lancet* 2, no. 7 (2014): e375.

[22] Ibid.

[23] World Health Organization, *Global Atlas of Palliative Care at the End of Life*, 71.

[24] Ibid., 62.

in palliative care takes place. On the other hand, research in low- and middle-income countries is severely lacking.[25] African specialists, for example, in end-of-life care affirm, "The level of health care coverage remains low in Africa, access to palliative care limited and research systems poor."[26]

These studies provide evidence that NCDs and the need for palliative care are issues to be addressed in global health, especially in low- and middle-income countries. Palliative care is an inter/multi-disciplinary approach grounded on an integral vision of the human person and his/her relations with his/her own body, fears, beliefs, and hopes as well as with family, friends, health professionals, community, and society. Studies also show that important actors for an adequate palliative care find it difficult to handle and even most health professionals lack specialized education in this area.[27] In general terms, experiences suggest that four areas must be addressed to develop palliative care services: efficient local and national health policies;[28] specialized education and training for health professionals, caregivers, family members, health workers, and communities;[29] broad availability of medication, including the access to opioid pain relief; and implementation of palliative care in all levels of care, from primary care[30] to tertiary and specialized care.[31]

[25] Ibid., 31.

[26] Eve Namisango, et al., "Possible Direction for Palliative Care Research in Africa," 517.

[27] Souza, et al., "Cuidados Paliativos na Atenção Primária à Saúde." See also World Health Organization, *Global Atlas of Palliative Care at the End of Life*, 27.

[28] World Health Organization, "Palliative Care."

[29] Liliana DeLima, "How Can We Monitor Palliative Care? Suggestions from the Latin American Association for Palliative Care," *International Journal of Palliative Nursing* 19, no. 4 (2013): 161.

[30] The Brazilian Public Health System has developed good initiatives around palliative care in primary care; see, for example, Souza, et al., "Cuidados Paliativos na Atenção Primária à Saúde."

[31] I shaped these areas based on WHO's orientations for effective approach in palliative care and suggestions of the Latin American Association for Palliative Care. See WHO, "Palliative Care"; DeLima, "How Can We Monitor Palliative Care?," 160–61.

The Art of Care as Attention to the Poor's Dignity and Justice

Jesus embraced the principles of the art of care, as he was the master of compassion and solidarity with the destitute sick. In Jesus' time, being sick was a reason for exclusion and marginalization: a sick individual was an unclean person, unworthy of participating in the society. Consequently, marginalization, suffering, and poverty were the natural paths of a sick person. Jesus' encounters with the destitute sick were moments of recognition of the other who suffered in a movement of compassion.

Although technically Jesus did not offer palliative care for the destitute sick, his relationship with the destitute sick offers a paradigm for reflection on palliative care in the context of global health and poverty. Thus, Jesus' encounter with the destitute sick was a revolutionary movement of compassion and *active care*. In a society in which the sick were not worthy of any care, such as the ten destitute people with skin diseases who met Jesus on his way (Luke 17:14-17), Jesus showed his compassion as a concrete act of care and offered them an opportunity of social inclusion. With this act, Jesus not only cared for the destitute sick, but also broke this institutionalized violence by showing that these people were worthy of care by integrating them into society. Palliative care in global health begins when we recognize the destitute sick as those for whom we are all responsible to care for and not only as recipients of crumbs from the table of rich nations. However, palliative care medication for chronic and non-communicable diseases are not considered cost-effective in low-income countries.[32]

Catholic tradition embraces this perception of care from the recognition of the face of the destitute sick, essential to support the urgency of palliative care. The biblical passage suggested above shows Jesus going beyond the healing aspect in caring for someone sick. Jesus' actions toward those who were sick incorporated the social dimension of care because he acted to promote quality of life and to reintegrate the marginalized sick into social life. Jesus was not only

---

[32] Paul Farmer, "Chronic Infectious Disease and the Future of Health Care Delivery," *The New England Journal of Medicine* 369, no. 25 (2013): 2424–36.

worried about the biological aspect of the destitute sick, but also about promoting a life with dignity to the human being and his/her participation in social life.[33] Based on this christological perspective, Latin American bishops say,

> Health is a biographic experience: covering the different dimensions of the human person and it has an intimate relationship with the particular experience that a person has with his/her own corporality, with his/her place in the world, and with the values on which he/she builds his/her existence. In short, we can say that health is a harmony between body and spirit, a harmony between person and environment, a harmony between character and responsibility.[34]

This harmony requires an approach able to integrate palliative care into global health inside socially just actions. Care and justice must walk hand in hand. The parable of the Good Samaritan (Luke 10: 25-37) shows care and justice as active social principles to be embraced by health care delivery. The action of the Samaritan toward the destitute sick embodies solidarity as a social principle[35] that cares and promotes justice without making distinction among people. Cost-effectiveness is not the logic of the Samaritan, but rather the recognition of dignity of the poor sick who need assistance and the neighbors responsibility to provide that. "This parable helps us think about solidarity and vulnerability inside the reality of the poor."[36]

If we fail to contemplate the suffering face of the destitute sick, care and justice are only an abstraction. Our contemporary society talks a lot about poverty, marginalized people, lack of opportunities, and health inequalities. Everyone who is talking about this reality of poverty and suffering with millions of early deaths has suggestions to address these issues. Many develop beautiful theories and systems to end poverty. However, those who are actually suffering are not

[33] Conferência Nacional dos Bispos do Brasil, *Campanha da Fraternidade 2012: Texto-Base* (Brasília: Edições CNBB, 2011), 181.
[34] Conselho Episcopal Latino-Americano, *Discípulos Missionários no Mundo da Saúde: Guia para a Pastoral da Saúde na América Latina e no Caribe* (São Paulo: Centro Universitário São Camilo Press, 2010), 8.
[35] John Paul II, *Sollicitudo Rei Socialis* 38.
[36] Conferência Nacional dos Bispos do Brasil, *Campanha da Fraternidade 2012*, 186.

mere numbers, statistics, nor a distant people we do not know.[37] In health care, the sick and the poor are totally anonymous, without face or voice. And they are dying every day. Many people create solutions for them but do not know who they are. These possible solutions are very arbitrary, non-democratic, and elitist because they come from people who are not victims of structural violence nor do they share life with the victims or listen to them. Listening to the poor, engaging them in dialogue, and promoting their participation are essential to caring and to promoting justice in a context of health inequalities. This is the reason that I have not presented here only numbers and evidence-based studies showing the need of palliative care in global health. I also presented Michelin, a real face, a voice in need of care and justice, a representative of the poor suffering from NCDs in low-income countries.

Catholic social teaching presents the preferential option for the poor as a principle to guide actions in global health toward care and justice for the poor.[38] The preferential option for the poor in health is a perspective that integrates care and justice. In addition, this option leads health professionals, policy makers, and global health activists to dialogue with the poor, listen to them, and engage them in actions of health care delivery, including palliative care. Experiences of community-based approaches—with community health workers in the process of caring for those who are sick and more vulnerable to diseases—have proven to be effective in health care delivery. Studies show that community health workers are an essential part of health care delivery in low and middle-income countries.[39] Palliative care strategies must count on the contribution of community health workers. They, along with community-based centers and health profes-

---

[37] Simone Weil affirms that one of the problems of our contemporary society is that we do not see those who are suffering. They are invisible in our society. She says that only when we can see them, can real transformation happen. And to see them, it is necessary to be touched by suffering. Simone Weil, "L'amour de Dieu et le Malhuer," in *Œuvres*, ed. Florence de Lussy (Paris: Quarto Gallimard, 1999), 691–716.

[38] John Paul II, *Sollicitudo Rei Socialis* 39; Francis, *Evangelii Gaudium* 198.

[39] Kyounghae Kim, et al., "Effects of Community-Based Health Worker Interventions to improve Chronic Disease Management and Care Among Vulnerable Populations: A Systematic Review," *American Journal of Public Health* 106, no. 4 (2016): e3-e28; Farmer, "Chronic Infectious Disease and the Future of Health Care Delivery," 2425.

sionals, interact directly with families in their homes and communities, providing a care that is also attentive to patients' and families' social and emotional needs.

Practical Recommendations:
Starting Points for a Conversation

How might a Catholic health care ministry committed to global health include palliative care in its agenda? While some of these recommendations are referenced in other chapters, I hope here to provide a way to engage with the complex realities of NCDs and the need for palliative care. These thesis statements below stand alone because, as Compton's chapter indicates, they need to be applied in conversation with local partners. Therefore, these recommendations serve as starting points for a conversation, rather than final conclusions:

- Cultivate a missionary spirit, in which Catholic health care ministry goes beyond national borders to serve in areas marked by poverty;

- Create interdisciplinary groups focusing on palliative care and Catholic ministry in global health;

- Invite community members to be part of these groups;

- Introduce Catholic social teaching in these discussions and seek for ways to apply them in global health;

- Create awareness around social issues and their relevance for health/health care;

- Analyze local realities, their social/health issues, and their main challenges for palliative care;

- Promote studies on palliative care and its impacts on health care assistance;

- In global health missions, choose a community-based approach of health care delivery to involve the participation of local members (see Compton chapter);

- Make dialogue a core methodological/pastoral approach;

- Listen to the locals, learn their perspective, engage them in decision-making processes and activities;

- Provide education on end of life to health professionals and local communities;

- Educate and cultivate Catholic social principles, such as solidarity, participation, justice, and option for the poor;

- Train community members to be health workers and to serve in palliative care teams;

- Develop strategies of palliative care that go beyond hospitals and clinics in order to include homecare, involving communities and families;

- Create advocacy groups that strive for the integration and expansion of palliative care in public health care systems.

Conclusion:
Expanding Palliative Care on the Global Health Agenda

Evidence-based studies, data, and narratives prove that the poor carry the burden of non-communicable and chronic diseases. They also show the urgent need for palliative care as part of the global health agenda in low- and middle-income countries. From this empirical reality, I suggest reflecting on care as attention to dignity and justice for the poor. Care and social justice together, including an active role of the poor and local communities, provide a foundation to develop strategies to embody palliative care into the global health agenda in low- and middle-income countries. Care and justice cannot be separated in bioethics, especially in the reality of the poor.[40]

Catholic principles that ground bioethics and actions in health care of Catholic organizations put the destitute sick at the center of Catholic health ministry. This tradition is clear in the way it connects care and justice to defend and promote the dignity of the human

---

[40] Olinto A Pegoraro, "O Lugar Bioético na História da Ética e o Conceito de Justiça como Cuidado," in *Bioética e Longevidade Humana*, ed. L. Pessini and C. P. de Barchifontaine (São Paulo: Loyola, 2006), 56.

being. There is a huge demand for palliative care in low- and middle-income countries. This is not speculation, rather, it is a fact. Therefore, Catholic organizations are encouraged to assume the responsibility of expanding palliative care into the global health agenda and to be partners of other organizations in delivering health care to the poor.

Chapter 20

Humanitarian Ethics: From Dignity and Solidarity to Response and Research

Dónal O'Mathúna

Imagine you are watching the news and reports of another disaster fill your screen. It is 2004; you watch footage of a massive tsunami generated by a magnitude 9.1 earthquake in the Indian Ocean claim more than 200,000 lives across the region within a matter of hours. It is 2005; Hurricane Katrina moves across the Gulf of Mexico, hitting New Orleans as a category three, flooding the city, destroying infrastructure, killing nearly 2,000 people, and leaving hundreds of thousands homeless. It is 2010; you watch footage of what is left after a magnitude seven earthquake strikes Haiti, killing over 200,000 and leaving almost a million Haitians homeless. It is 2017; Hurricane Maria makes landfall in Puerto Rico, leaving the island without power and food, and thousands are dead.

Many have died, and you are deeply moved by the images of the injured. You work in health care, and talk to your colleagues. A group of you feel like something needs to be done. Others agree, and you develop a plan to "do something." Flights are available to an airport just a few hours from the disaster, and you can rent a car to drive the rest of the way. Colleagues support your effort to help, and provide funds and cover the shifts you will miss. But others ask difficult questions. What are the actual needs of the victims? How will you decide between the injured when you cannot care for them all? What will you do about your own food, water, shelter and security? How will you coordinate with other groups on site? You and your team just want to help. People need help. What could be the problem?

❖ ❖ ❖ ❖ ❖

When a humanitarian crisis occurs, principles of social justice call for help to be provided. However, *what* help is given, *how* it is distributed, and to *whom* it is provided, can and should raise challenging bioethical questions. Some humanitarian responses have been criticized for assuming that good intentions are enough to justify the provision of whatever help we have. This chapter will address three types of bioethical challenges—without claiming that these are the only ones—in the midst of a humanitarian crisis. First, the help provided should be evidence-based, which also implies an ethical responsibility to generate valid evidence from research (and other sources as appropriate). Second, limited resources should be distributed based on explicit triage principles that are informed by social justice and Catholic social teaching—as exemplified by the work of Jesuit theologian Jon Sobrino. Third, humanitarian aid should be provided to all members of society, with a particular concern for those with heightened vulnerability. While each of these issues raises complexities that will be discussed in the chapter, it is important to acknowledge that each crisis raises a unique set of values and cultural challenges that must be balanced. Thus, humanitarian ethics arises in situations that are far from ideal, often offering only the possibility of ethical responses that can attend to the needs of vulnerable people at critical times. Catholic bioethicists can play a crucial role in educating and shaping their hospital and system staff in order to be prepared to respond to such disasters in the right way, at the right time, and with assistance that makes a difference without compounding matters of life and death with avoidable ethical lapses.

The Optics of Humanitarian Reponses

The term "humanitarian" is used in various ways. The Humanitarian Coalition provides a useful definition: a "humanitarian emergency is an event or series of events that represents a critical threat to the health, safety, security or wellbeing of a community or other large group of people, usually over a wide area."[1] Vulnerable populations are particularly at risk during humanitarian crises, which may involve or arise as a result of, "Armed conflicts, epidemics, famine, natural disasters and other major emergencies."[2]

Recent decades have seen an enormous growth in humanitarian action. In his book on humanitarian ethics, Hugo Slim claims that humanitarianism is based on the ethical premise that "every human life is good and that it is right to protect and save people's lives whenever and wherever you can."[3] For Slim, this ethical perspective is grounded in "a profound feeling of compassion and responsibility toward others who are living and suffering in extremis. It is a feeling of identification and sympathy that demands some reasonable and effective action as a response to suffering."[4]

Disasters sometimes do lead to extraordinary responses. For example, the 2004 Indian Ocean Tsunami led to record-breaking donations both globally and on the part of individual countries. Over $13.5 billion was donated to the humanitarian response.[5] The governments of 99 countries donated to the international relief project, 13 of whom had never done so previously.[6] What is more, these funds arrived quickly and allowed recovery to be initiated much sooner than is often the case.

All of this should be celebrated. So where is the bioethical problem? A social justice lens illuminates additional issues that are neither pleasant nor complimentary. While the 2004 Tsunami received much media attention, many other significant disasters do not. A review of 200 newspapers found that the 2004 Tsunami received more media

---

[1] Humanitarian Coalition, "What is a Humanitarian Emergency?," https://www.humanitariancoalition.ca/what-is-a-humanitarian-emergency?

[2] Ibid.

[3] Hugo Slim, *Humanitarian Ethics: A Guide to the Morality of Aid in War and Disaster* (Oxford, UK: Oxford University Press, 2015), 25.

[4] Ibid., 26.

[5] Tsunami Evaluation Committee, *Joint Evaluation of the International Response to the Indian Ocean Tsunami Synthesis* (London: Blackfriars, 2006), https://www.alnap.org/help-library/joint-evaluation-of-the-international-response-to-the-indian-ocean-tsunami-synthesis.

[6] Sophia Ayele, "The Indian Ocean Tsunami, 10 Years On," in *Oxfam Research Reports* (Oxford, UK: Oxfam, 2014).

coverage in six weeks than did ten other significant disasters over the whole previous year.[7] Additionally, some research found that although Western tourists made up one percent of the victims of the 2004 Tsunami, they were the focus of 40 percent of the media coverage of people impacted by the tsunami. This led one organization to conclude that "Western self-interest is the pre-condition for significant coverage of a humanitarian crisis."[8] Humanitarians can rush into emergencies and quickly set up programs, but, "When the funding dries up and the CNN cameras have moved on to the next crisis, the programs often collapse."[9] Failed programs leave complex ethical issues in their wake. Even the best of intentions can lead to inadvertent harm and the undermining of the dignity of those whom well-meaning people want to help.

Those well-meaning people are often motivated by media coverage, which impacts the economic response to particular aspects of the humanitarian crises that receive coverage. Unfortunately, economics guide media interest more than human suffering. Even when disasters are reported, more media reports address the economic and political dimensions of the disaster, instead of the human suffering. Yet, economics do not tell the complete story. Economic responses—even the economic response to the tsunami—fail often to address social and economic injustices present in the context prior to the disaster. Thus, a humanitarian response rooted in justice must move beyond the surface to explore the already present inequalities.

The Reality of Humanitarian Emergencies

Humanitarian emergencies or crises can be triggered by different factors. According to the International Disaster Database,[10] the number of weather-related disasters and related deaths were increasing

---

[7] Thomson Reuters, "Tsunami Coverage Dwarfs 'Forgotten' Crises—Research," *Thomson Reuters Foundation News*, March 10, 2010, http://news.trust.org//item/2005 0310000000-5sr0b/?source=search.

[8] Suzanne Franks, "The CARMA Report: Western Media Coverage of Humanitarian Disasters," *Political Quarterly* 77, no. 2 (2006): 281.

[9] Michael G. Wessells, "Do No Harm: Toward Contextually Appropriate Psychosocial Support in International Emergencies," *American Psychologist* 64, no. 1 (2009): 849.

[10] Centre for Research on the Epidemiology of Disasters, "The Human Cost of Weather Related Disasters," https://www.cred.be/index.php?q=HCWRD.

until around 2006, when they either peaked or leveled off.[11] However, the economic costs and the total number of people affected by weather-related disasters continue to increase. On average, weather-related disasters cost $153 billion US dollars per year, and affect 210 million people.[12]

These numbers do not include conflict-related disasters. The addition of conflict and violence into disaster settings elevates the challenges in humanitarian action. More people, about 300 million, live in the midst of violence and insecurity than are impacted by weather-related disasters.[13] As of May 2018, an unprecedented 65.6 million people have been forcibly driven from their homes.[14] Although conflict and war stir up images of combat-related deaths and injuries, civilians bear most of the burdens from the collapse of food supplies and health systems.[15] The problem has reached an unprecedented scale in the conflict in Syria with what has been called the weaponization of health care.[16] Health care workers, vehicles, and facilities have become the targets of attack in direct violation of the Geneva Convention which prohibits attacks on civilians and health care facilities. In addition to direct consequences, many health care workers have fled the country, further weakening people's ability to access health care.

In response to both conflict and weather-related disasters, the United Nations Office for the Coordination of Humanitarian Affairs (UNOCHA) reports that the amount of humanitarian aid donated has steadily increased from $3.7 billion in 2007 to $11.9 billion in 2017.[17] However, this total falls far short of what is needed, which

[11] Debarati Guha-Sapir, Philippe Hoyois, and Regina Below, *Annual Disaster Statistical Review 2016: The Numbers and Trends* (Brussels: CRED, 2016).

[12] Pascaline Wallemacq, "Natural Disasters in 2017: Lower Mortality, Higher Cost," *Cred Crunch* 50 (2018): 1–2.

[13] Jennifer Leaning and Debarati Guha-Sapir, "Natural Disasters, Armed Conflict, and Public Health," *The New England Journal of Medicine* 369, no. 19 (2013): 1836–42.

[14] United Nations High Commissioner for Refugees (UNHCR), "Figures at a Glance," 2018, http://www.unhcr.org/en-us/figures-at-a-glance.html.

[15] Leaning and Guha-Sapir, "Natural Disasters," 1836.

[16] Fouad M. Fouad, et al., "Health Workers and the Weaponisation of Health Care in Syria: A Preliminary Inquiry for *The Lancet*–American University of Beirut Commission on Syria," *The Lancet* 390, no. 10111 (2017): 2526.

[17] United Nations Office for the Coordination of Humanitarian Affairs, "Global Humanitarian Overview 2018," https://interactive.unocha.org/publication/global humanitarianoverview/.

was $23.5 billion in 2017. In 2007, 84 percent of the need was met, but 2017 saw only 50 percent of the financial costs covered.[18] While the response to the 2004 Indian Ocean Tsunami was exemplary, much of the aid promised during a crisis never materializes. Two years after the 2010 Haiti earthquake, only half the promised aid had been delivered.[19] Financial needs should not be the top priority, but a lack of financial resources makes difficult ethical decisions even more challenging.

The economic realities and governments' failure to deliver promised aid raise one type of concern that bioethics should play a role in addressing. However, the ethical dilemmas in humanitarian settings and disasters have rarely featured in bioethics, nor have issues of justice that underlie poverty and vulnerability to disasters.[20] Ethical problems in recent disasters have given rise to a new subfield, disaster ethics. Hurricane Katrina exposed the heightened vulnerability of some groups even in the wealthiest nations of the world. What might seem to have been an extreme weather event became deadlier when it interacted with a situation created by decades of human decisions. Many of these had components that impacted health and health care infrastructure, such as decisions to build levees in ways that cost less or avoided bureaucratic challenges.[21] Yet even in the rebuilding of New Orleans, some wanted to prevent the return of displaced poorer people so that profitable commercial development could occur.[22]

Disasters not only confront us with difficult ethical dilemmas, but they force us to reflect more deeply about the world in which we live. Disasters lead us to consider their origins. Some blame God, while others see only natural causes.[23] Sometimes human decisions lead to disasters, as with war or nuclear accidents. A closer examination

---

[18] Ibid.

[19] Tom Phillips and Claire Provost, "Haiti Earthquake: Two Years On, and Just Half of Promised Aid has been Delivered," *The Guardian*, January 11, 2012.

[20] Cheryl Macpherson and Muge Akpinar-Elci, "Caribbean Heat Threatens Health, Well-being and the Future of Humanity," *Public Health Ethics* 8, no. 2 (2015): 196–208.

[21] Byron Newberry, "Katrina: Macro-Ethical Issues for Engineers," *Science and Engineering Ethics* 16, no. 3 (2010): 535–71.

[22] Carole L Jurkiewicz, "Political Leadership, Cultural Ethics and Recovery: Louisiana Post-Katrina," *Public Organization Review* 9, no. 4 (2009): 353–66.

[23] Dónal P. O'Mathúna, "Christian Theology and Disasters: Where is God in all This?" in Dónal P. O'Mathúna, Vilius Dranseika, and Bert Gordijn, eds., *Disasters: Core Concepts and Ethical Theories* (Dordrecht: Springer, 2018), 27–42.

reveals that human choices contribute to many, if not all, disasters. The philosopher Jean-Jacques Rousseau reacted to the debate over whether God or nature caused the 1755 Great Lisbon Earthquake stating, "it was hardly Nature that had assembled there twenty thousand houses of six or seven stories. If the residents of this large city had been more evenly dispersed and less densely housed, the losses would have been fewer or perhaps none at all."[24] A report into Hurricane Katrina concluded that "This catastrophe did not result from an act of 'God'. It resulted from acts of 'People'. . . because of a large number of flaws and defects that had been embedded in the system."[25] Robert White, a geophysicist specializing in disasters, stated that "the deaths caused by 'natural' disasters can often be attributed almost in their entirety to actions taken by people, which turned a natural process into a disaster. In that respect there is nothing 'natural' about them."[26] Bioethics needs to consider more carefully how these underlying up-stream structural realities—the result of decades or centuries of human actions and decisions—factor into the massive scale of human mortality and ongoing morbidity and medical crises that attend humanitarian situations.

Humanitarian Disasters and the Limits of Bioethics

Humanitarian situations, and disasters in particular, differ from traditional issues considered by bioethics. First, bioethical discourse tends to proceed with unemotional detachment, applying ethical principles and theories in an objective, disinterested manner. Responses to disasters are highly emotional: horror at the suffering, particularly its suddenness and magnitude, can evoke a strong desire to help and admiration for the courage and sacrifice often exhibited by both victims and respondents. The tragedy of the situation always stares the responder in the face. However, many of the issues of suffering extend far beyond the clinical ethical questions that frequently take place in bioethics.

---

[24] Mark Molesky, *This Gulf of Fire: The Great Lisbon Earthquake, or Apocalypse in the Age of Science and Reason* (New York: Vintage, 2015), 331.

[25] Team Louisiana, "The Failure of the New Orleans Levee System During Hurricane Katrina, Appendix 6," 2006.

[26] White, "Who is to Blame," 19–20.

Second, bioethics has more traditionally focused on individual cases and dilemmas that occur within the confines of the clinical setting, particularly in high-income countries. Questions often focus on whether an individual is making an autonomous decision; less commonly does bioethics explore how those decisions impact others. Disasters trigger much bigger questions where the impact on others cannot be avoided, while the impact of community values on the individual's or individual impact on the community should not be ignored. In disasters, the bioethical questions center more on which person will receive the resources that are desperately short in supply; or how can someone work justly in a setting of chronic injustice; or whether providing much needed relief today is helpful if it cannot be provided later on.[27]

In the cholera outbreak in Haiti following the recovery efforts, global responders were faced with the dilemma of how best to treat and prevent cholera. The debate around how to control cholera in Haiti ultimately came down to a minimalist vs. maximalist approach.[28] The minimalists argued that it would be "too difficult" to control the spread of the disease, and opposed vaccinations in favor of water protection.[29] On the contrary, the maximalists argued that all possible ways to stop cholera be implemented or at least explored: improved sanitation, chlorine tablets, effective and safe vaccines, rehydration therapies, and antibiotics. Farmer reports that conversations tended to default to the ethical and public health position that academics and researchers had held for years and could not move beyond them to address the emergent situation at hand. What one side argued for may benefit one person in a particular location but may lead to harm to others.

---

[27] Lisa Schwartz, et al., "Ethics and Emergency Disaster Response. Normative Approaches and Training Needs for Humanitarian Health Care Providers," in Dónal P. O'Mathúna, Bert Gordijn, and Mike Clarke, eds., *Disaster Bioethics: Normative Issues When Nothing is Normal* (Dordrecht: Springer, 2014): 33–48.

[28] Paul Farmer, *Haiti After the Earthquake* (Philadelphia, PA: Public Affairs, 2011), 199.

[29] Louis Ivers and Paul Farmer, "Cholera in Haiti: The Equity Agenda and the Future of Tropical Medicine," *American Journal of Tropical Medicine and Hygiene* 86, no. 1 (2012): 7; WHO Publication, "Cholera Vaccines: WHO Position Paper-Recommendations," *Vaccine* 28, no. 30 (2010): 4687. Many of the "minimalist" public health practitioners cited unproven trials; however, Farmer and Ivers point to several successful trials in India, Vietnam, Bangladesh, Mozambique, and elsewhere included in the WHO report on cholera vaccines.

Thirdly, as noted in the cholera discussion, deeper questions of social (in)justice are inextricably interwoven with humanitarian disasters. Long-standing economic realities, governments' failures to deliver promised aid, global economic inequities, and political brinkmanship all play a role in creating the conditions that seed disasters. Bioethics rarely engages these deeper questions about social justice, particularly what we should do about poverty, and the ethical obligations of the rich to the poor. As such, traditional bioethics has been ill-equipped to wrestle with the ethical dilemmas in humanitarian settings and disasters or the issues of justice that underlie poverty and vulnerability to disasters.[30]

Disasters as X-Rays of Social Injustice

At the root of the problem is this: when we look at disasters honestly, we will find injustice at their core. Jon Sobrino, a Jesuit theologian, has written about his experience of prolonged civil war and devastating earthquakes in El Salvador. He argues that all disasters and humanitarian crises should force us to think about difficult issues and wrestle with serious questions about ourselves.[31] Doing so honestly should disturb us—and disturb us deeply. Writing a few weeks after the 2004 Tsunami, Sobrino says that the tsunami, like an earthquake, offers insight into our social reality.[32]

> The earthquake is not just a tragedy, it is an X-ray of the country. . . . Tragedies like an earthquake have natural causes, of course, but their unequal impact is not due to nature; it stems from the things people do with each other, to each other, against each other. The tragedy is largely the work of our own hands. We shape the planet with massive, cruel, and lasting injustice. We think of the planet as belonging to 25 or 30 percent of the human family; the rest—the poor, victimized majorities—have to wait for the leftovers, the crumbs that fall from the rich man's

---

[30] Macpherson and Akpinar-Elci, "Caribbean Heat Threatens Health."

[31] Jon Sobrino, *Where is God? Earthquake, Terrorism, Barbarity, and Hope*, trans. Margaret Wilde (Maryknoll, NY: Orbis, 2004).

[32] Jon Sobrino, "Tsunami: Exigencia de Conversion," in *Tsunami: Advertencia Para Los Que Viven* (El Salvador: UCA Editores, 2005), 24–29.

table. This ubiquitous inequality is evident even in normal times, and even more in an earthquake.[33]

Such disasters make visible what we in the West keep invisible on a day-to-day basis. It reveals that the majority of those who suffer and die in disasters do so because of human choices, not the random acts of nature (or God). The brunt of the suffering is inflicted on the poor, and much of the world's poverty exists because of injustices that the rich would rather not see or acknowledge. However, disasters bring this reality into our living rooms, into our consciences.

In other words, Sobrino argues that these crises represent a moment of reckoning with reality. Humanitarian crises force us to "be honest toward reality."[34] He notes that obviously disasters call attention to the need for compassion and mercy, but what is seldom insisted on is the need to pay attention to reality itself, to why this crisis was so devastating to this population. As in war, so with disasters: "the first casualty is truth."[35] Ignoring the truth stems from the lack of attention to underlying injustices that can be crucial to understanding disasters in the first place. During the 2004 Tsunami, much media attention was given to foreign tourists caught up in the disaster. Little if any discussion centered on the existence of these luxury resorts surrounded by extreme poverty. Yet the suffering of those living outside the gates of luxury was immense, before, during, and after the disaster. These are ethical issues that require an honest look at reality. "What the media say or don't say, and how they say or don't say it, helps to conceal the reality and effectively render it invisible."[36] Do disasters represent the opportunity to rebuild a false reality or an opportunity to reconsider reality for what it is?

The Limits of Charity and the Value of Solidarity

Another important bioethical issue is to examine humanitarian aid in light of how it impacts the recipient's dignity and helps to promote sustainability. In the last fifty years, Africa has received over

---

[33] Sobrino, *Where is God?*, 3–4.
[34] Ibid., 29.
[35] Ibid., 31.
[36] Ibid.

one trillion dollars in humanitarian aid, yet for much of Africa, things have gotten worse.[37] The most aid-dependent countries show the least amount of progress. According to one African economist, the problem with much aid is that rather than fostering dignity and independence, it fosters dependence, stifles innovation, and leads to corruption and conflict.[38] Aid itself has become a humanitarian disaster.

Rightly done, however, humanitarian aid can be quite constructive. For example, giving people cash as part of disaster relief was frowned upon for years, until it was tried and tested after the 2004 Indian Ocean Tsunami.[39] Rather than leading to wasteful spending, the cash was used carefully and effectively, and had the by-product of helping to stimulate the local economy. By providing assistance that develops practical skills, survivors can provide for themselves and their families, contribute to local communities, and develop economic independence. While in a certain sense this reinforces the charity aspects of humanitarian relief, nevertheless, providing cash led to an intervention in the community that offered direct assistance.

Humanitarian practices viewed through the lens of human dignity also illuminate questions about how funds have traditionally been raised for humanitarian aid using photographs and videos of suffering people, especially children. On one level, it seems to make sense to use such images to engage the hearts and minds of those with resources to give. These images illicit changes that tend to be short-lived, failing to address the deeper questions around why people are suffering in these ways. They foster emotional reactions that lead to short-term charity, not deeper compassionate responses that lead to solidarity between peoples. The realization that such portrayals can be demeaning for those in need and promote a view of dependence and inability to care for themselves is leading to change.[40] The alternative is to find ways that promote survivors' dignity even while accurately portraying their suffering.

---

[37] Robert D. Lupton, *Toxic Charity: How Churches and Charities Hurt Those They Help (And How to Reverse It)* (New York: HarperCollins, 2011).

[38] Dambisa Moyo, *Dead Aid: Why Aid is Not Working and How There is a Better Way for Africa* (New York: Farrar, Straus and Giroux, 2009).

[39] Ayele, "The Indian Ocean Tsunami."

[40] Philippe Calain, "Ethics and Images of Suffering Bodies in Humanitarian Medicine," *Social Science and Medicine* 98 (2013): 278–85.

The theme of family, community, and participation provides a useful counterbalance that highlights the social dimension absent in quandary ethics. In humanitarian settings, families and communities are especially important to take into consideration. Often community involvement may be more highly valued than in Western settings. Thus, rather than isolating the image of an individual in need, the communal setting reinforces the connections between victims, their families, and their neighbors whom we meet in and through solidarity.

Solidarity also captures the fellow-feeling that suffering can elicit, turning it into ethical action. Sobrino states that solidarity "seeks the living in order to rescue them, or the dead in order to bury them in dignity. In this primal solidarity, women stand always and everywhere as the focal point of life: caring for the children among the ruins, making and sharing whatever food there is in the refugee camps, always encouraging by their presence, never giving up, never tiring."[41] Going beyond even this, solidarity is "a feeling of closeness to other human beings."[42] It can overcome the differences that may have fueled years of suspicion and hatred, as was seen in how the 2004 Tsunami played a role in bringing to an end the violent conflict in Aceh, although the same did not happen in Sri Lanka.[43]

Participatory Research and Evidence-Based Interventions

Bioethics viewed through a social justice lens looks more deeply at causal factors contributing to a situation rather than just the ethical dilemmas faced by individuals. Such dilemmas exist, and humanitarian responders need training and support to address them. But much bigger ethical issues often are not examined. A social justice lens means that preexisting and chronic problems will not be ignored. An easy resolution may not be apparent, but the issues will be honestly discussed. For example, disaster responders are sometimes invited into jurisdictions only for the duration of an acute crisis—a hurricane or earthquake. However, this will create dilemmas over how to respond

---

[41] Sobrino, *Where is God?*, 6–7.
[42] Ibid., 8–9.
[43] Ayele, "The Indian Ocean Tsunami."

to non-disaster related needs, especially if these arise from injustices. Being aware of these may help responders to prepare better, but also determine ways they may be able to address those injustices.

Research should help to ensure that aid is examined within a social justice lens. The provision of cash noted earlier is one example of how research can lead to a change of practice. For example, when a foreign team arrives to provide free medical care, they can both meet important immediate needs and undermine long-term efforts to develop local health systems. Awareness of these factors could lead to better engagement and support of local systems, rather than undermining them. After Hurricane Mitch, many US teams travelled to Honduras to rebuild houses at a cost of about $30,000 each; local workers could have built the houses for $3,000 each, at the same time supporting employment and trade.[44] In conflict settings, things are even more complicated. Research has shown that introducing humanitarian aid into conflict zones is associated with increased violence as citizens are targeted and aid is stolen.[45] This highlights the messy political side of humanitarian responses. While there are no easy answers, being aware of the dilemmas can help to avoid inadvertent mistakes and possibly lead to alternative solutions.

For humanitarian aid to become more evidence-based, more research is required both to identify what is needed and to determine whether it is being effective or not. A social bioethics lens provides a basis for evaluating good evidence about what is needed and what will be effective. For this, research is needed into all aspects of disaster prevention and disaster responses. When aid is not evidence-based, junk gets sent, and things are done that cause more harm than good. For example, after the 2004 Tsunami, sleeping mats and hygiene kits were needed, but reporters found that international aid arrived including "winter jackets, expired cans of salmon, stiletto shoes, winter tents, thong panties, and even Viagra."[46] Our imaginary team faced

[44] Lupton, *Toxic Charity.*

[45] Reed M. Wood and Christopher Sullivan, "Doing Harm by Doing Good? The Negative Externalities of Humanitarian Aid Provision during Civil Conflict," *Journal of Politics* 77, no. 3 (2015): 736–48.

[46] Associated Press, "Useless Tsunami Aid Includes Thong Panties," *NBCNews.com*, February 11, 2005, http://www.nbcnews.com/id/6954302/ns/world_news-tsunami _a_year_later/t/useless-tsunami-aidincludes-thong-panties/.

with a humanitarian crisis in the opening vignette, might show up with the wrong skill set, or require so much support from other organizations that their net contribution is negative.

Research can identify important failings in the current situation and hopefully lead to better interventions and policies. Social justice should also remind researchers of the importance of considering the dignity and well-being of all people. The needs and views of those at risk of heightened vulnerabilities should be included and listened to in research. For example, participatory action research is an approach that engages throughout the research process with the communities where the research is being conducted.[47] Research in humanitarian settings is often challenged by how to ensure participants are adequately informed of what is involved and aware of potential adverse effects. A participatory approach means that these issues are actively discussed and responded to even while the research is being designed. This respects the dignity of participants and their communities and can help to avoid problems and ethical dilemmas. Being aware of the vulnerabilities existing in these communities will also help to ensure their concerns and needs are addressed.

Participatory approaches enhance the ethical power of research by respecting participants rather than seeing respect for autonomy or informed consent as simply a regulatory concern, as has happened in mainstream bioethics. This latter attitude has led to a tendency for research ethics to be seen as a bureaucratic hurdle to be overcome rather than a mechanism to support and promote ethical research that both respects participants and their communities and brings good through the production of better evidence to guide practice.[48] As high-quality research is conducted, reported, and used to inform practice, humanitarian aid can become more effective in meeting the needs of those it seeks to serve. Research that is conducted rigorously and ethically can bring to light the truth. Such truth is required in order to respond to reality as it really is, as Sobrino urges. This in-

---

[47] Dónal O'Mathúna, "The Dual Imperative in Disaster Research Ethics," in Ron Iphofen and Martin Tolich, eds., *SAGE Handbook of Qualitative Research Ethics* (London: SAGE, 2018), 441–54.

[48] Dónal O'Mathúna and Chesmal Siriwardhanam, "Research Ethics and Evidence for Humanitarian Health," *The Lancet* 390, no. 10109 (2017): 2228–29; and O'Mathúna, "Research Ethics."

cludes empirical research into the effectiveness of interventions and programs to ensure that only what works is implemented and that what is spent is spent well. It also includes qualitative research into the lives and experiences of those who live in the reality of poverty. When done honesty and truthfully, the media too can help to bring light to the needs of the vulnerable living in disaster-prone areas.

Beyond Good Will and an Open Wallet

Good will and an open wallet are not enough to sustain humanitarian aid that is just and dignifying. Traditional approaches to bioethics tend to search for the one right answer to dilemmas, while disasters are messy—here the best answer may not be very good, but only the least worst option.[49] Messy options may not sit well with those who have been trained in traditional bioethics or a more traditional Catholic approach to bioethics. However, moving beyond a purely principle-based approach to bioethics and incorporating the insights of Catholic social thought provides important avenues, and yet untapped resources, to address the structural inequalities that are compounded in the midst of humanitarian crises. A social justice perspective calls on us to dig deeper into underlying realities, and to develop solidarity with those we are moved to help.

Injustices can be deeply engrained and more exaggerated in low-income settings. Various groups can be openly discriminated against, and even prevented from receiving assistance after disasters.[50] The first step is to ensure that things are reported the way they really are. The pictures of both the injuries and the injustices may be difficult to view, but we have to allow ourselves to be affected first by the truth.[51] Social justice can give us eyes to see the world as it is, hearts that are motivated to do something about it, and minds to determine how it can be done effectively and with dignity.

---

[49] Dónal O'Mathúna, "Ideal and Nonideal Moral Theory for Disaster Bioethics," *Human Affairs* 26, no. 1 (2016): 8–17.

[50] Suresh Mariaselvam and Vijayaprasad Gopichandran, "The Chennai Floods of 2015: Urgent Need for Ethical Disaster Management Guidelines," *Indian Journal of Medical Ethics* 1, no. 2 (2016): 91–95.

[51] Sobrino, "The Indian Ocean Tsunami," 29.

Before boarding a plane to fly into the heart of a humanitarian disaster, health care professionals—especially those motivated by compassion and a desire to "do something"—should reflect carefully on the ethical problems their action might generate. Robert Lupton has proposed *The Oath for Compassionate Service* which provides practical proposals with which to conclude this chapter:[52]

- Never do for the poor what they have (or could have) the capacity to do for themselves.

- Limit one-way giving to emergency situations.

- Strive to empower the poor through employment, lending, and investing, using grants sparingly to reinforce achievements.

- Subordinate self-interests to the needs of those being served.

- Listen closely to those you seek to help, especially to what is not being said—unspoken feelings may contain essential clues to effective service.

- Above all, do no harm.

While the tendency for Catholic health care professionals may be to respond to the immediate needs, it is important to remember that only one facet of the crisis is often revealed. Sobrino's encouragement to come to understand the reality challenges us to ensure that responses promote justice as well as address the present crisis, and to cultivate relationships that allow institutions and individuals to address the complex realities of rebuilding from a humanitarian crisis.[53]

---

[52] Lupton, *Toxic Charity*, 8–9.

[53] The author would like to thank Etienne Casassa for his generous help translating the Sobrino (2005) article.

PART SIX

Reimagining Frontiers

The final section of the book addresses issues that push the development of Catholic bioethics in different ways. While each of the previous chapters have raised emerging issues in bioethics, these final chapters look for ways in which Catholic bioethics can better participate in ongoing secular bioethics conversations about the nature of health care and research practices itself. The issues raised in these chapters—research, the environment, genetics, and economics—will continue to affect the way in which health care functions as a global practice. The US, while not the leader in health outcomes, does contribute heavily to technological innovation through research. However, while theologians participated in the early development of bioethics within the US, they have rarely weighed in on the way in which research has developed, capitalizing on the health needs of the wealthy minority over the health needs of the majority.

Thus, for ethicists, theologians, and mission leaders the questions posed through this section ask: How can Catholic bioethics draw on the social tradition to participate in creating just structures that help shape future directions and implementation of biomedical research practices and genetic development? How does Catholic health care reflect on its role in the midst of the environmental crisis? What role should economics play in Catholic health care's ability to negotiate the tension between the margins and a ministry that demands justice?

Research guidelines, both secular and religious, fail often to consider the way in which research prioritizes technological innovation over the health needs of the majority. In chapter 21, "Research as a Restorative Practice: Catholic Social Teaching and the Ethics of Biomedical Research," Jesuit theologian Jorge José Ferrer critiques the technological prioritization that has resulted in what has been referred to as the 10/90 gap, in which 10 percent of the population benefits from 90 percent of the research. Social justice, Ferrer argues, offers an important corrective that can address the research gap and shift priorities that respond to the research needs of vulnerable communities. However, this aspect of CST is discussed infrequently within Catholic bioethics, even when issuing guidelines for research. This chapter proposes principles of CST that emphasize a restorative dimension to the practice of research.

In chapter 22, "Environmental Ethics as Bioethics," Jesuit theologian Andrea Vicini and Tobias Winright lead readers in a practice of contemplation—an important foundation for CST. Here, they challenge us to contemplate the reality of environmental challenges and the contexts from which they emerge. After reflecting on the various ways in which contemporary lifestyles contribute to the environmental crisis, they envisage the human impact of potential environmental changes. Drawing on the papal encyclicals and theological approaches, they argue—echoing Ron Hamel—that the boundaries of bioethics need to expand in order for bioethicists to play a prophetic role at the intersection of environmental ethics and bioethics.

From the macro issue of environmental concerns to the micro issues of genetics, the CST helps us rethink bioethics across the spectrum. Hille Haker, in chapter 23, "A Social Bioethics of Genetics," begins with the emphatic challenge of a mother who dismisses Haker's argument for a ban on germline editing. The mother, lamenting the loss of her child early in life, sees research—any form of research—as the last hope to cure the ills that caused her child to suffer. Haker, while sympathetic to the mother, exhorts caution around the new developments within reproductive genetic technologies (RGTs). She is critical of the traditional Catholic approach to RGTs that is framed within the context of protecting the embryo and magisterial teaching on sexual ethics. Instead, she argues for an interdisciplinary approach traced to Alfons Auer that engages modern social science, the humanities, and a contextual theological anthropology. Moreover, she argues that Auer's approach can be seen in Pope Francis's encyclicals and theological analysis. Drawing on this methodology, she argues that Catholic bioethics needs to engage in debates at the forefront of RGT development and to forward a social bioethics approach that can handle the complex question of scientific development and the concerns of future parents.

The final chapter, in a sense, asks the question that lies at the root of most, if not all, the ethical challenges analyzed in this book: What is the role of economics in creating and sustaining these injustices? Pope John Paul II identified "the all-consuming thirst for profit" as one of the overarching structures of sin in his 1987 encyclical *Sollicitudo Rei Socialis.* Yet Catholic bioethics has little if any capacity to wrestle with the role of economics as an operative driver of almost every ethical issue we face. In chapter 24, "For-Profit Health Care: An Economic Perspective," internationally recognized economist Charles M. A. Clark carefully outlines and wrestles with the economic implications of US health care as a commodity. More and more, Catholic health care systems flirt with—either at a system level or via subsidiaries—for-profit activities. How do for-profit assumptions align—or misalign—with Catholic identity and CST? Clark's chapter does not directly answer this question.[1] Instead, his economic analysis raises both a financial and theological question: What is the cost of being a Catholic health system that incarnates Catholic social teaching?

---

[1] For further analysis of this question, see M. Therese Lysaught, "Theological Foundations of Catholic Economic Thought: The For-Profit Question," in *Caritas in Communion: Theological Foundations of Catholic Health Care* (St. Louis, MO: Catholic Health Association, 2014).

Chapter 21

Research as a Restorative Practice: Catholic Social Teaching and the Ethics of Biomedical Research

Jorge José Ferrer, SJ

Reflection on the ethics of scientific research is a relatively recent development. Its genesis is linked to egregious abuses in research with human participants, such as those performed by Nazi scientists or the infamous Tuskegee syphilis study discussed in the earlier chapter by Sheri Bartlett Browne and Christian Cintron. Its scope has been enlarged to include the responsible use of nonhuman animals in research, as well as topics related to academic integrity and environmental responsibility. The ethics of conducting research is an integral part of scientific education today. However, theological voices are largely absent in this nascent field of study. Unsurprisingly, most of my secular colleagues cannot fathom the possible contribution of theology to the study of research ethics. More troublesome is the inability of Catholic colleagues to see the connection.

When I was invited to write this chapter, I mentioned to a friend and colleague that I was planning to work on a paper on the contribution of the Catholic social tradition (CST) to the ethics of scientific research. To my amazement, my friend was surprised by the topic of my investigation. He did not see any relation between the CST and the ethics of research. This reaction is noteworthy because my colleague is a biologist, with a PhD from a prestigious institution and with an interest and formal training in bioethics. He is also a practicing Catholic.

Even more troubling is that those who address issues of research ethics in the Catholic tradition do not seem, for the most part, to take into account the contributions of CST to the field. In this paper, I seek to correct that omission. In the first part of this chapter, I identify the reasons for such disconnection, while in the second part, I explore the potential contributions of our tradition of social thought to the field of research ethics.

Theological Ethics and Biomedical Research

In 2008, The National Catholic Bioethics Center and the Catholic Medical Association published *A Catholic Guide to Ethical Research.*[1] The focus of the Guide is clinical research. The document proposes four general principles, each one followed by a set of guidelines, for the ethical guidance of research in accordance with Catholic teaching and natural law ethics: (1) truth; (2) respect for human life at every stage of life from first formation to natural death; (3) respect for the integrity of persons; and (4) generosity and justice. These principles represent an attitude of social responsibility and consideration for the vulnerable. Guideline (a), for the first principle, clearly states that: "All research programs must be of value for the good society. Clinical research in particular should aim to relieve suffering and foster the health and well-being of humanity." The third principle, respect for the integrity of the person, emphasizes concern for vulnerable individuals: "Individuals who are vulnerable by virtue of their age, education, economic status, medical or psychological condition, or cognitive status must be particularly protected by all physicians and medical researchers." This concern for the vulnerable appears again in guideline (d), under principle four (generosity and justice): "Disadvantaged subjects should never be enrolled in clinical trials from which they cannot benefit at least indirectly. They should never compose the research population in a study primarily intended for the benefit of another, more advantaged population."

---

[1] The National Catholic Bioethics Center and the Catholic Medical Association, "A Catholic Guide to Ethical Clinical Research," *The Linacre Quarterly* 75, no. 3 (2008): 181–224.

While these principles and guidelines are congruent with CST, they express positions widely accepted in secular bioethics. They are accepted as fundamental tenets of the responsible conduct of research established in The Belmont Report (1978).[2] They are in no way explicitly linked to the distinctive principles of the CST. Despite the National Catholic Bioethics Center and the Catholic Medical Association being known for their devotion to the church's official magisterium, Catholic teaching about social justice and the option for the poor, for example, are not explicitly taken into account in this important document. The omission of issues such as the selection of research priorities or research in impoverished communities is striking. Such issues feature strongly in secular research ethics.[3] The guidelines proposed in this document are more distinctively Catholic only when they touch on issues related to the beginning and end of life, as well as the rejection and prevention of conception.

This restricted view of the ethics of research, however, can also be found in Catholic authors that represent what we may call—if labels may be used—more liberal interpretations of our tradition. An ample analysis of books in Catholic bioethics is not possible in this paper. An examination of two examples must suffice. The first example is Javier Gafo's *Bioética teológica*, a work published posthumously in 2003.[4] Gafo was a very influential author in Spain and Latin America, a pioneer in the field of bioethics in the Ibero-American context. Chapter 13 is devoted to human clinical trials. The chapter gives a good introduction to the topic of clinical experimentation. It gives a brief history of human experimentation, provides a general justification for such experimentation, and gives an overview of the ethical questions concerning clinical trials with human participants. Respect

[2] National Commission for the Protection of Human Subjects of Biomedical and Behavioral Research, *The Belmont Report: Ethical Principles and Guidelines for the Protection of Human Subjects of Research* (Bethesda, MD: The National Commission, 1978).

[3] Stephanie R. Solomon, "Protecting and Respecting the Vulnerable: Existing Regulations or Further Protections?," *Theoretical Medicine and Bioethics* 34, no. 1 (2013): 17–28; Ezekiel J. Emanuel, et al., "What Makes Clinical Research in Developing Countries Ethical? The Benchmarks of Ethical Research," *Journal of Infections Disease* 189, no. 5 (2004): 930–37; Charles Weijer and Ezekiel Emanuel, "Protecting Communities in Biomedical Research," *Science* 289, no. 5482 (2000): 1142–44.

[4] Javier Gafo, *Bioética teológica* (Madrid: Universidad Pontificia Comillas y Desclée de Brouwer, 2003), 329–56.

for the person of the human participant is presented as the basic ethical requirement concerning clinical experimentation. This principle is, of course, entirely congruent with the Catholic tradition.

When Gafo moves on to consider specific moral problems in the ethics of research, he analyzes informed consent, the proportion between risks and benefits, double-blind studies, and experimentation with vulnerable populations. The vulnerable groups considered are persons who lack capacity to consent, prisoners, minors, and mental patients: the classical vulnerable populations studied by secular bioethics. There is no special mention of impoverished populations or the social justice context in the determination of research priorities. Although Gafo was generally considered a progressive theologian, we can see that his reflection is as removed from the Catholic social tradition as that of the Guide previously mentioned.

A more recent work, published in the US, *Contemporary Health Care Ethics* by David F. Kelly, Gerard Magill, and Henk Ten Have, offers a more expansive consideration of social justice, however, one that is devoid of explicit reference to CST.[5] Their treatment of research ethics is informative and useful, as well as sensitive to the issues of social justice, such as the globalization and prevalence of the business model in clinical research. However, there is no explicit link to our rich Catholic tradition of social ethics despite both theological and magisterial critiques. From this brief review, we can see the gap between bioethics and the Catholic social tradition is real. However, we need to understand why it is there and how it can be overcome.

Understanding and Overcoming the Gap

Fortunately, we can see a shift of perspective in two books by Lisa S. Cahill, *Theological Bioethics*[6] and *Bioethics and the Common Good*.[7] Based on her 2004 Père Marquette lecture, *Bioethics and the Common Good* offers important insights that illuminate the bases for the gap between Catholic social teaching and Catholic bioethics. Analyzing

---

[5] David F. Kelly, Gerard Magill, and Henk Ten Have, *Contemporary Catholic Health Care Ethics* (Washington DC: Georgetown University Press, 2013), 257–70.

[6] Lisa S. Cahill, *Theological Bioethics* (Washington DC: Georgetown University Press, 2005).

[7] Lisa S. Cahill, *Bioethics and the Common Good* (Milwaukee, WI: Marquette University Press, 2004).

the decline of interest in the original controversies about proportionalism, Cahill identifies several shifts:

> The originating framework was double effect, a model primarily of individual decision-making about separate acts. One shift away from this moral worldview occurred when proportionalists looked toward the agent more than the act. Still another occurred insofar as they worked with a much more contextual understanding of agency. A third shift came about when developers of the proportionalist critique, such as feminist and liberation theologians, realized that ethics of acts and agency must be integrated with political, institutional and social ethics . . . since the 1980s Catholic ethicists have turned increasingly to the resources of Thomistic ethics . . . and of modern Catholic social teaching, even in taking up issues of sexual and medical ethics.[8]

The focus of traditional moral theology on individual actions and personal responsibility is not surprising.

Moral theology developed originally as a "science of confessors." The original moral textbooks—*Institutiones theologiae moralis*—were written to train priests to hear confessions. Attention to the social and political context of human actions was minimal or totally absent. Moreover, the advent of CST is relatively recent, if we take *Rerum Novarum* (1891) as its starting point. Even more recent are the contributions of political, liberation, and feminist theologies. In addition, moral theologians have tended to treat issues related to personal morality—such as sexuality and medical ethics—as distinct from social ethics. All these elements have contributed, in my opinion, to the gap between research ethics and Catholic social teaching. To these considerations, intrinsic to our own religious tradition, we need to add the cultural humus in which contemporary bioethics has developed, strongly rooted in the traditions of a liberal society, with its focus on issues related to individual freedom and its concomitant principle of respect for the autonomous choices of individuals. This mentality has exercised an inevitable influence on Catholic theologians working in bioethics, particularly in countries with a strong liberal ethos.

---

[8] Ibid., 21.

It is at this juncture that the Catholic social tradition becomes particularly relevant for the ethics of biomedical research. Let us examine the basic concepts from the CST that can enrich our reflection about the ethics of research. Although I will focus on the ethics of research with human participants, CST can and should be expanded to include the ethics of nonhuman animal research and environmental responsibility. I will proceed in two steps. First, I will identify the principles of Catholic social teaching that I consider most relevant for the elaboration of an ethics of scientific research with theological substance. I will conclude by referencing topics that I consider to be most urgent for an ethics of scientific research informed by the principles of our Catholic social tradition.[9]

Fundamental and Nonnegotiable Dignity of Every Person

Catholic theologians tend to confer a denser, ontological meaning to the notion of the person and her dignity than their secular peers, in conformity with the church's magisterium and the traditions of Catholic thought. A Catholic understanding of the person does not allow for an individualistic anthropology. The person has to be understood in the context of her community. Moreover, autonomy, even if it is understood in the restrictive sense of having the possibility of making autonomous choices, cannot be understood independently of the social contexts in which choices are made. Social factors—such as access to education or health care—condition the possibility of exercising truly autonomous choices. Therefore, it is not possible to protect and promote the dignity of persons and the exercise of autonomy if we do not guarantee that everyone's fundamental rights are respected and that every person has a life according to human dignity. Therefore, the dignity of the person requires a commitment to social justice and the common good.

---

[9] In the development of my argument, I want to acknowledge the influence of Alan J. Kearns, "Catholic Social Teaching as a Framework for Research Ethics," *Journal of Academic Ethics* 12 (April 2014): 145–59; and Thomas Massaro, *Living Justice* (Lanham, MD: Rowman and Littlefield, 2016), 81–124. In the search of periodical literature for this paper, Kearns's article was the only one found with a focus similar to mine. His vision, however, continues to focus on the protection of the individual participant.

Social Justice, the Common Good, and Solidarity

I take these three principles together because, in my opinion, they are intimately connected to each other. As Cahill points out, since Pius XI's encyclical *Quadragesimo Anno* (1911), popes and episcopal conferences have frequently spoken about social justice, but the concept has never been clearly defined. In my view, social justice refers to the creation of a society in which everyone has an opportunity to live a life according to human dignity. Following the Spanish philosopher Julián Marías, I would add that social justice has a restorative dimension in that it has the task of rectifying social situations that are the result of a previous injustice, which, if maintained, invalidates present efforts to act justly.[10]

From what has been said, it should be clear that there is an intimate connection between the notions of social justice and the common good. In my view, the requirements of the common good and of social justice are one and the same. We cannot achieve the common good without achieving social justice. Moreover, social justice and the common good must be considered today as principles that apply globally.

> The new economy and today's communication media link us all together in a way never before seen in human history. . . . These new global relationships make way for what Allen Buchanan calls *global basic structures,* a notion he defines as: "A set of economic and political institutions that have profound and enduring effects on the distribution of burdens and benefits among peoples and individuals around the world." We contend that this *global basic structure* is a sufficient basis on which to establish obligations of global justice, just as the traditional basic structure of the state has done at the national level. Indeed, we have already accepted the validity of requirements of justice in international commercial contracts and, at least, since Nuremberg, we establish international tribunals to judge offenses that are considered crimes against humanity.[11]

---

[10] Julián Marías, *La justicia social y otras justicias* (Madrid: Espasa-Calpe, 1979), 16.

[11] Jorge José Ferrer, "Multinational Biomedical Research in Impoverished Communities," in *Applied Ethics in a World Church,* ed. Linda Hogan (Maryknoll, NY: Orbis Books, 2008), 194–95; see also Allan Buchanan, "Rawls's Law of Peoples: Rules for a Vanished Westphalian World," *Ethics* 110, no. 4 (2000): 705.

These considerations lead us to the idea of solidarity. Solidarity refers, in a very basic sense, to the fundamental unity of all members of the human race, since we are all the product of the same evolutionary process, we share in one common human condition and our histories and economies are every day more intertwined. Moreover, this solidarity is increasingly evidenced by a growing ecological consciousness, commented on elsewhere in this volume. Many of these dimensions link us to other living beings, not only to humans. From a theological perspective, the grounds of solidarity run even deeper, since we have been created by the same Divine Creator and we are all called to share in the redemption realized by Christ. This fundamental human commonality is the ontological basis for the ethical principle of solidarity: We are all in the same boat, we need to help each other, and we will sail or sink together, at least in the long run, if we look at humanity as a whole. Solidarity requires that we care for the well-being of others, for the common good.[12]

Preferential Option for the Poor and the Vulnerable

The preferential option for the poor, the vulnerable, and the marginalized is at the heart of the Gospel. It is not an ideological innovation made up by liberation theologians under the influence of Marxist theorists. It goes back to Jesus himself and his healing and consoling ministry to the sick and marginalized. One can find its roots beautifully expressed in the Lucan parable of the Good Samaritan. The following of Jesus requires that we become neighbor to the one left half-dead on the road from Jerusalem to Jericho. It is also present in the parable of the rich man and the poor Lazarus, found in the same gospel. The rich man's sin is his insensibility toward the poor man who was sitting at his door. We can find the same idea in Matthew's narrative of the final judgment. Jesus identifies himself with the hungry, the naked, and the homeless, and wants to be served in them.

While it is true that the precise phrase "preferential option for the poor" was introduced into Catholic doctrine by the Latin American Church, it was coined in faithful continuity with the teaching of Jesus as well as the teachings of John XXIII, Paul VI, and the Second Vatican

---

[12] See Thomas Massaro, *Living Justice*, 88.

Council. It seems undeniable to me that this principle has an important potential impact for the ethics of scientific research, particularly at a time when business interests seem to rule the whole world of healthcare and scientific research in the biomedical realm.

Research as a Restorative Praxis

Social structures do not come down from heaven, according to a predetermined divine plan, nor are they predetermined by unchangeable natural laws. Social structures are the result of human decisions. It is true that once established, they tend to have a life of their own, but this does not mean that they cannot be changed. Social justice requires a commitment to repair the inequities that result from the ways in which we—or our forebears—have organized social relations and the distribution of power and wealth in society. Therefore, social justice has a restorative dimension in which the goal is the healing and reconstruction of society in order to create the conditions for every person to have the possibility of living a life in accordance with the requirements of human dignity. An ethics of scientific research guided by the aforementioned principles of CST will contribute to correct social structures that sustain inequities, both on the national and the global horizons. Scientific research inspired by the principles proposed by our tradition will necessarily be *a restorative human praxis*.

Selection of Research Priorities

The selection of research priorities should be guided by the commitment to the common good and social justice. This means that research cannot be guided only or mainly by financial interests. For example, many reports since the 1990s have focused on the 10/90 gap in health research. These reports have found that there is a discrepancy between disease burden and the availability of research funds. In other words, the health needs of the rich get more attention and funding than those of the poor. As Dónal O'Mathúna points out, the number might be overstated: "The important thing is not the numerical precision. . . . Yet the problem is real and of immense proportions. Eighteen million people die prematurely each year from medical conditions for which cures exist. This is roughly one third of all human deaths."[13]

The preferential option for the poor requires that the needs of the poorest and most needy sisters and brothers of Christ should receive preferential treatment. This principle demands that all of us—governments, industry, NGOs—make special efforts to find and provide funding for research that is not attractive to private investors, such as the drug industry, in terms of profit. Catholic universities and other church-sponsored institutions have the responsibility to foster and sustain research that meets the needs of the most vulnerable. Such research should include topics related to public health and an effort to ameliorate the conditions of communities affected by poverty. Social determinants of health are as important or more important than drugs, hospitals, and doctors: clean water, sanitation, nutrition, and education are the most basic requirements for good health. Poverty and inadequate access to education are extremely hazardous to public and individual health.

Research in Impoverished Communities

Clinical experimentation is on the rise in developing communities. It is a double-edged sword. While exclusion from research can be a form of unfair discrimination, inclusion brings with it the potential for exploitation, particularly when the participants are poor and vulnerable. Nevertheless, biomedical experimentation can bring great benefits, both direct and indirect, to a given population. Developing countries offer advantages to pharmaceutical companies. For example, they have an abundance of individuals deprived of medical care, the cost of doing business there is lower, and regulations and ethical screening tend to be weaker. As with any other vulnerable

[13] Dónal P. O'Mathúna, "Decision-making and Health Research: Ethics and the 10/90 Gap," *Research Practitioner* 8, no. 5 (2007): 164–72. For more recent statistics about the causes of death worldwide and their relationship to poverty, see World Health Organization, "The Top Ten Causes of Death," http://www.who.int/news-room/fact-sheets/detail/the-top-10-causes-of-death; Our World in Data, "What Does the World Die From?" https://ourworldindata.org/what-does-the-world-die-from; and Saving Lives Task Force, "Facts and Figures for Saving Lives," http://njpeaceaction.org/august9/articles_facts_and_figures_for_saving_lives.html.

population, ethical screening of both proposed and ongoing research needs to be tighter when we work in such settings because the danger of exploitation is greater.

We find in the literature different models proposed to safeguard the ethical quality of research with impoverished populations, not all of them satisfactory. In a 2004 paper, Ezekiel Emanuel and his associates proposed a cluster of principles with their corresponding benchmarks. They require that (1) a collaborative partnership be established between the researchers and sponsors from a developed country with the researchers, policy makers, and communities in the host country; (2) the study must have social value; (3) scientific validity; (4) fair subject selection; (5) favorable risk-benefit factor; (6) independent review; (7) informed consent; and (8) respect for recruited participants and study communities.[14]

Following the lead of Alex J. London, I would add that research in impoverished communities should (1) respond to the health needs of the community; and (2) contribute to the development of the community and its members, leaving them in a better situation than it was before the study started.[15] These requirements are congruent with the notion of social justice that we espouse. Social justice requires creating a society in which everyone has the opportunity to live a life according to human dignity. It also requires the rectification of situations of inequality that contradict such dignity, leaving some persons at a disadvantage.

Patents

Patents represent another important topic in which the principles of Catholic social teaching identified above can have an impact. The church's tradition does not condemn private property, but property is not an absolute right: every private property *has a social mortgage* according to John Paul II:

[14] Ezekiel Emanuel, et al., "What Makes Clinical Research in Developing Countries Ethical: The Benchmarks of Ethical Research," *The Journal of Infectious Diseases* 189, no. 5 (2004): 930–37.

[15] Alex J. London, "Justice and the Human Development Approach," *Hastings Center Report* 35, no. 1 (2005): 24–37.

> It is necessary to state once more the characteristic principle of Christian social doctrine: the goods of this world are originally meant for all. The right to private property is valid and necessary, but it does not nullify the value of this principle. Private property, in fact, is under a "social mortgage," which means that it has an intrinsically social function, based upon and justified precisely by the principle of the universal destination of goods.[16]

Patents are a form of intellectual property that, according to US law, "gives inventors exclusive rights to prevent anyone else from using, making, or commercializing their inventions without permission of the inventors."[17] There are some variations in patent law between the US and the European Union, but the basic concept is the same. The idea is to foster creativity and innovation, giving an economic incentive to the inventor in exchange for the public disclosure of his invention. After the patent expires, anyone can commercialize the invention. In principle, patents are an ethically justifiable form of property rights. However, it is subject to the social mortgage that limits all property rights according to Catholic social teaching. The common good—indeed, the global common good—takes precedence over property rights in many cases. The case of drug patents is a most obvious example, particularly in the case of life-saving medications and medical devices.

Animals and Ecological Responsibility

A final point needs to be mentioned, although we cannot develop it here. In the time of Pope Francis, the issue of the environmental responsibility of scientific research needs to be further developed by Catholic ethicists. In this context, a more developed and less anthropocentric theology of nonhuman animals, to whom we are certainly related in evolutionary terms, needs to receive greater attention from Catholic thinkers, both in dogmatic and in moral theology.

---

[16] John Paul II, *Sollicitudo Rei Socialis* 42.

[17] Adil E. Shamoo and David B. Resnik, *Responsible Conduct of Research*, 3rd ed. (New York: Oxford University Press, 2015), 175.

Conclusion

There is a gap between the Catholic social tradition and Catholic bioethical reflection, particularly in the area of research ethics. We have shown the urgency of overcoming such a divide. The principles of Catholic social teaching can greatly transform and enrich the ethics of scientific research. Catholics ethicists in the field of bioethics are called to renew their work in the light of our rich social tradition. Such renewal has the potential to invigorate research ethics beyond the realm of Catholic moral theology and Catholic bioethics. The principles of Catholic social teaching address fundamental issues for the preservation and enhancement of all life on Earth. They require us to transform biomedical research into a restorative praxis. But theologians and bioethicists are not the only ones called to action. Catholic universities, hospitals, and research centers are called to be the main actors in the transformation of research into a powerful restorative praxis in the twenty-first century.

Chapter 22

Environmental Ethics as Bioethics

Andrea Vicini, SJ, MD, and Tobias Winright

The planet Earth needs care. Humankind shares the living conditions on the planet with many other living beings and things, from animals to plants, soil to stones, water, and gases and air. How can individual citizens and believers, nations, and peoples care for Earth? Which type of care is needed? Which ethical approach is helpful? In these pages, we discuss the contributions of, and argue for an expanded engagement with, theological bioethics in promoting just sustainability[1] that relies on the richness of ethical resources characterizing Catholic social thought.[2]

Environmental ethics is attentive to the multiple ways in which people live and situate themselves in the environment. So, too, ought Catholic social bioethics. Hence, to lay out our bioethical framework, first, we consider how human beings might respectfully appreciate nature in its variety and richness (what the spiritual tradition has defined as one's ability to contemplate) and how this appreciation of the natural environment might lead to action to protect the whole

---

[1] See Christiana Z. Peppard and Andrea Vicini, eds., *Just Sustainability: Technology, Ecology, and Resource Extraction*, Catholic Theological Ethics in the World Church (Maryknoll, NY: Orbis Books, 2015).

[2] See Tobias L. Winright, ed., *Green Discipleship: Catholic Theological Ethics and the Environment* (Winona, MN: Anselm Academic, 2011). See also Tobias Winright, "Verdant Virtues: Serving and Protecting People and Planet," *Health Progress* 97, no. 3 (2016): 50–52.

creation.[3] Second, contemplation and action lead to the examination of, at least in the form of imaginative journeys, today's environmental challenges and contexts. Third, we articulate the contribution of Catholic social bioethics to address these diversified challenges by stressing its commitment to promote the common good and by emphasizing its prophetic role.

Contemplation and Action

Contemplation could be a starting point for defining how to care. In such a case, as citizens and believers, we contemplate what we have received and what has been entrusted to our care: the Earth. We contemplate ourselves and other people. We contemplate all sorts of living beings within what appears to us as an infinite space and an ungraspable time. As believers, we contemplate the divine presence in our world and history.

Contemplation includes both passivity and activity. We might stand on our planet with awe and serenity while enjoying the beauty that surrounds us. As the psalmist so eloquently asked, "When I look at your heavens . . . the moon and the stars that you have established; / what are human beings that you are mindful of them, / mortals that you care for them?" (Ps 8:3-4). We could also experience fear and trembling at the uncontained and uncontainable wildness with its at times destructive power and its ability to harm and to destroy, as when natural catastrophes occur. According to the ancient writer of Ecclesiastes, "For no one can anticipate the time of disaster. Like fish taken in a cruel net, and like birds caught in a snare, so mortals are snared at a time of calamity, when it suddenly falls upon them" (Eccl 9:12).

Maybe there is something in common with these opposite experiences and feelings. What is common is our vulnerability. Whether we are in peaceful awe or shaken by fear of what could happen to us, to others, and to those things that populate our civilized lives, we realize how small and vulnerable human beings are. We risk being

---

[3] The readers who are familiar with the spiritual tradition will recognize the importance of contemplation and action as the ways to express one's "being" and one's "doing" in both Ignatian and Franciscan spirituality.

overwhelmed, even by the majestic beauty of nature and, certainly, by the uncontainable strength of natural phenomena.

Moreover, our perceived vulnerability and our feeling overwhelmed can further increase if we contemplate what we should do to protect our planet with the beauty and diversity of the various continents and oceans, as well as the atmosphere that allows life to happen. We wonder, or even obsess, about the many ways in which we are threatening the quality of life on our planet. Impotence and being overwhelmed seem to accompany our vulnerability.

However, human beings are able to act. Unfortunately, even when we think we are choosing not to act, that choice is still an act. When Joshua instructed the people of Israel to "choose this day whom you will serve" (Josh 24:15), even the choice not to serve God would have been an act. If we focus on action, contemplation might empower us. In fact, contemplation and action have always formed a key part of how we think about the practice of medicine. Daily health problems of particular communities and individual patients are contemplated, discussed, and then acted on for the betterment of both the community and individual. The environmental challenges and the health consequences likewise require the resources of health care and bioethics to further contemplate and act on the challenges we face.

By engaging in contemplation and action, we could feel energized by today's challenges and what is ahead of us. How do we think about access to clean water across the globe? In what ways can we consider how to provide energy for development and how we limit our energy consumption? When will we express our concern about our limited resources and the process of resource extraction of minerals? Have we examined sufficiently food production and food availability? How will we deal with the consequences of global warming and its global health effects?

Contemplatively Imagining Our World Today

In an imaginative journey around the world, we visit mines by witnessing the terrible working conditions of many people—children, adolescents, and adults—in the depths of the Earth. We discover how they are exploited. We visit sites where fracking is taking place, and we realize how it harms the land and the cultures nearby. We explore sites where oil is extracted and where it is refined, with the risk of causing environmental disasters when the extraction goes wrong. We see how oil is shipped and, finally, we follow it up to the gas pump and to our cars. We visit the North Pole and the South Pole, and we are shocked by the extent and the fast pace of the progressive melting of the ice caps because of global warming,[4] with its most visible consequences for those people on Pacific islands, like Kiribati, who are forced to relocate because their countries are threatened by rising water levels.[5] We journey to the Amazonian rainforest and are appalled by the extent and pace of deforestation. Finally, we are shocked by the damages caused by wild fires, waste, drought, along with air and water pollution. We should care for our planet. Why does it seem that humankind does not bother to care?[6]

In our journey across the globe, we can visit many more places where we witness the suffering of people, of many living creatures and non-living things, and of the whole Earth. How is this journey shaping our awareness and assessment of the care that our planet needs? In this demanding journey, to care means being able to see where our hope will lead us to intervene by joining others who are already addressing these challenges, injustices, and struggles in solidarity with them. Our hopeful care will lead us to join them and to act.[7] In his encyclical *Sollicitudo Rei Socialis*, Pope John Paul II wrote that solidarity as a duty and a virtue "is not a feeling of vague compassion or shallow distress at the misfortunes of so many people, both near and far. On the contrary, it is a firm and persevering determination to commit oneself to the common good; that is to say to the good

---

[4] See the documentary by Jeff Orlowksi, *Chasing Ice* (2013). See also http://earth visioninstitute.org/extreme-ice-survey/.

[5] See Brookings Institution and London School of Economics Project on Internal Displacement, *On the Front Line of Climate Change and Displacement: Learning from and with Pacific Island Countries* (Washington, DC: The Brookings Institution, 2011); Maryanne Loughry and Jane McAdam, "Kiribati: Relocation and Adaptation," *Forced Migration Review* 31 (2008): 51–52.

[6] See James F. Keenan, SJ, *Moral Wisdom: Lessons and Texts from the Catholic Tradition*, 3rd ed. (Lanham, MD: Rowman and Littlefield, 2016), 29, and 42–44.

[7] For a similar journey, see the National Geographic documentary *Before the Flood*, where the actor Leonardo DiCaprio meets scientists, activists, and world leaders to discuss the dangers of climate change and its possible solutions. Fisher Stevens, *Before the Flood* (2016).

of all and of each individual, because we are all really responsible for all."[8] In Catholic social bioethics, this solidarity encompasses other human persons, especially the vulnerable, but also the natural world.

Broadening the Ethical Framework

Some authors suggest we rely on the so-called four principles of bioethics—autonomy, beneficence, nonmaleficence, and justice— proposed by Tom Beauchamp and James Childress since 1979.[9] This principlist approach has been the dominant one in bioethics until recently. Among others, Maura Ryan and Mary Jo Iozzio are not satisfied with the four principles approach because these principles presuppose an isolated individual, separated from her relational context, and offer a simplified understanding of justice as solely giving to one her due.[10] Philip Keane proposes "an integrated notion of social justice. Such a notion helps foster a dynamic vision of an integrated society in which we are all responsible, even co-responsible, for one another."[11] An "integrated notion of social justice" leads us to search for what is good for everyone. The ethical tradition suggests we name it "the common good," to highlight its inclusivity and its comprehensiveness. As Gary Gunderson and James Cochrane affirm, "The common good requires that individual interest find meaning amid generalized interests."[12] Hence, possible tensions can be anticipated between individual and collective interests. However, protecting biological diversity and the whole environment by assuring the conditions for life on the planet for both current and future generations could be considered "a collective enterprise for the common good."[13]

---

[8] John Paul II, *Sollicitudo Rei Socialis* (1987), 38.

[9] See Tom L. Beauchamp and James F. Childress, *Principles of Biomedical Ethics*, 7th ed. (New York: Oxford University Press, 2013).

[10] See Mary Jo Iozzio, "Health Care and the Common Good: A Catholic Theory of Justice," *Theological Studies* 62, no. 1 (2001): 186–88; Mary Jo Iozzio, "Justice Is a Virtue Both in and out of Health Care," *Irish Theological Quarterly* 63 (1998): 151–66; Maura A. Ryan, "Beyond a Western Bioethics?" *Theological Studies* 65, no. 1 (2004): 158–77.

[11] Philip S. Keane, *Catholicism and Health-Care Justice: Problems, Potential, and Solutions* (New York: Paulist Press, 2002), 13.

[12] Gary Gunderson and James R. Cochrane, *Religion and the Health of the Public: Shifting the Paradigm* (New York: Palgrave Macmillan, 2012), 11.

[13] Ibid.

To identify the common good for our planet is not an easy task. It is a process. We strive to define and then pursue what is the common good for humankind and for all creatures on Earth. Sustainability might be identified as one of the possibilities and strategies in striving to achieve the common good. Hence, sustainability is more than a commodity. Sustainability encompasses specific ecological dimensions with their social and economic implications. Sustainability implies interconnectedness and relationality, and influences moral discernment, decision-making, actions, and practices. Sustainability is a good. As such, it needs to be acknowledged, protected, and promoted as part of humankind's common good.

Within Catholic bioethics, Philip Keane suggests, "The classic Catholic concept of the common good argues for a deeper vision of society, a creative participative vision that holds that all people must strive for a level of goodness that is larger than any one individual, and indeed larger than the sum total of the goods of all individuals taken separately."[14] For Lisa Cahill, the common good includes equal access of all people to basic necessities and a variety of social goods and, among them, education, environmental innovation, and innovative scientific research.[15]

The Common Good

The common good is important and even urgent, but it is difficult to identify, define, and promote what is good for everyone, everything, everywhere. Can we agree that to protect Earth from the consequences of global warming is part of the common good? Can we pay attention to the warning of many scientists? In such a case, the

[14] Keane, *Catholicism and Health-Care Justice*, 12. Keane echoes the Second Vatican Council's definition of the common good: "the sum total of social conditions which allow people, either as groups or as individuals, to reach their fulfillment more fully and more easily. The resulting rights and obligations are consequently the concern of the entire human race. Every group must take into account the needs and legitimate aspirations of every other group, and even those of the human family as a whole." Second Vatican Council, *Gaudium et Spes* (Pastoral Constitution on the Church in the Modern World) 26.

[15] See Cahill, "Catholics and Health Care," *Journal of Catholic Social Thought* 7, no. 1 (2010): 29–49, at 31–32. See also David Hollenbach, SJ, *The Common Good and Christian Ethics* (New York: Cambridge University Press, 2002).

further step is to decide how to intervene, and how to do it together in our pluralist and multicultural world. For example, we need innovative and alternative ways to produce energy efficiently that gradually reduce fossil fuels and minimize their negative impact on the quality of air and on the percentage of CO_2 in the atmosphere—without doing it at the expense of jobs and people's health and well-being. In Catholic social thought, the common good and the individual good are not supposed to be at odds with each other. Rather than either/or, the common good entails a both/and.

Searching for the common good requires that we interact and dialogue with one another by listening to each one's argument, particularly to the voices that are always missing because of race and gender discrimination, or countless inequalities.[16] Hence, the pursuit of the common good is a fascinating and demanding process. In theological bioethics, as Lisa Cahill affirms, this process presupposes participation, requires justice, and can lead us to change.[17]

Participation, Justice, and Change

Participation, justice, and change indicate three values that should be pursued and, at the same time, offer insights into how these values should be pursued. In other words, citizens join and collaborate in caring for the planet in ways that respect their diversity. Moreover, people's strategies for action aim at promoting justice and fulfilling just requirements and practices. Finally, change presupposes the assessment that both participation and the promotion of just behaviors and practices are not yet entirely realized and implemented. Groups, communities, and nations are not yet fully joining in sharing their human, intellectual, religious, and social capabilities, nor in fulfilling their obligations to future generations.

---

[16] In James F. Keenan, ed., *Catholic Theological Ethics, Past, Present, and Future: The Trento Conference* (Maryknoll, NY: Orbis Books, 2012); see Antonio Moser, "Trent: The Historical Contribution and the Voices That Went Unheard," 96–106; Anne Nasimiyu-Wasike, "The Missing Voices of Women," 107–15; Bryan Massingale, "The Systemic Erasure of the Black/Dark-Skinned Body in Catholic Ethics," 116–24.

[17] See Lisa Sowle Cahill, *Theological Bioethics: Participation, Justice, and Change* (Washington, DC: Georgetown University Press, 2005).

The Principle of Subsidiarity

For Philip Keane, "whenever a social reform can be justly accomplished by a smaller, simpler agency, this is what should happen."[18] In Catholic social teaching, this is called the principle of subsidiarity. Lisa Cahill reminds us that the principle of subsidiarity aims at promoting the common good in two ways.

First, as Pope Pius XI affirmed in his 1931 encyclical letter *Quadragesimo Anno*,[19] "groups, organizations, and structures of government at the local level have the right to determine and manage local, community needs."[20] In this first sense, the principle promotes reciprocity between smaller and larger social collectives and sources of authorities.

Second, as Pope John XXIII affirmed thirty years later in his 1961 encyclical letter *Mater et Magistra*,[21] "when local communities, property owners, or investors are unable or unwilling to respect the concrete requirements of justice, the government or higher authority should intervene to rectify the situation."[22] As a consequence, governments have the duty to intervene for the benefit of their citizens.

Prophetic Care for Our Planet

The urgency to realize the common good might require raising prophetic voices in the public arena, embodying prophetic practices, and being prophetic witnesses. As biblical scholar Walter Brueggemann puts it, "prophetic imagination" leads to "effecting change in social perspective and social policy."[23]

How can bioethics help us in our life journey and in the journey of humankind on behalf of the current and future generations? Like Lisa Cahill, we think that bioethics can be a public discourse as well as a theological one. As such, it aims at empowering citizens and

---

[18] Keane, *Catholicism and Health-Care Justice*, 23.

[19] Pius XI, *Quadragesimo Anno* 79.

[20] Cahill, "Catholics and Health Care," 33.

[21] John XXIII, *Mater et Magistra* 54.

[22] Cahill, "Catholics and Health Care," 34.

[23] Walter Brueggemann, *The Prophetic Imagination*, 2nd ed. (Minneapolis, MN: Fortress Press, 2001), xii.

believers. Internationally, agreements, conventions, and documents can be ways in which solidarity and just social transformations can be articulated and might lead to change.

International official documents and agreements exemplify one modality of articulating scientific discourse and promoting the bioethical care of the planet. They assess, analyze, and set priorities. But, are they prophetic? Do they stimulate engagement and commitment? In other words, to promote sustainability, should bioethical discourse be prophetic in inspiring, positive, and constructive ways to act?

A Prophetic Role for Bioethics

In her 2014 presidential address at the American Academy of Religion, Jewish bioethicist Laurie Zoloth made a passionate and strong case for the prophetic role of theological bioethics by stressing its three duties: first, it ought to warn us; second, it should lead us to imagine the future; and, third, it must offer us a choice of interrupting and restarting our lives as moral individuals, citizens, and scholars. In this world, and at this time, climate change threatens the possibility of life on our planet. As she urges, climate change is "the most important issue in bioethics and the central moral imperative of our time."[24] To strengthen her prophetic voice and commitment, she turned to the biblical account of creation and to biblical narratives describing the natural struggles that affect, then and now, vulnerable populations. Finally, she forcefully claimed,

> *We must be interrupted; we must stop.* To make the future possible, we need to stop what we are doing, what we are making, what we are consuming, what we think we need, what makes us comfortable. We need to interrupt our work—even our good work—to attend to the urgency of this question. . . . Is our society unable to stop careening toward the deep trouble of the coming storm because we have not fully attended, because we cannot stop?[25]

---

[24] Laurie Zoloth, "2014 AAR Presidential Address: Interrupting Your Life: An Ethics for the Coming Storm," *Journal of the American Academy of Religion* 84, no. 1 (2016): 3–24, at 5.

[25] Ibid., 16 (original emphasis). Concretely and in a provocative way, she proposed that every six years the American Academy of Religion should pause and, to reduce

Prophetic Practices

Bioethical discourse and bioethical public engagement support multiple prophetic practices. While Pope Francis, with other authors, is vocal in asking for individual behavioral choices that aim at containing consumption and that are sustainable, other scholars disagree. For them, only technological innovation will be able to provide the needed solutions to avoid any environmental collapse.[26]

Individual practices that promote sustainability, however, should not be easily and quickly dismissed as irrelevant because of their limited impact on the global scale of the ecological issues (e.g., in the case of water and energy consumption) compared, for example, to the energy consumption and pollution caused by the industrial complex around the world.[27] Individual commitment of citizens, families, groups, associations, and even towns should be praised.[28] If the total sum of these contributions, in quantitative terms, is minimal, its qualitative bearing is very valuable. Personal and communal behavioral changes highlight how people can be virtuous and act in virtuous ways. They participate in defining prophetic behaviors.

As Jacquineau Azetsop suggests, education should aim at training transformational leaders, that is, "people who have a passion for the kingdom of justice, peace and love; a sensitivity for changing circumstances; a capacity of discerning the emerging dilemmas of their respective milieu in cooperation with others; and the skills to identify systems of oppression that perpetuate structural violence and to act

---

its carbon footprint, choose "to not meet at a huge annual meeting in which we take over a city." Ibid., 23.

[26] As examples, see Ted Nordhaus and Michael Shellenberger, *Break Through: From the Death of Environmentalism to the Politics of Possibility* (Boston: Houghton Mifflin, 2007); Ted Nordhaus and Michael Shellenberger, *Break Through: Why We Can't Leave Saving the Planet to Environmentalists* (Boston: Mariner Books, 2009). See also http://www.thebreakthrough.org/.

[27] "A change in lifestyle could bring healthy pressure to bear on those who wield political, economic and social power." Francis, *Laudato Si'* (On Care for Our Common Home), 206. Hereafter LS.

[28] "There is a nobility in the duty to care for creation through little daily actions, and it is wonderful how education can bring about real changes in lifestyle" (LS 211). Moreover, "We must not think that these efforts are not going to change the world" (LS 212).

upon them."[29] Concrete practices nourish our hope. Should we be hopeful?

David Goodstein asks, "Is there any hope for a truly sustainable long-term future civilization?"[30] Lisa Cahill argues that

> hope is not detached from our life in community, nor does it grow independently of human efforts. Christian hope is a practical virtue, one that requires imagination and commitment. Hope feeds on action, undertaken with courage to change difficult situations. Hope does not require guarantees of future success or even a balance of success over failure. Hope comes from solidarity in action that makes a difference, enabling participants to realize that a different future is possible.[31]

For Cahill, hope "comes from concrete initiatives to serve the poor and underserved."[32] Hence, she invites us to identify, examine, and appreciate some of these initiatives to strengthen our hope and to support our commitment. In focusing on sustainability, we can identify more practices that inspire and strengthen our hope. Probably, each one of us could name practices that, locally or globally, embody solidarity in action and give us hope. And because Cahill's reference to practices serving the poor and underserved brings to mind the corporal works of mercy, we believe Conor M. Kelly offers an imaginative proposal for developing corporal works of justice as analogs to the corporal works of mercy in connection with food insecurity and accessibility, ethical consumption, migration and displacement, health care as a universal good, mass incarceration and related racial disparities, and gun violence and war.[33]

---

[29] Jacquineau Azetsop, SJ, *Structural Violence, Population Health and Health Equity: Preferential Option for the Poor and Bioethics Health Equity in Sub-Saharan Africa* (Saarbrücken: VDM Verlag Dr. Müller, 2010), 302.

[30] David Goodstein, "Energy, Technology and Climate: Running out of Gas," in *Expanding Horizons in Bioethics*, ed. Arthur W. Galston, et al. (Norwell, MA: Springer, 2005), 233–45, at 243.

[31] Cahill, "Catholics and Health Care," 43.

[32] Ibid.

[33] See Gerard Mannion, "Catholic Social Thought: Topic Session," *CTSA Proceedings* 71 (2016): 85–86.

Conclusion

Theological bioethics can help us to contemplate both the frightening, damaging progress of human-made environmental destruction and the astonishing, resilient beauty of our planet and of the universe. Solidarity aims at promoting the common good, with privileged attention to the environmental challenges that humanity, and particularly the poor, face today and in the future. Prophetic discourses and practices shape both the bioethical reflection and actions, and the lives of believers. Prophets speak the truth on behalf of those who cannot do that on their own—the voiceless, the poor, the minorities, the marginalized, the vulnerable, and all those who, for many, do not count in the public arena. Prophetic bioethical education committed to promote social justice contributes to train citizens and professionals engaged in promoting social justice and just sustainability.

Will our solidarity and our engagement to promote the common good be sufficient to care for our planet and to protect it for future generations? In the case of climate change, maybe it is already too late to avoid many of its consequences for the planet and for the people living on the shores of our oceans. But our creative commitment might be able to slow down the fast changes affecting the global climate. We will answer with our personal and collective choices. We hope we will be up to the challenges. The care for our planet is entrusted to us. Our many journeys can have good endings, for us and for those who will follow us.

Chapter 23

A Social Bioethics of Genetics

Hille Haker

The 2015 National Academy of Science International Summit Meeting discussed the new CRISPR technique that may one day allow for genetic interventions in human embryos, altering the DNA make-up of a human embryo and all future generations.[1] This technology is emerging; its effects are unknown. At the summit, I recommended keeping the long-established ban on germline editing. The goal of society, I held, should be "to promote a better life for all, and to ensure that everybody can live a life in dignity and freedom. . . . Can this be achieved by germline gene editing? My view is no."[2] This position was critiqued by another bioethicist, John Harris, and in the discussion of the panel, the critics were confronted by a parent and representative of the American Association of Tissue Banks. She took the microphone and told her story as the mother of a child who died six days after his birth due to a lethal birth defect. She said, challenging

---

[1] CRISPR stands for stands for Clustered Regularly Interspaced Short Palindromic Repeats. Developed in the last decade, it is a gene editing technology that utilizes specialized proteins to precisely cut and paste DNA into the human genome. More efficient than previous gene-editing techniques, it raises ethical questions primarily with regard to human gene transfer interventions into somatic and germline cells.

[2] Committee on Science, Technology, and Law; Policy and Global Affairs; National Academies of Sciences, Engineering, and Medicine; S. Olson ed., *International Summit on Human Gene Editing: A Global Discussion* (Washington, DC: National Academies Press, 2016). International Summit on Human Gene Editing: A Global Discussion: Meeting in Brief.

the audience tearfully, that her son suffered every day of his life. "If you have the skills, the knowledge—to fix these diseases, then fricking do it!"[3]

This story captures the dilemma of the new reproductive genetic technologies (RGTs): on the one hand, there is the cry of the parent who urges medicine to develop therapies so that other parents need not be faced with the death of an infant; on the other hand, RGTs may involve more and more research on human embryos; they may result in violations of future children's rights; and they may shift once more the priority of health care toward a particular group of prospective parents while ignoring the cries of those parents whose children die, too, but die from easily preventable diseases.

❖ ❖ ❖ ❖ ❖

RGTs offer people options for procreation that are radically new in human history. As is well known, assisted reproduction is not offered within Catholic health care. Nonetheless, Catholic voices are crucial to illuminating the deeper ethical issues surrounding RGTs. If Catholic ethics wants to play a role in the public debate, it must address the emerging questions associated with RGTs.

In this chapter, I will comment only on some issues regarding RGTs, as a glimpse into a complex area of research.[4] First, I will comment on the new developments in genetics; second, I will critique the Catholic approach to bioethics rooted in the Vatican's approach to sexual ethics; and third, I will argue for a critical ethics in and for the sciences and humanities, here spelled out as a social bioethics of genetics and human reproduction.

---

[3] Organizing Committee Summit Meeting Gene Editing, "On Human Gene Editing: International Summit Statement," https://vimeo.com/149190913.

[4] For more thorough analyses, see Hille Haker, "Reproductive Rights and Reproductive Technologies," in *The Routledge Handbook of Global Ethics*, ed. Heather Widdows and Darrel Moellendorf (London: Routledge, 2014), 340–53; Hille Haker, *Ethik der genetischen Frühdiagnostik. Sozialethische Reflexionen zur Verantwortung am menschlichen Lebensbeginn* (Paderborn: Mentis, 2002); and Hille Haker, *Hauptsache gesund? Ethische Fragen der Pränatal- und Präimplantationsdiagnostik* (München: Kösel, 2011).

Genetics in Human Reproduction: Gene Editing

The modern RGTs are part of a much broader scientific paradigm that goes back to the beginning of modern genetics in the nineteenth century. They have changed considerably over the last decades, and the new possibilities, e.g., prenatal and preimplantation genetic diagnosis, are generally embraced by prospective parents and the societies that have introduced them. Nevertheless, the history of human genetics renders genetics in connection with reproduction a sensitive issue. Historian of eugenics Daniel Kevles warns, correctly in my view, that the CRISPR technology allows the eugenic dreams of the early twentieth-century finally to come true—more likely used as "bottom up" consumer eugenics than state-driven improvement of the "gene pool."[5]

In contemporary bioethics, *reproductive autonomy* serves as the supreme principle of RGTs. It is defined as a consumer/client/patient right and physician/health care professional obligation to respect the client's freedom.[6] The principle of autonomy implicitly (or explicitly) assumes that a client, for example, the prospective parents or a pregnant woman, is sovereign, free, and able to choose among several goods. This ethics thereby mirrors the idealized image of the modern *citizen* and *consumer* that liberalism has depicted throughout modern philosophy. Feminist ethics as well as theological bioethics critique this emphasis on autonomy, arguing that it ignores the

---

[5] Daniel J. Kevles, "The History of Eugenics," *Issues in Science and Technology* 32, no. 3 (2016): 45. For disability studies, see Hans S. Reinders, *The Future of the Disabled in Liberal Society: An Ethical Analysis* (Notre Dame, IN: University of Notre Dame Press, 2000); and Peter Blanck and Eilionóir Flynn, *Routledge Handbook of Disability Law and Human Rights* (London: Routledge, 2017).

[6] See Hille Haker, "Transcending Liberalism—Avoiding Communitarianism: Human Rights and Dignity in Bioethics," in *Oltre L'individualismo. Relazioni e Relazionalità per Ripensare l'idendità*, ed. Ardian Ndreca Lorealla Congiunti and Giambattista Formica (Rome: Urbaniana University Press, 2017), 85–100. In the context of human reproduction, the liberal ethics is spelled out most clearly in Allen Buchanan, Dan Brock, Norman Daniels, and Daniel Wikler, *From Chance to Choice. Genetics and Justice* (Cambridge: Cambridge University Press, 2001). For a critical response, see Jurgen Habermas, *The Future of Human Nature* (Cambridge, UK: Polity, 2003); and Hille Haker, "On the Limits of Liberal Bioethics," in *The Contingent Nature of Life: Publication of the European Science Foundation Conference, Doorn April 2005*, ed. Christoph Rehmann-Sutter, Marcus Duewell, and Dietmar Mieth (Berlin: Springer, 2008), 191–208.

relatedness and interdependency of persons, proposing instead a feminist ethics of care, or a theological ethics of sacramental love.[7]

New developments in genetic research, however, require a new look at RGTs. Gene and genome editing allow for a more efficient and more precise modification of any organism's genetic makeup—a fact that is only beginning to sink in with the general public. In non-human genetics, for example, the so-called *gene-drive technology* has emerged over the last few years. "Gene drive" means that gene editing is used to enhance the passing of specific, "modified" characteristics from the "parent" generation to their "offspring," resulting in a preferential genotype that ultimately will change the phenotype of the given organism. Gene drives may, for example, modify the DNA of mosquito populations which are responsible for the transmission of malaria, enhance food production, or preserve diversity of species affected by dramatic reduction or even extinction.[8]

Regarding medical research on gene editing in *humans*, there are basically three major fields: drug development as personalized medicine; somatic cell therapies; and gene editing that modifies the human genome on the germline level. The last application means that the offspring's cells will now express the genetic modifications. Many people seem to resonate with the summit meeting's statement by the mother who lost a child. Early committee reports of different national and international scientific academies mostly follow the approach of liberal bioethics.[9] They address technical questions and echo an ethics

---

[7] See, among others, Catriona Mackenzie and Natalie Stoljar, *Relational Autonomy: Feminist Perspectives on Automomy, Agency, and the Social Self* (New York: Oxford University Press, 2000); and Eva Feder Kittay and Ellen K. Feder, eds., *The Subject of Care: Feminist Perspectives on Dependency* (Lanham, MD: Rowman and Littlefield, 2002). For a critical discussion from the perspective of feminist ethics, see Hille Haker, "Reproductive Rights and Reproductive Technologies," 2014.

[8] For a good overview, see Committee on Gene Drive Research in Non-Human Organisms, *Gene Drives on the Horizon: Advancing Science, Navigating Uncertainty, and Aligning Research with Public Values, Recommendations for Responsible Conduct*, ed. Engineering Board on Life Sciences; Division on Earth and Life Studies; National Academies of Sciences and Medicine (Washington, DC: National Academies Press, 2016). This important report concludes that the governance models are insufficient to include the low-income countries where gene drive is being tested.

[9] For an overview, see these comprehensive reports: National Academy of Sciences and National Academy of Medicine, *Human Genome Editing: Science, Ethics, and Governance* (Washington, DC: National Academies Press, 2017); Nuffield Council on Bioethics, *Genome Editing: An Ethical Review* (Nuffield Council on Bioethics, 2016);

of reproductive autonomy, mostly ignoring any *structural* discussion of consumer-oriented RGTs, the *social* desirability of germline editing research, feasible *alternatives*, including nonmedical options, the *effects* on social and global health care justice, or the effects on ethnic minorities,[10] and disability groups. Justice is mainly discussed as unequal access to the benefits of the new technologies.

Vatican Bioethics after Vatican II

Given the implications for and involvement of RGTs with embryos and human reproduction, Catholic bioethics approaches these technologies through a lens primarily shaped by Catholic sexual ethics. Not surprisingly, Catholic bioethics prohibits any research that involves the destruction of human embryos, rendering *research* into germline modification using human embryos illicit. Yet the Vatican is far less categorical when it comes to the application of germline therapy than with respect to abortion: *"in its current state*, germ line cell therapy in all its forms is morally illicit."[11] Mirroring its liberal counterpart, most of the conversation regarding the development of RGTs centers around the Vatican's teaching and leaves little room to engage in social ethics questions around future RGT developments.

John Paul II promoted a sexual ethics that continued Paul VI's understanding developed in *Humanae Vitae*. He understands "human procreation" as mirroring divine creation in human self-giving love. It differs both from the biological understanding of human reproduction and from the social understanding of self-realization of couples, connecting procreation with the *sacrament* of marriage.[12] From the

---

and European Academies Scientific Advisory Council, *Genome Editing: Scientific Opportunities, Public Interests and Policy Options in the European Union* (Halle [Saale], Germany: German National Academy of Sciences, 2017).

[10] Sheldon Krimsky and Kathleen Sloan, *Race and the Genetic Revolution: Science, Myth, and Culture* (New York: Columbia University Press, 2011); and Keith Wailoo, Alondra Nelson, and Catherine Lee, *Genetics and the Unsettled Past: The Collision of DNA, Race, and History* (New Brunswick, NJ: Rutgers University Press, 2012).

[11] Congregation of the Doctrine of Faith, *Dignitas Personae* (On Certain Bioethical Questions), 26 (emphasis added).

[12] John Paul II, *Theology of the Body: Human Love in the Divine Plan* (Boston: Pauline Books and Media, 1997). The concept of marriage and procreation is stated in Paul VI's *Humanae Vitae* and often cited in bioethical texts like, for example, *Dignitas Personae*, 6.

1970s on, the Vatican rejected any technical intervention into the sexual act, criticizing that it denigrates the sacramentality of marriage. Furthermore, it held that the claimed reproductive autonomy exacerbates the categorical misunderstanding of human life as "chosen" rather than "given," ultimately replacing the gift of life with the arbitrary design of life.

The Vatican's position argues that reproduction and parenthood have become "projects" under the conditions of modern family planning, rendering the care for and living with children as a choice that aims at one particular form of the "good life."[13] But it does not at all follow that such choices deny the "givenness" of human life. In fact, several models of (Western) parenthood exist side-by-side. The Vatican claims that the sacramental model of marriage and parenthood provides a theological hermeneutics that gives meaning to marriage *and* sexuality, including procreation. But it argues further that this understanding of sexual and reproduction ethics is normatively binding, prescribed by natural law and ultimately, divine law. This means that a particular theological interpretation of sexuality defines reproductive rights and responsibilities.

John Paul II's approach to sexuality is reflected in his approach to questions in bioethics. *Dignitas Personae* sees John Paul II's approach to bioethics in the twentieth-century question of Catholic social teaching (CST). In an astonishing parallel, he compares the Catholic solidarity with impoverished European workers in the nineteenth century with the now-required protection of "another category of persons being oppressed," i.e., the human embryo. But this is a striking statement, prioritizing the embryos' right to life over any other— or any other group's—right. Social ethics, this means, is now to begin with sexual ethics and bioethics, and both are to prioritize the protection of human embryos.[14]

---

[13] Elisabeth Beck-Gernsheim, *Reinventing the Family: In Search of New Lifestyles* (Malden, MA: Polity Press, 2002); and Onora O'Neill, "The 'Good Enough Parent' in the Age of the New Reproductive Technologies," in *The Ethics of Genetics in Human Procreation*, ed. Hille Haker and Deryck Beyleveld (Aldershot: Ashgate, 2000), 33–48.

[14] Congregation of the Doctrine of Faith, *Dignitais Personae* 37, quoting John Paul II. For a critique, see Hille Haker, "Catholic Sexual Ethics—A Necessary Revision: Catholic Responses to the Sexual Abuse Scandal," in *Concilium 47/3, Human Trafficking*, ed. Hille Haker, Lisa Cahill, and Elaine Wainwright (London: SCM Press, 2011).

Catholic Social Ethics: Dissent and Renewal

Alfons Auer[15] was a member of the international expert commission that advised Paul VI on the issue of contraceptives. Like many theologians, he was an outspoken critic of the encyclical *Humane Vitae*; after his publication of the "Ten Theses against *Humanae Vitae*" in 1968, however, he and his approach to Catholic moral theology, quickly referred to as the Auer School of Catholic ethics, was dismissed by the Vatican. Nevertheless, Auer began to move theological ethics beyond Paul VI's and John Paul II's natural law ethics that failed to integrate science adequately into its theological framework. He argued that theology must recognize modern natural and human sciences as an independent source of knowledge, taking them seriously in a first step of ethical evaluation. In a second step of ethical evaluation, Auer held, the insights from the sciences and humanities are to be assessed in view of the philosophical analysis of moral norms. Only then, in the third step, are these insights to be contextualized and integrated into the Christian perspective, especially its theological anthropology that says more about the ultimate existential meaning of life than explaining it in scientific and cultural-anthropological terms.

Auer's ethics became the leading school of theological ethics in Germany. Auer's student and social ethicist Dietmar Mieth developed it further into an ethics in the sciences and humanities. Over the years, Mieth, who was the founding director of one of the first bioethics centers in Germany, together with his students from multiple disciplines analyzed issues surrounding assisted reproduction, the Human Genome Project, and the new biotechnologies. Mieth's approach is a decidedly social bioethics: it converses with scientists who practice assisted reproductive technologies (ART) and genetics but also with scholars from the humanities who explore the personal and social

---

[15] Alfons Auer, "Nach dem Erscheinen der Enzyklika 'Humanae Vitae'. Zehn Thesen über die Findung sittlicher Weisungen," *Theologische Quartalschrift* 149 (1969):75–85; Alfons Auer, *Autonome Moral und christlicher Glaube* (Düsseldorf: Patmos, 1971). For a more thorough analysis of Auer's work, see Hille Haker, "Christian Ethics in Germany—Tendencies and Future," in *Modern Believing: Church and Society, 50/1,* ed. Ian Markham, Paul Badham, and Rob Warner (Oxford, UK: The Modern Churchpeople's Union, 2009), 16–28.

experiences of love, sexual ethics, and family planning. Correlating these interdisciplinary insights with the philosophical principles of moral respect and justice on the one hand, and the given or developing political and legal frameworks for research and clinical medicine on the other, Mieth and his colleagues engaged in ethical analyses compatible with any other, non-theological approach. Theology's genuine form of reason is situated in the hermeneutical-ethical reflection, offering, among others, one particular narrative of human existence, captured as the gift of unconditional acceptance by God, and the called-for response in one's own responses to others.[16]

Like the German theologians, US Catholic bioethicists also departed from John Paul II's insistence on seeing social ethics as primarily invested in the protecting of human embryos; but they kept closer ties with the tradition of Catholic social teaching than the Auer School in Germany. Both schools, however, pointed, for example, to global health disparities, global health discrimination against women, the lack of participatory justice in medical research decisions, global epidemics, and the pandemic of HIV/AIDS. Methodologically, however, US contributions on social bioethics mostly left the natural law tradition untouched, taking it (rather than the Kantian tradition of dignity and respect, as is the case in the Auer School) as the normative foundation underlying Catholic ethics.[17]

In a contrast to John Paul II and Benedict XVI that has not escaped his critics, Pope Francis has recently explicitly endorsed an interdisciplinary, integrative method of social ethics. Francis not only promotes a practical-pastoral ethics—he also embraces social ethics as an ethics in dialogue with the sciences and humanities. This interdisciplinary, integrative approach is explicitly taken up in the encyclical *Laudato Si'*, concerning the problem of climate change. The

---

[16] For Mieth's approach to social ethics and bioethics, see, among others, Dietmar Mieth, *Moral und Erfahrung II*, vol. 76, *Studien zur Theologischen Ethik* (Fribourg i. Ue: Universitätsverlag Fribourg/Herder, 1998); Dietmar Mieth, *Moral und Erfahrung I. Grundlagen einer theologisch-ethischen Hermeneutik*, 4 ed. (Freiburg i. Ue: Fribourger Universitätsverlag, 1999); and Dietmar Mieth, *Was wollen wir können? Ethik im Zeitalter der Biotechnik* (Freiburg i. Br: Herder, 2002).

[17] See Lisa Sowle Cahill, Hille Haker, and Eloi Messi Metogo, *Human Nature and Natural Law* (London: SCM Press, 2010). This issue brings together scholars who have addressed the natural law theory in thorough works, either as proponents or critics.

question today is whether this turn will also affect other areas, including bioethics, mediating the dialogue with the sciences and humanities *and* philosophical ethics with an explicit theological ethics that prioritizes the care for the wounded and the suffering. Regarding RGTs, this ethical approach cannot mean that we should just go ahead with any new technology and "fix the fricking diseases," no matter what the price for the future children and their offspring may be. The list of diseases that are targeted by researchers goes far beyond lethal genetic conditions. It remains to be seen whether it can be argued convincingly that the new RGTs will trade the freedom and integrity of future children for their health—and whether this is a price our societies are willing to pay.

Catholic Social Bioethics Revisited

In Western societies, RGTs have become part of the health service while *also* being a considerable factor of the economy. The size of the global ART market generated revenue of $22.3 billion in 2015 and is expected to reach $31.4 billion by 2023.[18] Furthermore, RGTs have shaped the understanding of "healthy children" along the lines of genetics. Prenatal diagnosis of Down syndrome, for example, results in the termination of most pregnancies when the tests are offered, reflecting not only personal choices but also medical and social expectations. Genetics, this means, creates its own social norms, whether intended by scientists or not.

Today, the question becomes whether the notion of "responsible parenthood" includes the genetic modification of one's offspring—a prospect that was explicitly rejected as "against human dignity" by several international regulatory bodies and UN documents in the 1990s and 2000s.[19] Once germline gene editing is on the table, new questions follow: Should human embryos be modified for health

---

[18] These numbers stem from https://www.gminsights.com/pressrelease/assisted-reproductive-technology-market.

[19] See UNESCO, *Universal Declaration on Bioethics and Human Rights*, 2005; and Council of Europe, *Convention for the Protection of Human Rights and Dignity of the Human Being with regard to the Application of Biology and Medicine: Convention on Human Rights and Biomedicine*, 1997.

purposes only or also for purposes of enhancement? Who should be allowed to seek such modifications? Who should decide? And what procedures are needed before deciding when the research is safe enough to be tested in vivo? Catholic bioethics must respond to these questions, independent of the practices Catholic hospitals offer. We need thorough studies that discern the goals and means of RGTs and that assess the targeted diseases, social contexts and social priorities, technical alternatives, underlying anthropology, and principles that guide our responses to "what we ought to do." Bringing together the insights of the sciences, humanities, and moral philosophy that integrates rights and responsibilities, and a critical hermeneutics that turns to experience and theological tradition as a source for ethical insights, these studies will offer deeper insights than any single discipline is able to provide.

First, science and humanities: Ethics needs to analyze the insights from the sciences *and* humanities in order to understand how genetics, love and sexuality, family planning and human reproduction, health and well-being, models of parenthood, etc. are reflected upon in the different disciplines. Germline gene modification cannot be seen merely as a technical "fix" of human diseases: if it turns out that it will result in social changes that go far beyond the intended repair of a gene, ethics must contribute to raising the public awareness of these effects.

Second, philosophical-ethical analysis: Normative judgments regarding actions and practices (including the practice of research) concerning RGTs, policies, and legal regulations must pass the test of responding to the many faces of suffering, human rights violations, and the striking structural injustice in reproductive services. Normative reasoning about how to protect and promote freedom and justice becomes the subject of philosophical-ethical deliberation as an integral part of theological ethics, and as a critique of moral harms and injustices.

Liberal bioethicists argue that (a) human gene/genome editing that aims to modify the genetic make-up of future children is *good* because prospective parents and future children will benefit from it; and (b) it is within the realm of the prospective parents' *right* to pursue their reproductive interests. Both claims do not respond to the argument that germline gene editing research depends on ever-more human embryo research and may well violate the rights of future children.[20]

Many ethicists follow a consequentialist, utilitarian approach to bioethics. From a utilitarian perspective, the development of gene editing technologies must be compared with alternative methods, and RGTs must be weighed against the reproductive rights of all prospective parents. For example, improvements regarding maternal and infant mortality rates, prematurity, and basic health care would have a greater benefit to a greater number of prospective parents and their future children than the modification of genetic conditions. If justice is the overall principle of this approach, it cannot be reduced to access rights to RGTs. Furthermore, the argument for reproductive rights must not only apply to a particular group of prospective parents and only to particular reproductive rights. Rather, justice must be spelled out in all its facets, including social justice and global health care justice. Scientists and ethicists who address questions of justice merely as *access rights* to gene editing and RGT ignore that social justice requires not only to *prevent* new injustices but to *correct* already existing social inequalities, disadvantages, and discrimination. Research *policies*, too, require *priorities decisions*, but those individuals and groups who are *at present* marginalized are often marginalized in medical research, too, as Ferrer notes in the previous chapter. Distributive justice requires prioritization between competing goals.

Framing RGTs primarily as a question of personal "reproductive rights" ignores multiple factors that are in play in human reproduction. Social bioethics cannot escape the question of justice, to wit, whose lives, whose rights, and whose interests count, and whose rights are ignored in the current frameworks of research as well as in the bioethics discourse.[21] Health care practitioners, including

---

[20] For an argument that explicitly embraces the principle of autonomy yet critiques the parental or societal intervention into the genetic make-up of future children because of *their* right to autonomy, see Habermas, *The Future of Human Nature*.

[21] In contrast the UN 2030 Agenda for Sustainable Development, see https:// sustainabledevelopment.un.org/post2015/transformingourworld with an alternative approach, in which new technologies are *embedded* in a broader agenda instead of being an "autonomous" social practice.

nurses, ethicists, and chaplains, are the first responders to medical ills—and yet, their voices and their experiences with suffering are rarely heard in the discussions.

The fundamental principle of Catholic—as of any—social bioethics must indeed be human dignity, spelled out in the various kinds of human rights. Dignity is not grounded in the utilitarian principle of the best-possible consequences for the greatest number, nor in the liberal principle of autonomy; to the contrary, it is grounded in the recognition that every human being is vulnerable to luck, moral harm, and structural vulnerability, to which agents and institutions are called to respond.[22] Human dignity is to be correlated to the overall framework of human rights, which are indivisible and not to be reduced to reproductive rights only. Health care rights, women's rights, disability rights, antidiscrimination rights, and rights of children are also addressed in the human rights framework. Unless Catholic bioethics attends to this framework, it cannot provide answers to the many questions raised by the new developments in RGTs.

A comprehensive human rights approach critiques the concern for human embryo protection as the primary "new social question," as John Paul II claimed. But Catholic bioethics does also not follow the (neo-)liberal and often neocolonial approach to biotechnology and biomedical research.[23] *Beginning* rather than ending the work of discernment of responsibility in view of human rights, Catholic social ethics can turn to numerous so-called middle principles of contextual practical reasoning, helpful for the studies of social bioethics: *phronesis* (prudence), rooted in *remembrance, docility, caution, foresight,* or the regard for *circumstances,* may support the concrete normative assessments and the weighing of prospective actions and practices in the field of bioethics.

---

[22] Hille Haker, "Vulnerable Agency: A Conceptual and Contextual Analysis," in *Dignity and Conflict: Contemporary Interfaith Dialogue on the Value and Vulnerability of Human Life,* ed. Jonathan Rothschild and Matthew Petrusek (Notre Dame, IN: Notre Dame University Press, 2019).

[23] The fight about the patents for CRISPR is only one sad fact that the economic dimension matters as much, if not more, for the research institutions as the ethical rhetoric wants us to believe, see https://www.the-scientist.com/bio-business/flux-and-uncertainty-in-the-crispr-patent-landscape-30228.

Third, discernment of the Christian tradition: In addition to the normative questions, Catholic social bioethics discerns and interprets its own tradition regarding human existence and relationships. Its genuine theological horizon of meaning allows for an interpretation of the "deeper meaning" of human existence and is a constitutive source of and for ethical reflection. Ethically speaking, this tradition serves as a reminder that to love God is to respond to the other without setting conditions for their right to exist, even though human finiteness may limit responsible actions. In this, theology offers a realist, not an idealist, notion of human responsibility.

In sum, Catholic social bioethics is interdisciplinary in its *descriptive* analyses, philosophical in its *normative* claims, and *hermeneutical* in offering its own interpretations of the theological tradition. Presupposing that every historical situation is non-ideal, a critical theological ethics will attend to the experiences of *limits* and *failures* of human actions, both regarding the care for others and the care for oneself; it will critically discern *ideological* social visions by attending to how they increase rather than reduce social exclusion; it will attend to the *violations* of human rights and the effects of *refused responsibilities and solidarity*; and it will *prioritize remedies* for structural or institutional forms of *injustice*. Asking how we should proceed with respect to RGTs will not yield easy answers. Thorough analyses are needed in order to respect the freedom of research—but more urgently, in order to do justice to all parents who are faced with the threat of their children's preventable illness or death.

Conclusion:
The Tasks for a Critical Theological Ethics

What can theologians and practitioners in health care contribute regarding the new RGTs? I have pointed to one critical area, germline genetic modification that needs further ethical assessment. Catholic bioethics can indeed counter the myth of the "genetically perfected child" that underlies the new genetic pursuit, ignoring all burdens it may place on future children. Germline genetic modification is not only risky, it also normalizes RGTs for multiple groups of prospective parents, and it opens the door to genetic enhancement on the level of germlines. Social bioethics must discuss the scientific research but also the social vision for the future of parenthood, creating new standards of the "good enough child." It is here that health care practitioners and theologians are critical.

But the critical social bioethics I depict requires much more, namely, a radical revision of magisterial sexual ethics. Theologians need to keep in mind how hard-won the reforms of the Vatican II Council were at the time. Catholic bioethics will *defend* scientific innovations against the dystopian depiction that modern—and postmodern—life merely expresses a culture of death. Moreover, it will insist on the freedom to reason and to act in accordance with one's moral convictions—freedom is the most important insight of the gift of human reason. Ultimately, Catholic social bioethics will need to recognize the indivisible human rights, for example, reproductive rights *as well as* the rights of future children—and acknowledge that sometimes moral agents are faced with tragic dilemmas. Scientific and social analyses, philosophical argumentation, and theological interpretations of human existence are integrative elements of theological ethics. Together, they inform the critical social bioethics. All Christians contribute to ethical discernment, reflected systematically by theological scholarship. Likewise, every moral agent engages in the discernment of rights and responsibilities, reflected systematically by ethical scholarship. Regarding genetic diseases targeted by gene editing, the sciences are certainly the experts in the understanding of diseases, but the critical social bioethics will caution against hyping every new technology, as if it were the ultimate savior of human illness, finitude, and suffering.

The humanities analyze how societies deal with illness and diseases or how they construct what counts as disease in the technical-medical sense. But ultimately, human subjectivity can neither be reduced to the scientific point of view nor can it be reduced to a sociological or cultural point of view. Ethics must therefore attend to the experiences of those who are easily considered undesirable, as persons with a "wrongful life," especially when they belong to the groups targeted by the new RGTs. A critical theological ethics will take its own tradition as a source to understand such misrecognition and exclusion; in addition, theology offers a myriad of narratives of suffering *and* healing, among them the literal healing but also the transformation of the experience of illness through the care and solidarity of others. Pope Francis's turn to social-ethics scholarship may pave the way for a fresh start, urging for solidarity with those whose living conditions are a far cry from a decent life that modern societies and technologies have long promised to offer them—and long failed to deliver to them.

Chapter 24

For-Profit Health Care: An Economic Perspective

Charles M. A. Clark

The provision of health care, at least in the West, has its origins in the role healing played in Jesus' earthly mission and in passing this mission on to the church, especially in his pronouncement on the "judgment of the nations" (Matt 25), linking salvation to care for the sick. For the first nineteen centuries, churches met this call with individual acts of mercy and health care institutions operated and run by religious communities or secular charities. The development of modern medicine in the twentieth century, however, transformed health care into a capital-intensive industry: human capital in terms of years of training; manufacturing capital in terms of equipment and buildings; financial capital in terms of funding health care. All of this is well beyond what charity and religious organizations could provide. Most countries eventually turned health care into a public good, financed largely or completely with government revenues. This approach views health care as a right and not as a commodity. The United States developed a mixed health care system, with government-supported institutions and financing alongside non-for-profit and for-profit health care institutions.

Catholic health care works, struggles, and survives in this mixed context. For-profit dynamics change the market context for Catholic providers and create significant tensions—and temptations—for them, as witnessed in the earlier chapter by Michael Panicola and Rachelle Barina. Therefore, it is crucial for those engaged in ethics and mission within Catholic health care to understand these dynamics. The purpose of this chapter is to examine the for-profit part of our health care system, especially the arguments that health care is a commodity in which consumer choice is paramount and the use of the profit motive as a way to ration the provision of health care. These arguments will then be evaluated, using in part the lens of Catholic social thought.

Follow the Money:
Sources and Expenditures in the US Health Care Sector

In 2016, the United States spent $3.3 trillion on health care, which accounted for 17.9 percent of the Gross Domestic Product (GDP). This is larger than the retail sector and a little smaller than the total of state and local government spending.[1] In economics, we evaluate a sector based on the value or benefits we obtain from this spending. One benefit of health care spending is employment. In 2016, health care employed just over 15.4 million workers—nearly 1 in 10 jobs (9.9 percent).[2] A second benefit is improved health outcomes, addressed below. However, unlike many industries, which rely mostly or completely on consumers spending their own money, the source of health care funding is varied, with only 10.6 percent coming directly from consumers. As we see in table 1, most spending on health care comes from private insurance (33.7 percent) and government programs

---

[1] Gross Domestic Product (GDP) is the main measure of the size of the economy. It measures the total of final goods and services produced in a given year. Data comes from Centers for Medicare and Medicaid Services, *National Health Expenditure Accounts: Methodology Paper, 2016* (Washington DC: US Department of Health and Human Services, 2016), https://www.cms.gov/Research-Statistics-Data-and-Systems/Statistics-Trends-and-Reports/NationalHealthExpendData/downloads/dsm-16.pdf.

[2] Bureau of Labor Statistics, *Employment by Major Industry Sector*, https://www.bls.gov/emp/tables/employment-by-major-industry-sector.htm (this does not include social assistance).

(37 percent). This spending source is significant if the goal is to apply "market efficiency"[3] to allocating health care in America.

Table 1	
Health Care Expenditures by Source of Funds	
Health Expenditures	**% of total**
Private Health Insurance	33.7
Medicare	20.1
Medicaid	16.9
Out of pocket (consumers)	10.6
Other Third-Party Payers and Programs	7.7
Investment/R&D	4.7
Dept. of Defense/VA	3.2
Public Health Activity	2.5
CHIP	0.5

Source: Center for Medicaid and Medicare Services (CMS)

What patients/consumers get for the trillions spent on health care is found in table 2. The largest health care expenditure is for treatment in hospitals, followed by clinic and physician visits and prescription drugs. The fourth largest expenditure is "Total Administration and Total Net Cost of Health Insurance Expenditures," which accounted for 8.3 percent of the total and which has grown 224.5 percent since 2000. This money does not go for actual health care but to manage paying for health care.

[3] Market efficiency, in theory, means the distribution of resource that is Pareto Optimal (allocation in which no change can be made without making at least one person worse off). However, in practice, efficiency is measured in profits and stock prices.

Table 2

Health Consumption Expenditures in 2016

Health Consumption Expenditures	2016 ($millions)	% of Total	2000–2016 growth
Total Hospital Expenditures	1,082,479	34.0%	160.5%
Total Physician and Clinical Expenditures	664,882	20.9%	130.7%
Total Prescription Drug Expenditures	328,588	10.3%	171.5%
Total Administration and Total Net Cost of Health Insurance Expenditures	**263,652**	**8.3%**	**224.5%**
Total Other Health, Residential, and Personal Care Expenditures	173,486	5.5%	171.3%
Total Nursing Care Facilities and Continuing Care Retirement Communities	162,685	5.1%	91.3%
Total Dental Services Expenditures	124,373	3.9%	100.2%
Total Home Health Care Expenditures	92,364	2.9%	186.0%
Total Other Professional Services Expenditures	91,980	2.9%	151.0%
Public Health Activity	82,187	2.6%	90.9%
Other Non-Durable Medical Products Expenditures	62,201	2.0%	97.0%
Total Durable Medical Equipment Expenditures	50,952	1.6%	102.5%
Total	**3,179,830**		**147.3%**

Source: CMS

Most significant is the net cost of health insurance—the difference be-tween "private health insurance expenditures and benefits incurred" (money spent—money spent on actual health care) which includes "administrative costs, additions to reserves, rate credits and dividends, premium taxes and fees, and net underwriting gains or losses."[4] Net

---

[4] CMS, 2016, 25.

costs of health care reflect profitability (market efficiency), but for society, it is a measure of *inefficiency*. It is money that is not going to improve health. As we see in table 3, private insurance has a significantly higher gap between expenditures and benefits. We should note that both Medicaid and Medicare's net cost were below 2 percent up until 2000 and have risen as both move closer to a market-orientated model.

Table 3	
Net Cost of Health Insurance by Type, 2016	
Type of Insurance	% of Expenditures
Private	11.5%
Medicare	5.4%
Medicaid	6.4%

Source: CMS

Health care spending as a percent of GDP has risen significantly since 1960, from 5 percent to the currently just under 18 percent. The rate of growth has experienced two periods where it has slowed down substantially, the 1990s and from 2010 to 2016 (due to AHCA).

Table 4							
Growth in Health Care Spending as % of GDP in United States, 1960–2016							
	1960	1970	1980	1990	2000	2010	2016
% GDP	5.0%	6.9%	8.9%	12.1%	13.3%	17.3%	17.9%
Change		38.0%	29.0%	36.0%	9.9%	30.1%	3.5%

Source: CMS

This growth in health care spending indicates that health care is a normal good, meaning that people will buy more of it as their income rises. Yet the growth in health care spending in the US is atypical of spending on health care in other advanced capitalist economies. In graph 1, we see that countries with higher per capita income tend to spend more as a percent of their GDP on health care, at least up until per capita GDP of $50,000, at which we see a leveling off. The US, however, is way off the trend line, spending at nearly twice the rate as other OECD (Organization for Economic Cooperation and Development) countries.

Graph 1

Health Care Spending of OECD Countries, 2016

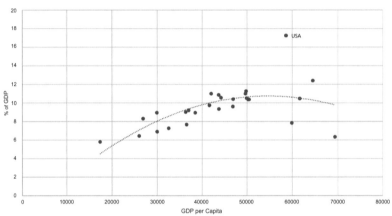

Source: OECD

While all the advanced capitalist economies have a mixture of public and private spending on health care, no country has as large a private health care sector as the US (graph 2). The US spends close to what other rich countries spend on public health care, yet alone spends even more on private health care. The reasons for the high costs of health care in the US are: prices of labor and goods (including pharmaceuticals) and administrative costs (8 percent in the USA, compared with 3 percent in Canada, 2 percent in the UK and Sweden, and 1 percent in France and Japan).[5]

[5] Irene Papanicolas, Liana R. Woskie, and Ashish K. Jha, "Health Care Spending in the United States and Other High-Income Countries," *JAMA* 310, no. 10 (2018): 1024–39, at 1026.

Graph 2

Public and Private Health Care Spending, 2016

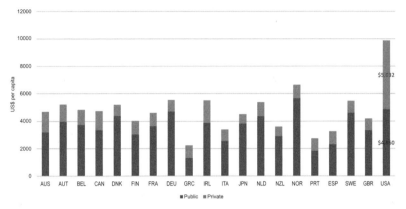

Source: OECD

Along with spending the most, the US gets much less value for its money. First, only about 90 percent of the population is covered by our health care system, whereas all other rich countries have coverage ratios of 99 to 100 percent. Furthermore, the US has poorer health outcomes than other rich countries. This is seen using the broadest measure of health outcomes: life expectancy. Graph 3 presents the relationship between health spending per capita and life expectancy in 2015. It shows that while the United States spends nearly double what its comparable countries spend, its life expectancy is the fourth lowest. As we saw in graph 1, the US deviates greatly from the trend line for rich countries. This holds for many health outcomes.[6] Clearly the US does not efficiently provide health care.

[6] Maternal and infant outcomes differences are particularly striking: the United States has 26.4 maternal deaths per 100,000 live births compared with 9.2 for the UK, 7.3 for Canada, and 4.2 for Denmark; and the US has an infant mortality rate of 5.8 (1000 live births) to 5.1 for Canada, 3.9 for the UK, and 2.1 for Japan. Papanicolas, et al., "Health Care Spending in the United States and Other High-Income Countries," 1030. For more on these disparities, see the chapters by Sheri Brown and Christian Cintron, and Aana Vigen earlier in this volume.

Graph 3

Health Care Spending and Life Expectancy, OECD 2015

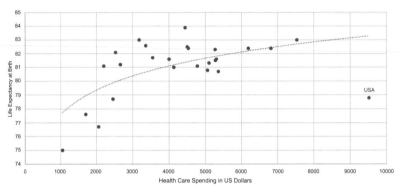

Is Health Care a Commodity?

Providing health care goods and services is clearly a major part of the US economy. To evaluate for-profit health care, however, one needs to ask the question: Is providing health care more like buying a pair of sneakers at Footlocker or is it more like allocating tax dollars for national defense? In both cases, material resources are being allocated, but the character of the goods and services provided are fundamentally different. For-profit health care providers argue that health care is a commodity and that the efficient production and use of health care is best promoted with markets (supply and demand) determining pricing and use. But if health care does not have the characteristics of a commodity, then the argument in favor of for-profit health care is substantially weakened. To answer the question, "Is health care a commodity?" we need to examine if health care providers (supply) and patients (demand) will make better decisions if they are trying to maximize their income or will they make better decisions if they use some other criteria. For example, if two individuals each want to buy the last pair of sneakers, market efficiency dictates that the sneakers go to the person willing to pay the highest price (this reflects that they value the sneakers more); however, if the two individuals get into a car accident on the way to the store, do we find it acceptable for the ambulance to only pick up the person who has health insurance? Do we believe emergency ambulatory care is a commodity—like sneakers—or do we believe that other criteria should be operative in these sorts of decisions? In this section, I work through these distinctions.

Health Care as an Economic Good (Commodity)

The argument for market efficiency starts with individuals choosing to buy a commodity and other individuals looking to sell that commodity. Sometimes the supply and demand of health care fits this model. A person whose allergies are acting up will go to the local drugstore or supermarket and purchase an antihistamine. We will leave aside for now the issue of knowledge acquisition (how do they know that allergies are the problem and that antihistamines will work?) and instead look at it in isolation. The shopper chooses to buy a commodity, making the judgment that its value to them is equal to or greater than its cost, and the seller willingly sells the commodity, making the valuation that it is in their interest to sell at the posted price. Treating health care as a commodity gives the consumer and producer greater agency (people choose what they want), thus allocating health care goods and services more optimally. Here health care production and consumption are understood as individual acts. In neoclassical economic theory, all economic actions are seen as solely individual actions,[7] with the market as the primary mediator between individuals. As such, they are construed as *private* goods.

Health Care as a Social Good

However, more so than most goods, health care decisions, both on the supply and the demand sides, are not carried out by isolated individuals maximizing their utility or profits, subject only to their budget constraints and prices. The knowledge necessary to produce and to select health care goods and services is in almost all cases beyond the individual consumer, and is instead institutionalized in medical professionals, research entities, and regulatory agencies that

---

[7] This is called methodological individualism.

monitor and certify these units. As medical knowledge expands, this becomes even more the case.[8]

Furthermore, the production and consumption of health care goods and services often affects others outside the circle of exchange (buyer and seller). The purchase of health care, and the non-purchase of health care, has great social costs and benefits. A person might diagnosis their aliment as a stomach virus when in fact they have typhoid, they might to go to their job working in a school cafeteria because they have made a cost/benefit calculation that missing a day's pay costs more than they can afford and end up infecting hundreds. Each year the flu is more widely spread because millions of people make individual decisions that are either inaccurate or that only consider their own situation, or both.

Thus, a case can be made that health care is a *social* good. On the one hand, health care is best produced and allocated by health care professionals and institutions, which not only have superior knowledge, but which can also keep in mind social costs and benefits. Here health care is a public good, administered collectively. On the other hand, health is an essential aspect of human flourishing. Excluding people from the provision of health care can be seen as a denial of their right to live. Viewing health care as a human right does not eliminate considering costs and benefits when making health care provisioning decisions, but instead forces a wider understanding of costs and benefits and the nature of the goods in question

Private Good/Public Good Distinction

The key distinctions between private and public goods relate to the issues of exclusion and rivalry. A pure private good is one for which it is both possible and desirable to exclude others from an individual's consumption of a good or service, and their consumption

---

[8] Keep in mind that the development of medical knowledge is not ethically neutral and takes place in the same social and political structures that have generated current levels of injustice. Paul Farmer has noted that as science and technology develop, structural violence deepens rather than lessens because we are now choosing how we use and allocate such resources. See *In the Company of the Poor: Conversations with Dr. Paul Farmer and Fr. Gustavo Gutierrez* (Maryknoll, NY: Orbis Books, 2013), chap. 5.

prevents others from consuming the same thing. It is possible and desirable that I exclude others from eating my slice of pizza, and no one can eat the same slice that I am eating. A pure public good is one in which it is not possible or desirable to exclude others, and one person consuming it does not limit others consuming. A good example here is breathable air. Some goods, like education, are mixed: it is possible to exclude some people from education, but it is not desirable as all people are made poorer when many people are excluded from education. Health care that affects public health (like vaccines) are clearly public goods, as their effectiveness is based on very high level of coverage (as is the case with herd immunity). Health care that has individual benefit without much social benefit, like elective plastic surgery, might be more of a private good.

These positions have significant implications for public policy. If health care *is* a commodity, then health care will be treated as a private good, ideally provided by for-profit companies, with free markets balancing the quantity supply and quantity demand of health care (collectively or for each good and service that comprises a part of the health care industry) by adjusting prices, with suppliers of health care and consumers/patients adjusting their offers to sell and offers to buy accordingly.[9] There is a long and rich body of economic analysis supporting these ideas, from Adam Smith's concept of the "invisible hand" (1776) to the rigorous theoretical elaboration by Kenneth Arrow and Gerard Debreu (1954).[10]

However, if health care in general, or the production and consumption of particular health care goods and services, have the characteristics of a social good, we should expect a strong government presence in the allocation and production of health care goods and services. Opponents of this position suggest that this approach would lead to

---

[9] We must also keep in mind, of course, that all markets have some aspect of government involvement, and that a perfectly free market, defined as one without any government involvement, is a myth and not an historical or potential reality. Property rights do not define or enforce themselves. Libertarian fantasies should never be mistaken as serious economic analysis.

[10] Adam Smith, *An Inquiry into the Nature and Causes of the Wealth of Nations* (Oxford: Oxford University Press, 1976 [1776]); and Kenneth J. Arrow and Gerard Debreu, "Existence of an Equilibrium for a Competitive Economy," *Econometrica* 22, no. 3 (July 1954): 265–90.

health care "rationing"—this is a great misunderstanding. All health care is rationed, just as every good and service sold or provided in the economy is rationed. Health care as a public good uses a different method of rationing than health care as a private good, but it is rationed nonetheless.

An examination of the health care systems in advanced capitalist economies shows that there are many ways and levels of government involvement in the provision of health care. If health care is deemed a human right ensuring universal access becomes a government obligation. How this is achieved is a question of expediency.

Markets, Profits and Health Care

The case for using the profit motive to guide health care provisioning starts with first arguing that health care goods and services are private goods. However, it does not end there. Relying on markets to provide the efficient creation and use of goods and services also requires that markets are competitive; competition is how the "invisible hand" of the market directs individual self-interest toward the common good. Without effective competition, and other factors discussed below, markets become a means for exploitation and the misallocation of resources. High profits earned in a free and open market can be an important signal that a company is doing a very good job, but in a market without competition, or where consumers have insufficient information, high profits are a sign of market failure.

Provisioning and Profits

Economics is about social provisioning: what gets produced; how production is carried out; and how the benefits of production get distributed. We categorize all solutions of the economic problem into three categories: tradition, command, and market. We should keep in mind, however, that no society uses exclusively one type of solution; every real society has used a combination. The traditional solution is to follow the past practice of our parents and grandparents, so that if my father was a wheat farmer I will become a wheat farmer. Traditions, however, must start somewhere, and they usually start with the command solution, which is some authority dictating what gets produced, who will do the producing, and to whom will go the benefits of production. The market solution is often seen as a non-solution: individuals make their own decisions and "the market mechanism" adjusts prices to balance quantity supply and quantity demand. In the real world, markets have always required supporting values and attitudes (part of tradition) and extensive government support and protection (command) to create the social space for individuals to trade (markets).

The case that markets are the most efficient way to coordinate the individual decisions of economic actors (buyers and sellers) into an optimal and stable equilibrium has been a central issue in the history of economics. It suggests that free individuals and flexible prices will result in order rather than chaos while promoting economic growth and raising living standards. This argument was developed to counter government policies that interfered with the free flow of goods and money and were really designed to support the interests of one group or industry at the expense of other industries, or the commonwealth as a whole. In the classic words of Adam Smith:

> every individual necessarily labours to render the annual revenue of the society as great as [one] can. [One] . . . neither intends to promote the public interest, nor knows how much [the individual] is promoting it. . . . [One] intends only his own gain, and he is in this, as in many other cases, led by an *invisible hand* to promote an end which was no part of his intention. . . . By pursuing his own interest, he frequently promotes that of the society more effectually than when he really intends to promote it. I have never known much good done by those who affected to trade for the public good.[11]

The pursuit of profits is what drives a market economy, as owners of capital (money or productive assets) direct their capital to where it will get the highest return. Profits are supposed to go to those who produce what consumers want at the lowest costs (profit being the difference between price and costs). Profits serve three purposes in

---

[11] Smith, *An Inquiry,* 456.

a market economy: (1) they provide the necessary financial surplus to fund investment; (2) they are a signal to market participants on where to direct investment and efforts; and (3) they are an incentive to holders of wealth to use their wealth in a productive manner.

Within the Catholic social tradition, profits can be seen as a necessary part of how markets work. As John Paul II wrote, "The Church acknowledges the legitimate *role of profit* as an indication that a business is functioning well. When a firm makes a profit, this means that productive factors have been properly employed and corresponding human needs have been duly satisfied."[12] But importantly, within CST profit is a secondary outcome that should always serve more crucial ends. John Paul II continues, "Profit is a regulator of the life of a business, but it is not the only one; *other human and moral factors* must also be considered which, in the long term, are at least equally important for the life of a business."[13] Benedict XVI added to this perspective: "Once profit becomes the exclusive goal, if it is produced by improper means and without the common good as its ultimate end, it risks destroying wealth and creating poverty."[14] The singular focus on profits, much like the singular focus on humans as self-interested maximizers, distorts our understanding of the purpose and function of business in our economy and society.[15]

Perfect Competition

In theory, markets collect all the information of buyers and sellers and balance this information so that the resulting prices will balance social costs and social benefits. One way this balance is demonstrated is in supply and demand graphs that depict market equilibrium. The demand curve represents all offers to buy a good (benefits) and

---

[12] John Paul II, *Centesimus Annus* (Vatican City: Vatican Publishing House, 1991) 35.

[13] Ibid. (original emphasis).

[14] Benedict XVI, *Caritas in Veritate* (Vatican City: Vatican Publishing House, 2009) 29.

[15] For an overview of how the Catholic social tradition views the purpose of business, which is to promote human flourishing, see Pontifical Council for Justice and Peace, *Vocation of the Business Leader: A Reflection*, 2014, https://www.stthomas.edu/media/catholicstudies/center/ryan/publications/publicationpdfs/vocationofthe businessleaderpdf/PontificalCouncil_4.pdf.

the supply curve represents all offers to sell (costs of production). Demand curves slope downward because as prices fall consumers are willing and able to purchase more of a good, and supply curves slope upward because sellers are willing to sell more of a good when its prices go up and less when they go down. When the

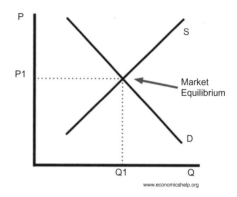

curves intersect the market is in equilibrium, with offers to sell equaling offers to buy, so that there is no excess supply or demand (goods wasted, unmet wants).

However, the argument that markets are efficient is based on a specific type of market structure. Economists do not argue that a private monopoly or that slave markets were efficient to the extent that they equate social costs and social benefits. Only the so-called perfect competition market structure has sufficient competition (invisible hand effects) to, at least in theory, produce these optimal results. In table 5, we see the five main characteristics (assumptions that underlie the simple perfect competition model) and how the health care industry deviates from these conditions.

The health care industry is becoming increasingly concentrated; by 2016 "90 percent of all metropolitan areas had highly concentrated hospital markets."[16] Concentration is also increasing in primary care physicians and specialist physicians.[17] Furthermore, advanced technology creates high capital costs, which become an extremely high entry barrier. One extreme example is the $150 million machine needed for "proton-bean therapy" which is used mostly for prostate cancer.[18] Market discipline requires easy entry. Theoretically, this discipline could come from concentration in the insurance industry (which is

---

[16] Brent D. Fulton, "Health Care Market Concentration Trends in the United States: Evidence and Policy Responses," *Health Affairs* 36, no. 9 (September 2017): 1530–38, at 1530.

[17] Ibid.

[18] Katherine Hobson, "Cost of Medicine: Are High-Tech Medical Devices and Treatments Always Worth It?" *US News and World Report*, July 10, 2009.

Table 5	
Does Health Care Industry Fit Perfect Competition Model?	
Assumption necessary for Markets to produce economic efficiency	**Health Care Industry Reality**
1. Large number of buyers and sellers (each is a price taker).	1. Increasing concentration due to mergers of providers and insurers into large networks.
2. No significant economies of scale (no competitive benefit to being large).	2. Significant economies of scale in health care for producers and insurers.
3. No entry or exit barriers (new producers can enter markets easily).	3. Government regulation is a significant entry barrier, as is the high capital requirements.
4. Homogenous product (which includes known demand).	4. Extreme uncertainty on demand side.
5. Perfect information (about costs, benefits, prices).	5. Consumers do not have medical or price knowledge to make rational choices.

even more concentrated) acting as a "countervailing power."[19] For this to happen the insurance companies with market power can check the market power of hospitals and other concentrated parts of the health care industry and pass on the benefits to patients. Leemore S. Dafny provides evidence that increased concentration in the insurance industry has instead led to higher premiums and lower rates paid to health providers,[20] concluding that "economic research demonstrates that insurance industry consolidation in the past has not tended to improve the lot of consumers."[21] This is not surprising, as

[19] John Kenneth Galbraith, *American Capitalism: The Concept of Countervailing Power* (Boston: Houghton Mifflin, 1952).

[20] It is worth noting that lower provider rates often hurt patients, leading to cost shifting, often to areas covered by out-of-pocket expenses.

[21] Leemore S. Dafny, "Health Insurance Industry Consolidation: What Do We Know From the Past, is it Relevant in Light of the ACA, and What Should We Ask?" *Testimony to Senate Committee on the Judiciary, Subcommittee on Antitrust, Competition Policy and Consumer Rights* (September 22, 2015), 2.

the insurance industry is part of FIRE (Finance, Insurance and Real Estate), that is, Wall Street in common parlance, where market outcomes disproportionately favor shareholders.

Health Care Is a Market Failure

However, one of the biggest barriers to effective market discipline in the health care industry is the difficulty of patients/consumers obtaining basic price information before, or even after, they make their health care choices.[22] Markets do not work efficiently for most health care goods and services.

Many scholars date the beginning of health economics to the publication of an article written by Kenneth Arrow titled "Uncertainty and the Welfare Economics of Medical Care."[23] Arrow, along with Debreu mentioned above, provided the first mathematical proof of equilibrium in a market economy (what is needed to get Adam Smith's "invisible hand" to work).[24] Arrow highlighted that health care does not fit the requirements of an efficient market. The most obvious divergence is that a market is efficient when producer supply matches consumer demand (equilibrium), yet consumers cannot have a rational demand for health care because the need for it is highly uncertain (we do not know what we need or when we are going to need it) and is based on expertise that comes from third parties (usually medical professionals). For most health care goods and services, you cannot have a standard price-and-quantity-demand relationship. No matter how much the price of a heart transplant falls, the quantity demand for it will not go up for most people, and for the few that need a heart transplant the price is not the determinant factor in their choosing to get one (if you can even call it a free choice). Furthermore, necessary health care, especially for the poor, is often beyond the

---

[22] Government Accounting Office, 2011.

[23] Kenneth J. Arrow, "Uncertainty and the Welfare Economics of Medical Care," *American Economic Review* 53 (December 1963): 941–73; and Kenneth J. Arrow, "Uncertainty and the Welfare Economics of Medical Care: Reply (The Implications of Transaction Costs and Adjustment Lags)," *American Economic Review* 55 (March 1965): 154–58. For a history of the field of health economics, see Luis Pina Rebelo, *The Origins and the Evolution of Health Economics: A Discipline by Itself?* 2007, https://ideas.repec .org/p/cap/wpaper/162007.html.

[24] Arrow and Debreu, "Existence of an Equilibrium for a Competitive Economy."

budgets of many, thus their needs and wants are not included in a market allocation. As we saw in table 5, the requirements for an efficient market do not hold for most health care goods and services. We should not be surprised that trying to use market discipline to make health care more efficient in the US has produced the exact opposite: higher prices and less optimal outcomes.

Evaluation of For-Profit Health Care

The large presence of for-profit health care institutions is one reason why health care costs are higher in the United States than in other rich countries. For-profits tend to have higher administrative costs, which include a return for money invested in health care capital: physical (buildings and equipment); human (education of medical professionals); financial (higher borrowing costs and taxation); as well as intellectual property (patents for drugs). While public money is often a major contributor to the investment in health care buildings, equipment, research and development, and education, a higher share of the benefits of these are privatized in higher incomes to investors and managers of these institutions than in not-for-profit institutions or in other countries. These factors all work against those already marginalized in society. Thus, it is left to the non-for-profits to bear this responsibility to either keep their tax-exempt status or in the case of Catholic health care to fulfill its mission.

Table 6 presents the breakdown of community hospitals by for-profit, not-for-profit and public status. In table 7, we can see the differences between for-profit and not-for-profit health care institutions.

Regardless of for-profit or not-for-profit status, health care institutions work hard to increase profitability. This is done more through cherry-picking patients and using market power to raise prices than by lowering costs. Market discipline has not brought down health care costs because for-profit institutions are only viable (competing against not-for-profits) by serving the patients who can most afford their services. A recent study by NYSHealth (2016) showed that hospitals with low rates of Medicaid and Medicare patients charged significantly higher prices in the same markets, and that low and high prices were not necessarily good indicators of quality of care.

Table 6	
Types of Hospitals, 2016	
Community Hospitals	4,840
Not-for-Profits	2,849
For-Profits	1,035
State and Local	956
Catholic	654

Source: AHA; CHA

Table 7		
Some Differences Between For-Profit and Not-For-Profit Health Care Institutions		
	For-Profit	**Not-For-Profit**
Ownership	Corporations owned by investors	Corporations without owners or owned by "members"
Surplus	Distribute % profits to owners	Cannot distribute surplus to those who control organization
Taxation	Pay property, sales and income taxes	Mostly exempt from taxes
Source of Capital	Equity capital from investors; Debt; Retained earnings; Return on equity payments from 3rd party payers	Charitable contributions; Debt; Retained earnings; Government grants
Purpose	Has legal obligation to enhance the wealth of shareholders.	Has legal obligation to fulfill a stated mission, must maintain economic viability to do so.

In a survey of 149 studies comparing for-profit and not-for-profit health providers, Rosenau and Linder found that a higher percent of the studies found that not-for-profits provided better access, quality, efficiency, and charity care (graph 5).[25] Herrera et al. looked at fifteen studies from both high- and low-income countries to see if there was a difference between for-profit, not-for-profit, and public health providers.[26] They concluded that for-profit institutions had worse results than not-for-profits, but that they did not have enough data to compare public providers with private providers.

Graph 5

Summary of 149 Studies on Performance of
For-Profit vs. Nonprofit Providers

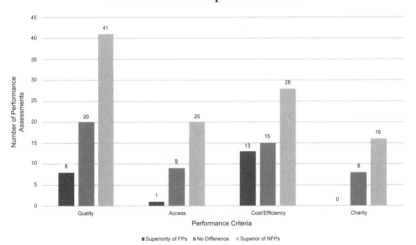

Source: Rosenau and Linder, 2003.

In an analysis of Thomson Reuters 100 Top Hospitals, Foster found Catholic and other church-owned systems "provided higher quality performance and efficiency to the communities they served than

[25] Pauline V. Rosenau and Stephen H. Linder, "Two Decades of Research Comparing For-Profit and Nonprofit Health Provider Performance in the United States," *Social Science Quarterly* 84, no. 2 (June 2003): 219–41.

[26] Cristian A. Herrera, Gabriel Rada, Lucy Kuhn-Barrientos, and Ximena Barrios, "Does Ownership Matter? An Overview of Systematic Reviews of the Performance of Private For-Profit, Private Not-For-Profit and Public Healthcare Providers," *PLoS One* 9, no. 12 (2014): e93456.

investor-owned systems" and that "investor-owned systems have significantly lower performance than all other groups."[27]

Interestingly, a 2014 study published in *JAMA* found that hospitals that made the switch from non-profit to for-profit status generally improved their financial performance without changing quality or mortality rates or the proportion of poor or minority patients.[28] The study window gathered data from two years before and after conversion. It would be interesting to see if these results hold up in the long run once the for-profit mentality is infused throughout the culture of the institutions; changing culture and patient clientele can be a slower process.

Homo Economicus or Homo Communicus?

As we stated above, health care goods and services, like all goods and services produced in the United States, are rationed. Health care provision uses resources and human effort, and these need to be directed and paid for. The United States uses profits and the price mechanisms much more than other developed countries, and by any measure other than profitability, our health care system is less efficient (costs more, produces less). Furthermore, the institutions that rely most on profits are the costliest parts of the system. One reason for this is the role that the insurance, pharmacology, and health care companies have played in shaping the US health care system, especially in how they shape the government's role in this sector. Another part of this story, however, is the distorted view of what it means to be human and how best to promote human flourishing.

The economic argument that markets are more efficient than governments for providing health care or any other good or service starts with a view of the human person, called "rational economic man" or *homo economicus*. This perspective views people as self-interested and autonomous actors, with the "invisible hand" of the market turning their individual greed into efficient outcomes. We

[27] David Foster, "Differences in Health System Quality Performance by Ownership," Research Brief (Thomson Reuters, 2010).

[28] Karen E. Joynt, E. John Orav, and Ashish Jha, "Association Between Hospital Conversions to For-Profit Status and Clinical and Economic Outcomes," *JAMA* 312, no. 16 (2014): 1644–52.

have seen that health care as a good or service does not fit the market model well. Moreover, the CST offers a very different view of the human person, emphasizing that all humans have dignity and an inherent social nature, and that human flourishing is based on participation (working with others).[29] While buying and selling in a market context are one form of social participation, it is not a privileged form, superior to all others. Thus, while CST endorses the right to property and economic freedom, all rights come with responsibilities, and are part of an overall set of human rights. Given the role health care plays in a person's ability to participate in the communities in which they live, access to health care must be universal, and not based on one's income or position in society.

With this different starting point, an analysis of health care provision must look beyond the profitability of health care institutions (how the market measures efficiency) and instead evaluate them based on universal access and outcomes. This is not to say that health care spending should be unlimited, and that everyone needs to get everything they want. Society, and individuals, have many needs to support human flourishing. But these are social decisions, and the excesses of some cannot be the cause of the exclusion of others.

Health care has always been more a vocation and a mission based on caring and *caritas* than a business directed to maximizing profits. In a modern economy providing health care consumes a considerable amount of a community's time, talent, and treasure, all of which can be used for other purposes; thus the health care sector is also competing against businesses that are directed mostly to generating profits, as well as competing for other public goods (roads, military, education). These resources need to be used efficiently as waste hurts everyone in the long run. But our understanding of efficiency needs to be grounded in the mission of caring. Using profitability as the sole or primary criteria to measure efficiency in health care spending runs the risk of distorting the mission and debasing the vocation.

---

[29] See Charles M. A. Clark, "Where There Is No Vision, Economists Will Perish," *Econ Journal Watch* 11, no. 2 (May 2014): 136–43.

Contributors

Editors

M. Therese Lysaught, PhD, is professor at the Neiswanger Institute for Bioethics & Healthcare Leadership at Loyola University Chicago Stritch School of Medicine and Loyola's Institute of Pastoral Studies. Her first book, *Gathered for the Journey: Moral Theology in Theological Perspective* (Eerdmans, 2007, coeditor David Matzko McCarthy), was awarded third-place honors in Theology by the 2008 Catholic Press Association. She is also the coeditor of the classic text *On Moral Medicine: Theological Perspectives in Medical Ethics*, 3rd edition (Eerdmans, 2012, coeditor Joseph Kotva), and author of *Caritas in Communion: Theological Foundations of Health Care Ethics* (Catholic Health Association, 2014).

Michael McCarthy, PhD, is assistant professor at the Neiswanger Institute for Bioethics & Healthcare Leadership at Loyola University Chicago Stritch School of Medicine. Dr. McCarthy codirects the Physician's Vocation Program, which seeks to ground the formation of medical students in the *Spiritual Exercises* of St. Ignatius Loyola. His research focuses on integrating liberation philosophy and theology as an epistemological approach for understanding the task of bioethics. He has published and presented on the role of justice in bioethics, the importance of spirituality in patient care and medical education, the intersection of the humanities with the formation of the "well-rounded" physician, and clinical ethics.

Contributors

Armand J. Andreoni, MBA, served as community benefit officer and director of Community Benefit and Strategic Analytics for Loyola

University Health Systems (LUHS). He had been director of Strategic Planning for LUHS for over twenty years. Early in his career he coauthored a monthly column in *Hospitals, Journal of the American Hospital Association*. He is currently working as a consultant to Proviso Partners, a nonprofit community group advising on grant development, organizational structure, and planning.

Rachelle Barina, PhD, is vice president of Mission Integration Wisconsin and System Ethics at SSM Health, a Catholic health care organization operating in Wisconsin, Missouri, Oklahoma, and Illinois. Her academic interests arise from contemporary challenges experienced within Catholic health ministry. She has an academic appointment in the Albert Gnaegi Center for Health Care Ethics at St. Louis University and publishes frequently in the areas of bioethics and Catholic health care ethics.

Jana Marguerite Bennett, PhD, is professor of religious studies at the University of Dayton. She is a moral theologian with a wide range of research interests and publications, including books on singleness (*Singleness and the Church: A New Theology of Single Life*, Oxford University Press, 2017; *Water is Thicker than Blood: An Augustinian Theology of Marriage and Singleness*, Oxford University Press, 2008) and a book on technology use and theology (*Aquinas on the Web? Doing Theology in an Internet Age*, Bloomsbury, 2012). She is the author of several essays on disability and technology, and is a coeditor for the *Journal of Disability and Religion*. She also coedits catholicmoraltheology.com, a website that features work from twenty North American theologians on a range of subjects.

Sheri Bartlett Browne, PhD, is a historian, biographer, and board-certified Catholic chaplain. She is professor of history and women's studies at Tennessee State University in Nashville and recently earned an MA in Health Care Mission Leadership from Loyola University Chicago. As a health care chaplain, she has worked for Vanderbilt University Medical Center and Monroe Carell Jr. Children's Hospital at Vanderbilt, primarily in pediatric intensive and palliative care. Dr. Browne's historical and health care research analyzes the impact of racial-ethnic, socioeconomic, and gender inequalities on women's lives and well-being.

Michelle Byrne, MD, MPH, is a second-year Family Medicine resident at the Northwestern McGaw Family Medicine in Humboldt Park, Chicago. Her training focuses on care for the urban underserved, leadership, and advocacy. Prior to medical school, she worked in health policy and operations in Washington, DC, as a member of President Obama's inaugural intern class, and in a startup pediatric practice in Kansas City while obtaining her MPH. During medical school at Loyola University Chicago, she coordinated the free health clinic program, served as a representative advising the Consortium of Universities for Global Health, and completed research on gun violence interventions in the hospital setting. Throughout medical school she coordinated the medical school's free health clinic and worked as a live-in volunteer at a Catholic Worker house for migrant women and children from Central and South America.

Lisa Sowle Cahill, PhD, is J. Donald Monan, SJ, Professor at Boston College. Dr. Cahill is a past president of the Catholic Theological Society of America (1992–93) and the Society of Christian Ethics (1997–98), and is a fellow of the American Academy of Arts and Sciences. In addition to her numerous academic essays, she is the author of multiple books, including *A Theology and Praxis of Gender Equality* (Dharmaram Publications, 2018); *Blessed Are the Peacemakers: Pacifism, Just War, and Peacebuilding* (Fortress, 2019); and *Global Justice, Christology and Christian Ethics* (Cambridge University Press, 2013). Her *Theological Bioethics: Participation, Justice, and Change* (Georgetown University Press, 2005) and *Bioethics and the Common Good* (Marquette University Press, 2004) refocused the discourse at the intersection of theology, social justice, and bioethics. Dr. Cahill received her MA and PhD degrees from the University of Chicago Divinity School.

Christian Cintron, PhD, works in Mission Integration for Trinity Health. He completed his doctoral studies at Loyola University Chicago in 2017. His research interests include social, biomedical, health care, and public health ethics. His dissertation focused on the relationship between the Catholic social tradition, neo-Arisotelian and communitarian traditions, and public health ethics as they help us reimagine the good life for the aging population in the United States. He has held teaching appointments at Sacred Heart University, Fairfield University, and Georgetown University.

Charles M. A. Clark, PhD, is professor of economics and finance and senior fellow, Vincentian Center for Church and Society at St. John's University in New York. He is the author of *Economic Theory and Natural Philosophy* (1992), *Pathways to a Basic Income* (with John Healy, 1997), *Basic Income: Economic Security for All Canadians* (with Sally Lerner and Robert Needlham, 1999), and *The Basic Income Guarantee: Ensuring Progress and Prosperity in the 21st Century* (2002); and the editor of *History and Historians of Political Economy* (1994), *Institutional Economics and the Theory of Social Value* (1995), *Unemployment in Ireland* (with Catherine Kavanagh, 1998), and *Rethinking Abundance* (with Helen Alford, Steve Cortright, and Mike Naughton, 2005). Dr. Clark is past president of the Association for Evolutionary Economics and past president of the Association for Institutionalist Thought.

Bruce Compton is senior director of international outreach for the Catholic Health Association of the United States. Mr. Compton is responsible for assisting and supporting CHA-member organizations in their outreach activities in the developing world. His duties include facilitating collaboration among CHA-member organizations and others, seeking to enhance the impact of international ministries. Mr. Compton lived in Haiti from 2000 to 2002 and continues to work in support of health missions in the developing world after his return to the US in his capacity as founding president and chief executive of Springfield, Illinois–based Hospital Sisters Mission Outreach, a ministry organization bringing surplus medical supplies from Midwest hospitals to medical missions in the developing world.

Robert J. DeVita, MBA, served as a health care leader for medical school faculty practices in Wisconsin, Virginia, and Tennessee, before leading startup HMOs for Blue Cross and Blue Shield in Tennessee, and Security Health Plan of Marshfield Clinic in Marshfield, Wisconsin, for whom he afterward served as chief administrator. He continued his career as a senior health care leader for two nonprofit, faith-based health care systems in Wisconsin (Ministry Healthcare and Wheaton Franciscan Healthcare, now Ascension Health of Wisconsin). In April 2012, he was asked to come out of retirement to become the founding CEO for the newly formed and successfully launched startup health insurance cooperative Common Ground

Health Care of Wisconsin, headquartered in Brookfield, Wisconsin. Bob continues serving as a volunteer advisor and on boards of directors for nonprofit health care organizations. He is a member of the adjunct faculty of the Lubar School of Business at University of Wisconsin—Milwaukee MBA program where he teaches graduate courses in health care leadership.

Daniel P. Dwyer, PhD, is executive director, Theology and Ethics, for Providence St. Joseph Health System. An executive, ethicist, and educator with more than thirty years of experience in the health care field, he has worked in many environments including health care systems, hospitals, clinics, and medical colleges. Prior to working for St. Joseph Health, he served as senior vice president of Mission Integration for Trinity Health, and director of Mission and Community Health for Sisters of Mercy Health System.

Jorge José Ferrer, SJ, ThD, served as director of Eugenio María de Hostos Bioethics Institute at the Medical Sciences Campus of the University of Puerto Rico from 2012 to 2018. He has previously taught at the Gregorian University (Rome), Comillas Pontifical University (Madrid), and held visiting appointments at Georgetown University and Seattle University. He has authored, coauthored, and edited numerous publications in the area of bioethics, most recently a co-edited collection of essays on the theoretical foundations of bioethics for the Ibero-American cultural context: *Bioética: el pluralismo de la fundamentación* (Madrid, Universidad Pontificia Comillas, 2016, with Juan Alberto Lecaros and Róderic Molins). As of fall 2018, he holds The Anna and Donald Waite Endowed Chair, a visiting chair for Jesuit scholars, at Creighton University.

Robert J. Gordon, DMin, is manager of Pastoral Care at St. Bernard Hospital and Health Care Center, Chicago. He began his career as an on-call chaplain in 1988 at St. Bernard while also serving as a full-time director of religious education for twenty-four years in the Archdiocese of Chicago. Robert continues as a sixth-grade catechist at his home parish of St. Francis of Assisi, Bolingbrook, Illinois. In 2015, he was appointed manager of Pastoral Care. He received a doctor of ministry degree in Spirituality from Catholic Theological Union.

Hille Haker, PhD, is the Richard McCormick, SJ, Chair of Moral Theology at Loyola University Chicago. Dr. Haker has been the president of *Societas Ethica*, European Society of Research in Ethics (2015–2018), a member of the European Group on Ethics in Sciences and New Technologies (EGE) of the European Commission (2005–2015), and coeditor of the international theology journal *Concilium* until 2015. Her books on medical ethics include *Ethics of Genetics in Human Procreation* (H. Haker/D. Beyleveld, eds.; Aldershot [Ashgate], 2000) and *Medical Ethics in Health Care Chaplaincy* (W. Moczynski/H. Haker/ K. Bentele, eds. Berlin [Lit] et al., 2009).

Ron Hamel, PhD, served as senior director of Ethics for the Catholic Health Association of the United States (CHA) for seventeen years. He has lectured widely to health care professionals, has served on numerous hospital ethics committees, was a member of the Health Care Ethics Commission of the Archdiocese of Chicago, serves as resource ethicist to the American Association of Nurse Anesthetists, and is currently president of SSM Health Ministries and a member of the SSM Health Board of Directors. In October 2001, he received the Kevin O'Rourke award from the Gateway Catholic Ethics Network in St. Louis for his contributions to Catholic health care ethics. Dr. Hamel has authored numerous articles, columns, and chapters in health care ethics and has edited several books.

Lena Hatchett, PhD, is associate professor of medical education, Loyola University Chicago, and principal investigator for Proviso Partners for Health. As a community-based participatory researcher and health equity coach, her research evaluates the policy, systems, and environmental change strategies that connect community health and the local food economy. Dr. Hatchett works locally to build a culture of health in low-income communities of color in Proviso Township. In partnership with the Illinois Proviso Partners for Health, local businesses, schools, community organizations, and resident partners, she supports three social enterprises in the local food economy. Nationally, she guides the implementation of Community of Solutions model and skills as co-lead on the Leadership Team for the Robert Wood Johnson Foundation 100 Million Healthier Lives Initiative. Dr. Hatchett is currently training organizational leaders from Loyola University Chicago, the Institute of Medicine Chicago, the Alliance for Health Equity, and the Cook County Department of Public Health.

Kelly R. Herron, MAPS, is chief mission officer at St. Joseph Mercy Oakland, Trinity Health. Kelly is a member of the Human Trafficking business resource group of Trinity Health, where she serves colleagues across the Trinity Health system as they respond to the needs of people who have been trafficked while ensuring quality programming and training on the topic. Kelly loves system design in collaboration with others to reach the most marginalized people in a community or within an organization. For twenty years, she has taught and served on boards in southeastern Michigan that seek to alleviate the suffering of people living on the margins of society.

Sharon Homan, PhD, is president of the Sinai Urban Health Institute, a biostatistician, and a maternal child mental health epidemiologist. Additionally, she serves as the director of the Chicago Gun Violence Research Collaborative. Previously, Sharon served as professor and chair of the Department of Biostatistics and Epidemiology and associate dean for research at the University of North Texas School of Public Health in Fort Worth, Texas. Her prior experience includes public health leadership and faculty positions with Rockhurst University (academic vice president), the Kansas Health Institute (vice president for public health), and Saint Louis University (professor of biostatistics).

Mark G. Kuczewski, PhD, is the Fr. Michael I. English, SJ, Professor of Medical Ethics and director of the Neiswanger Institute for Bioethics & Healthcare Leadership at Loyola University Chicago Stritch School of Medicine. He is a past president of the American Society for Bioethics and Humanities (ASBH). He has been an articulate spokesperson for the just and equitable treatment of immigrant patients. His writings argue for a prohibition on forced medical repatriation and the severing of any relationship between health insurance and immigration status. He is a member of the Advisory Board of the Undocumented Patients project of the Hastings Center and has recently served as the project manager to revise the admissions policy of the Loyola University Chicago Stritch School of Medicine to include Dreamers. This has resulted in Stritch becoming the first medical school in the nation to welcome applications from Dreamers of DACA status.

Antoinette Lullo, DO, is a family medicine physician and faculty member at Hinsdale Hospital Family Practice Residency Program in Hinsdale, Illinois. She graduated with a doctor of osteopathy degree from Midwestern University Chicago College of Osteopathy. Dr. Lullo subsequently completed fellowships in Family Medicine at the Cook County-Loyola-Provident program and Maternal Child Health at West Suburban Hospital, focusing on high-risk obstetrics, surgical obstetrics, and newborn care. She went on to work at the Parental Child Center (PCC), serving as the codirector of the Maternal Child Health Fellowship program focused on providing care for underserved poor communities in Chicago. From 2012 to 2016, she served as one of the medical directors at Centro de Salud Santa Clotilde in Peruvian Amazon with her husband through the support of Mission Doctors Association.

Alexandre Martins, MI, PhD, is a Brazilian bioethicist and theologian, a religious priest of the Order of Saint Camillus, and an assistant professor in the Theology Department and College of Nursing at Marquette University. He serves on the Latin American Regional Committee of the Catholic Theological Ethics in the World Church. He has published several articles and books, including *Introdução à Cristologia Latino-Americana: Cristologia no Encontro com a Realidade Pobre e Plural da América Latina* (São Paulo: Paulus, 2014), *A Pobreza e a Graça: Experiência de Deus em Meio ao Sofrimento em Simone Weil* (São Paulo: Paulus, 2013), and *Bioética, Saúde e Vulnerabilidade: Em Defesa da Dignidade dos Vulneráveis* (São Paulo: Paulus, 2012). He also translated Paul Farmer's important book *Pathologies of Power* into Portuguese and has worked with Partners in Health in Haiti.

Virginia McCarthy, MDiv, serves as the director of Health Sciences Division Ministry at Loyola University Chicago. Her academic interests include contextual and immersion-based learning, health disparities, gun violence, migration, and the value of reflection in higher education. She is a fellow in the Chicago Gun Violence Research Collaborative and continues work in gun violence research and prevention through the University-Hospital Committee, Loyola Stands Against Gun Violence.

Brian Medernach, MD, is assistant professor at the Stritch School of Medicine at Loyola University Chicago as well as assistant director of the Center for Community and Global Health. He and his wife Dr. Antoinette Lullo, DO, served in the remote region of the Peruvian Amazon jungle in the town of Santa Clotilde in coordination with Mission Doctors Association. There he completed a diploma course in Tropical Medicine and Hygiene at the Gorgas Institute of Tropical Medicine in Lima, Peru.

Carly Mesnick, LPCC-S, is manager of the Crime and Trauma Assistance Program (CTAP) at Mount Carmel Health System in Columbus, Ohio. CTAP provides trauma specific counseling to victims, survivors, and cosurvivors of crime and traumatic events at no cost to those served. Carly develops programming that delivers optimal care of those affected by crime or traumatic events throughout the continuum of care, in an atmosphere sensitive to each person's physical, emotional, social, and spiritual needs. Her work focuses on trauma-informed care practices within healthcare and specializes in the research, training, and development of specific treatment models to treat victims and survivors of human trafficking. She serves on many internal and external committees to assist in the fight against human trafficking while presenting as a source for how trauma specifically affects this population and their daily functioning within our communities.

Cory D. Mitchell, DBe (candidate), MA, is a graduate of the Health Care Mission Leadership program at the Loyola University Chicago and current doctoral candidate at the Loyola University Chicago Neiswanger Institute for Bioethics & Healthcare Leadership. Having served in the US Navy, as a research intern at Johns Hopkins University's Bloomberg School of Public Health, and as a program specialist intern at the National Institutes of Health Institute on Aging, Cory has significant experience working with vulnerable populations, including veterans and the homeless. As an African American, his research interests are Catholic health care, health disparities, and theological ethics.

Abraham M. Nussbaum, MD, MTS, is the chief education officer at Denver Health and associate professor of psychiatry at the University of Colorado School of Medicine, where he also serves as an assistant dean in Graduate Medical Education. He earned a medical degree and completed psychiatry residency at the University of North Carolina, and a master's degree in theology at Duke Divinity School. He has authored three psychiatric textbooks and a memoir, *The Finest Traditions of My Calling: One Physician's Search for the Renewal of Medicine* (Yale, 2015), which *The New York Times* called "dazzling and instructive." He lives in Denver, where he coaches the Blessed Sacrament boys' basketball team.

Dónal P. O'Mathúna, PhD, is associate professor in ethics, School of Nursing & Human Sciences, Dublin City University, Ireland, and the College of Nursing, The Ohio State University, Columbus, Ohio. His research interests are in both health care ethics and evidence-based practice. He is the principal investigator on funded research projects examining research ethics in disasters and humanitarian crises. He has contributed to ethics initiatives with the World Health Organization, UNICEF, and the UN agency for disaster risk reduction (UNISDR). He has spoken and published widely, and coedited *Disasters: Core Concepts and Ethical Theories* (Springer, 2018).

Michael Panicola, PhD, is a principal at Third View Advisors in St. Louis, Missouri, which he founded after having worked previously in Catholic health care for two decades serving in progressively expansive roles with responsibilities ranging from business/clinical ethics and community health improvement to his most recent role as the senior vice president of Mission, Legal, and Government Affairs for SSM Health. Panicola has also served as a professor of moral theology and health care ethics at Saint Louis University and published extensively in health care and theological journals, including serving as the lead author of *Health Care Ethics: Theological Foundations, Contemporary Issues and Controversial Cases*, 2nd edition.

Cristina Richie, PhD, is assistant professor in the Department of Bioethics and Interdisciplinary Studies at the Brody School of Medicine, East Carolina University, with an adjunct appointment in the

School of Public Health. She is the author of *Principles of Green Bioethics: Sustainability in Health Care* (Michigan State University Press, forthcoming) and over twenty-five peer-reviewed journal articles. In 2013, she won the Catholic Health Association (CHA) Annual Theology and Ethics Colloquium graduate student award for her essay on green bioethics. Dr. Richie is an associate fellow at the Center for Bioethics and Human Dignity at Trinity International University and the head of the North Carolina Unit of the UNESCO Chair in Bioethics.

Alan Sanders, PhD, is vice president of Ethics Integration and Strategy at Trinity Health. He has served in a mission and ethics role in Catholic health care for over ten years, with previous experience in teaching and biotech research. In his current role, Alan leads Trinity Health's national Champions education program in both ethics and spiritual care, presents for Trinity Health's formation program, and facilitates Trinity Health's Catholic identity assessment. He has authored numerous articles on clinical, organizational, and social ethics, and has developed Trinity Health's system-wide approach to these three ethical realms. Alan also serves as a member of the Pennsylvania Catholic Health Association board, as well as other hospital boards and committees.

Abigail Silva, PhD, MPH, is assistant professor in the Department of Public Health Sciences at Loyola University Chicago. She is an epidemiologist and health disparities researcher with a practice and research portfolio that includes using data, particularly local-level data, to inform policies and interventions. Dr. Silva recently served as a faculty fellow in the Chicago Gun Violence Research Collaborative. She is also currently involved with Loyola Stands, a university-hospital committee that is working toward identifying and implementing interventions to address gun violence in the community of Maywood and surrounding areas.

Andrea Vicini, SJ, MD, PhD, STD, is associate professor of moral theology in the School of Theology and Ministry at Boston College. A native of Italy who earned his medical degree from the University of Bologna, Fr. Vicini worked as a pediatrician before joining the

Society of Jesus and becoming a priest. He is coeditor of *Just Sustainability: Technology, Ecology, and Resource Extraction*, part of the Catholic Theological Ethics in the World Church book series, as well as *Genetica umana e bene comune* (Human Genetics and the Common Good; Cinisello Balsamo: San Paolo, 2008). He served as a fellow in the Center of Theological Inquiry at Princeton University in 2015–2016.

Aana Marie Vigen, PhD, is associate professor of Christian social ethics at Loyola University Chicago. She is the author of *Women, Ethics, and Inequality in U.S. Healthcare* (Palgrave, rev. ed., 2011). She coauthored and coedited *God, Science, Sex, Gender* (with Patricia Beattie Jung; University of Illinois, 2010) and *Ethnography as Christian Theology and Ethics* (with Christian Scharen; Continuum, 2011). Dr. Vigen has also contributed several invited chapters to interdisciplinary anthologies. She is presently working on a book on prenatal genetics and the perspectives of new mothers of color and of medical professionals.

Brian Volck, MD, MFA, is a pediatrician, theologian, and writer. He served as assistant professor of pediatrics in the Division of Hospital Medicine at Cincinnati Children's Hospital Medical Center until 2017. He has provided pediatric care at an Indian Health Service hospital on the Navajo Reservation, at an inner-city community health center in Kentucky, at a storefront pediatric office, and at a university-affiliated combined internal medicine-pediatrics teaching practice. He has participated in medical education and direct service medical teams to Central America and the Navajo Reservation. He was a member of the American Academy of Pediatrics' Committee on Native American Child Health (2009–2015), and US Planning Chair for the Fifth and Sixth International Meeting on Indigenous Child Health. His memoir, *Attending Others: A Doctor's Education in Bodies and Words*, was published in 2016. He has a collection of poetry, *Flesh Becomes Word*, released in October 2013, and is coauthor of *Reclaiming the Body: Christians and the Faithful Use of Modern Medicine*. His essays, poetry, and reviews have appeared in *America*, *The Christian Century*, Double-Take, and IMAGE, *Comment Online*, the Ekklesia Project, *Front Porch Republic, Good Letters*, and *The Other Journal*. His current project is a book on the intersection of health, history, and culture in the Navajo nation.

Tobias Winright, PhD, holds the Hubert Mäder Endowed Chair at the Albert Gnaegi Center for Health Care Ethics at Saint Louis University and is associate professor of theological ethics in the Department of Theological Studies. He has coedited and contributed to *Can War Be Just in the 21st Century?: Ethicists Engage the Tradition* (Orbis, 2015), coauthored *After the Smoke Clears: The Just War Tradition and Post War Justice* (Orbis, 2010), edited *Green Discipleship: Catholic Theological Ethics and the Environment* (Anselm Academic, 2011), coedited *Violence, Transformation, and the Sacred: "They Shall Be Called Children of God"* (Orbis, 2011), and coedited *Environmental Justice and Climate Change: Assessing Pope Benedict XVI's Ecological Vision for the Catholic Church in the United States* (Lexington, 2013).